Living with HIV

Living with HIV
A Patient's Guide

Mark Cichocki, RN

SECOND EDITION

McFarland & Company, Inc., Publishers

Jefferson, North Carolina

LIBRARY OF CONGRESS CATALOGUING-IN-PUBLICATION DATA

Names: Cichocki, Mark, 1961–, author.
Title: Living with HIV : a patient's guide / Mark Cichocki, RN.
Description: Second edition. | Jefferson, North Carolina : McFarland &
Company, Inc., 2017 | Includes bibliographical references and index.
Identifiers: LCCN 2016055223 | ISBN 9781476664958 (softcover : acid free paper) ∞
Subjects: LCSH: HIV-positive persons. | AIDS (Disease)—Patients. |
Self-care, Health. | MESH: HIV Infections—popular works. |
Self Care—popular works.
Classification: LCC RA643.8 .C53 2017 | DDC 616.97/92—dc23
LC record available at https://lccn.loc.gov/2016055223

BRITISH LIBRARY CATALOGUING DATA ARE AVAILABLE

ISBN (print) 978-1-4766-6495-8
ISBN (ebook) 978-1-4766-2774-8

Front cover images © 2017 Shutterstock

Printed in the United States of America

*McFarland & Company, Inc., Publishers
Box 611, Jefferson, North Carolina 28640
www.mcfarlandpub.com*

To all the physicians, social workers, and medical assistants
I have worked alongside for the past twenty years.
Your commitment to our patients has been an inspiration
and the driving force in my professional life.
The respect you have shown me has been humbling,
the lessons you have taught me have been priceless,
and the friendship we have shared has always been a blessing.

Contents

INTRODUCTION:
WHY IS THIS BOOK NEEDED?

Judith Rabkin, Ph.D., author of the book *Good Patients, Good Doctors*, summed it up in one sentence: "The patient's first major task after learning he or she is HIV positive is self-education."

Self-education not only enables people to go on with their lives, but allows them to make informed decisions regarding their own HIV care and empowers them, making them critical members of the healthcare team and, in a sense, a part of the HIV scientific community.

Historically, medical information was solely the domain of physicians, healthcare professionals, and scientists. The doctor was in charge, and the patient submitted to the physician's recommendations and orders. Take, for instance, the term compliance. Twenty years ago, doctors would prescribe a therapy and then monitor how *compliant* the patient was with respect to that therapy. By definition, to comply means to conform to someone's wishes. Simply put, the patient was expected to conform to the doctor's decision, regardless of his or her own wishes.

Times have changed, and today medicine is no longer just for the physician. People living with HIV are at the grassroots of a movement that has taken the hierarchy out of the doctor-patient relationship. Patients and doctors now work together as equals in developing care plans, assessing needs, and creating treatment regimens that meet the common goals of patient and medical professional. Take our example from the previous paragraph. Today, patients no longer comply with their doctors' wishes, they *adhere* to a given therapy. Webster's Online Dictionary defines the word adhere as the action of joining or uniting. Today doctors and patients unite or work together to develop care plans and medication therapies for the person living with HIV. This partnership is possible because of the determination and desire of patients to learn about their HIV. People living with HIV and AIDS are dedicated to the process of self-education.

But all that being said, does education improve prognosis and quality of life? The answer is a resounding *yes!* In fact, scientific studies have proven time and again that educated and knowledgeable patients fare much better than those who aren't. In one study, researchers at RAND, a research institute in Santa Monica, California, found that the educated patient is much better able to adhere to treatment regimens than the patient with less education. Experts attribute this improved prognosis to the fact that greater understanding of a disease process contributes to an increased desire to take an active role in one's own healthcare. In stark contrast to twenty years ago, patients no longer submit to their doctors' wishes. Instead, they take an active role in their own care.

HIV is a very complex and ever changing disease. How is a lay person supposed to learn about and understand such a complicated disease? And what is the most effective way for a person to learn about their illness? The effectiveness of any patient education tool depends on many factors, ranging from the educator's own experiences and qualifications to patients' preconceived ideas about their illness and their own health. But most important, the success of health education depends on the patient's willingness and ability to learn. Ideally, people living with HIV could sit down with a medical practitioner, nurse or other educator and take as much time as they need to learn about their disease process. Unfortunately, staffing shortages, financial factors, and time constraints put much of the education burden on the person living with the disease; in other words, it's all about self-education. So in order to self-educate properly, people need the right tools with which to learn. People need resources that are current, accurate and in a form that is conducive to learning. *Living with HIV: A Patient's Guide, 2d ed.* is the tool people have been looking for.

Your desire and willingness to learn about your disease is evident by the fact you're reading this text. And you won't be disappointed. The following chapters will take you through the entire HIV lifespan—from prevention to diagnosis and beyond. HIV affects the entire person, both the physical and the emotional. This book provides you with the information you need to address both. Choosing a doctor can be confusing and frightening. This book will walk you through the process of finding a doctor that is right for you. Medications have become the key component of a long healthy life. This text will prepare you for your first HIV medication regimen by helping you work through side effects, by helping you to adhere to your medication regimen, and by providing you the information necessary to help choose the regimen that's right for you. And when the time comes for you to address the inevitability of any chronic illness, this book will walk you through end-of-life issues such as advanced directives, living wills, and hospice.

For those of you newly diagnosed, you're frightened of what the future holds. For those of you who have been living with HIV for years or decades, you need to take the next step in understanding your illness. And for those of you caring for a loved one, you want to be there for support when he or she needs you most. This book will help all of you achieve the educational goals you have set for yourself. You have in your hand an up to date resource that will help you take control of your life and your illness. Knowledge is power, and having opened this text, you have taken a very important first step in living your life with HIV.

Now let's get started.

1

THE HISTORY OF HIV AND AIDS

In July 1981 millions of people around the world watched the royal wedding of Prince Charles and Lady Diana Spencer. That same year martial law was declared in Poland, the first IBM personal computer was introduced, and NASA launched the first space shuttle. While Pope John Paul II struggled for his life after an unsuccessful assassination attempt, small groups of gay men in New York and California were losing their battle with a rare and fatal form of cancer called Kaposi's sarcoma. Still others were presenting to emergency departments in Los Angeles and New York City with a seldom seen pneumonia called *Pneumocystis (carinii) jirovecii*. As people watched the nationally televised attempt on President Ronald Reagan's life, the greatest public health threat of the twentieth century was emerging, to the notice of almost no one.

HIV Is Older Than You Think

Publicly, the HIV/AIDS epidemic began in 1981. However, searching for the true origin of HIV and the reason for its sudden emergence as an epidemic has become a topic of intense research and investigation. There are many theories ranging from a polio vaccine that went bad to the radical belief that suggests HIV is the result of a top secret germ warfare program. One thing HIV experts agree upon is that the virus actually appeared decades before it made the nightly news in 1981. Statistical analysis of the most aggressive form of the virus, HIV-1, indicates that the earliest evidence of HIV-1 was between 1910 and 1930. The evidence also suggests the virus spread throughout Africa for up to 70 years before it was recognized. While examining infected blood and tissue about 1959 and 1960, researchers found that there were already examples of HIV-1 that had undergone small genetic changes, creating "sub-types" of HIV-1. Understanding that the genetic changes take time to occur, researchers felt that the presence of sub-types of HIV-1 suggested the virus had been around prior to 1959, maybe even decades prior. Yet it wasn't until 1959 that researchers found strong evidence that HIV-1 was causing illnesses in people.

Research has shown that the spread of HIV-1 sub-types can be traced geographically. Knowing that fact allows experts to trace the origin of HIV-1 and how it has spread from place to place and population to population. For instance, the predominant type of HIV in the U.S. and Europe can be traced to a specific sub-type found in Africa, a type that made its way to the U.S. via Haiti in the 1960s. Using the same method, experts have concluded that the first victim of AIDS was a man from a town formally known as Leopoldville, an area known today as Kinshasa, the capital of the Democratic Republic of the Congo. He initially presented to a local clinic with symptoms that resembled sickle cell anemia. Sickle cell is a hereditary blood disorder characterized by oddly shaped blood cells; a condition commonly found in the Congo at that time. Because sickle cell was a common disease in the area, nobody questioned the diagnosis.

In the mid–1990s, in an effort to date the emergence of HIV and AIDS, leading HIV researcher David Ho and his colleagues at the Aaron Diamond Research Center examined blood samples taken from the man decades earlier. The researchers found evidence of HIV, but what intrigued Ho was that the HIV found appeared to be an ancestor of the HIV infecting people in the 1990s. To Ho, this provided more evidence that HIV entered the human species just prior to 1959, refuting earlier theories suggesting its emergence closer to 1935.

While we have some idea when HIV first infected man, no one knows for sure how HIV came to be. There are several theories that try to explain how HIV emerged as the greatest epidemic of the 20th century. Let's look at some of the most debated.

Researchers around the world start looking for the origin of HIV soon after it was determined to be the cause of AIDS. Searching desperately for a cause and origin of the deadly virus, experts found a very close cousin of HIV in monkeys and chimpanzees: Simian Immunodeficiency Virus, or SIV for short. In 1995, scientists studied blood from a woman who died of AIDS and found her HIV to be a unique variant possessing characteristics of both HIV and SIV, suggesting that SIV somehow changes over time and becomes HIV. But how could SIV, a virus that has existed more than 30,000 years, become HIV? And what's more, how could a virus in a monkey get into the bloodstream of a human? Experts believe that different sub-types of SIV can exist in a single monkey. Once in the same host, these sub-types can combine to form a single type of virus, a type that is able to move from species to species. Once in a human, SIV becomes HIV. But again, there are questions. Specifically, how does the virus get from a monkey to a human? There are a few theories.

The "Hunter Theory"

The most widely accepted theory is referred to as the "hunter theory." For most African tribes, monkey meat is a large part of the diet. Monkeys are hunted, butchered, and eaten by the local population. Experts theorize that eating the meat or brains of SIV infected monkeys introduces the virus into the human species. The act of butchering exposes people to a large quantity of potentially infected blood. Any small cuts or breaks in the skin allows the infected blood to enter the human host. The SIV sub-type changes over time to become HIV, the virus that now runs rampant around the world.

The Polio Vaccine

In his book titled *The River,* journalist Edward Hooper suggests that HIV could have been introduced into the human species during testing of the world's first polio vaccine. The polio vaccine, referred to back then as "Chat," needed to be grown in living tissue cultures.

According to Hooper's theory, infected monkey tissue was used to grow the "Chat" polio vaccine. That infected monkey tissue allegedly contaminated the vaccine itself. The vaccine trials included one million local residents, some of whom could have been infected with the contaminated vaccine. Experts doubt this occurred based on testing of a single vial of "Chat" found in a lab tucked away for future study. The vial was tested and was found to be free of HIV and SIV, debunking the Polio Vaccine Theory. Proponents of the theory contend that only one vial out of thousands was tested. Any one of thousands of the polio vaccine vials could have been contaminated, meaning it is possible that the theory has not been ruled out entirely.

Contaminated Needles

In the late '50s, disposable needles and syringes hit the market, drastically reducing infection and the spread of disease from person to person. However, the cost of these disposable systems were out of reach for some parts of Africa where millions of people were immunized in a relatively short time. It was not uncommon for medical staff in those areas to use the same needle and syringe on many people to keep immunization costs low. But in doing so, thousands of people could have been infected with SIV/HIV. Once in humans, the virus would spread to even more people through various ways.

Colonialism: The "Heart of Darkness" Theory

In the 19th and early 20th centuries, most of the Congo was under colonial rule. Their rule was notoriously cruel and violent with hard labor camps, little food or water, and disease and sickness. Because the conditions were so deplorable, sickness ran rampant, especially immune system weakness and disease. Any worker suffering from an infection like SIV or HIV was just pushed aside and left to die. In addition, because food was so scarce it was not unusual for the healthier workers to capture and kill local wildlife, including SIV-infected monkeys, and butcher them for food. With so much underlying illness and suppressed immunity, any SIV that was spread from monkeys to man was most likely going to take hold and in theory contaminate and infect a large group of workers. Many of the colonial guards became infected due to a high incidence of female workers being raped and sexually assaulted by their colonial captors. Ironically, when those colonial soldiers went home they took the SIV/HIV with them, infecting women on a different continent.

Conspiracy Theory: "Germ Warfare" Theory

The conspiracy theorists of the world speculate that HIV was actually developed from SIV as a weapon against marginalized groups such as African Americans and gay men. One theory is that the virus was spread to millions of people via the smallpox vaccine. Another claim was that the CIA infected tens of thousands of gay men during Hepatitis B vaccine trials and subsequent systematic immunization with the approved Hepatitis B vaccine. The proponents of this theory choose to ignore the real facts and scientific research for a more spectacular and devious plot against certain groups of disenfranchised people. We know HIV is a slow progressing infection, sometimes taking seven to ten years to make a person sick or die. It seems obvious that if HIV were a biological weapon, it wouldn't be a very fast way to kill off the enemy. Not to mention the cost to the U.S. to care for all those with HIV while they waited for the devious plot to do its job. Yet conspiracy theorists find this HIV theory very plausible even today, when people are living long healthy lives with HIV.

AIDS Makes Its Worldwide Debut

Despite evidence that HIV was around in the late 1950s, the AIDS epidemic didn't officially burst onto the scene until 1981. In June of that year a report from the Centers for Disease Control (CDC) discussed an emerging epidemic among gay men, characterized by shortness of breath, chest pain, fevers and a productive cough requiring hospitalization. Bronchial biopsy of five patients confirmed the diagnosis: *pneumocystis carinii pneumonia* (PCP), a rare but potentially fatal lung infection. Known today as *pneumocystis jirovecii pneumonia,* it became the hallmark symptom of an epidemic that was about to change the world forever. What concerned experts most was the fact that pneumocystis pneumonia typically occurred almost exclusively in people with severely weakened immune systems such as people being treated with chemotherapy for cancer. However, the gay men presenting with pneumocystis had no previous history of illnesses like cancer that would severely weaken their immune systems. Experts were also surprised to find that all the patients presenting with PCP also had *cytomegalovirus* (CMV) infections and oral *candida* (yeast or thrush) infections, both infections that occur mainly in people with very weak immune systems.

Another source of concern was the fact that all the patients presenting with PCP were gay men, suggesting the cause of the weakened immune systems and the pneumocystis was related to sexual lifestyle or was sexually transmitted. This fact alone was especially concerning because the CDC realized that any disease transmitted sexually could potentially become a public health nightmare very quickly.

When news of the pneumocystis outbreak hit the *New York Times*, the public immediately made it an issue of morality because of its connection to the gay community. At that time, homosexuality already was a source of social stigma and prejudice. In the court of public opinion, the fact that a fatal, contagious, sexually transmitted disease had been linked to the gay population justified prejudice. People infected with the mysterious disease were immediately labeled as a risk to public safety and were deemed as sexual deviants, perverted, and immoral. Unlike other terminal illnesses that garner public support and empathy, HIV became the "gay plague," much like leprosy a century before. A combination of fear and ignorance gave birth to AIDS prejudice and discrimination, problems that are alive and well even today.

The "Gay Cancer"

While the CDC struggled to find a cause for the sudden increase in pneumocystis among gay men, another rare disease was emerging among the same population. Kaposi's sarcoma

(KS), a cancer normally seen in about 2 of every 3 million people, was mysteriously appearing in young, gay men in alarming numbers. In a five-week period in 1981, 41 cases of Kaposi's sarcoma were diagnosed, all of them in gay men. Most alarming was that a majority of those men would be dead within 24 months. Doctors investigating the outbreak found all of the victims of the KS outbreak had severely weakened immune systems, had suffered other infections (such as herpes and CMV), were recreational drug users, and admitted to having multiple sex partners. Once again the public made KS an illness of immorality and labeled KS the "gay cancer," stereotyping gay men as promiscuous drug addicts, fueling discrimination against gay men and by extension those living with HIV and AIDS.

Understanding the climate of prejudice against gay men and the gay lifestyle, men found the best defense against gay prejudice in the '80s was to keep their sexual preference private. Hiding one's sexuality, commonly referred to as "being in the closet," served as protection from the stereotypes and prejudices that faced gay men. By trying to blend in with the traditional male stereotype, gay men were able to live a secret life. That all changed with the emergence of KS. Characterized by dark lesions on the skin, men were identified as being gay simply by the presence of the dark KS lesions. The movie *Philadelphia* was based on such a premise. In the film, an attorney was fired, and his illness and sexuality were called into question, when his boss noticed the attorney's KS lesions. The movie's premise reflected real life. When the media made public the connection between KS and AIDS, men could no longer hide their sexual lifestyle or their illness. The dark lesions of KS became the face of AIDS.

The Term AIDS Is Born

Over the course of the next year, deaths related to pneumocystis and KS began to climb. And while an exact cause was still a mystery, the CDC determined that the mysterious illness was blood borne. It was in 1982 that the CDC renamed the disease Acquired Immune Deficiency Syndrome, or AIDS for short. While the media ran with AIDS-related stories almost every night, then–President Ronald Reagan had not yet commented on the emerging public health crisis. In fact, President Reagan's press secretary, Larry Speakes, made light of the illness at a press conference in 1982:

> **Q:** Larry, does the President have any reaction to the announcement the Centers for Disease Control in Atlanta that AIDS is now an epidemic and has over 600 cases?
>
> **Mr. Speakes:** What's AIDS?
>
> **Q:** Over a third of them have died. It's known as "gay plague." [Laughter] No, it is. I mean it's a pretty serious thing that one in every three people that get this has died. And I wondered if the President is aware of it?
>
> **Mr. Speakes:** I don't have it. Do you? [Laughter]
>
> **Q:** No, I don't.
>
> **Mr. Speakes:** You didn't answer my question.
>
> **Q:** Well, I just wondered, does the President…
>
> **Mr. Speakes:** How do you know? [Laughter]
>
> **Q:** In other words, the White House looks on this as a great joke?
>
> **Mr. Speakes:** No, I don't know anything about it, Lester.
>
> **Q:** Does the President, does anyone in the White House know about this epidemic, Larry?
>
> **Mr. Speakes:** I don't think so. I don't think there's been any…

Q: Nobody knows?

Mr. Speakes: There has been no personal experience here, Lester.

Q: No, I mean, I thought you were keeping…

Mr. Speakes: I checked thoroughly with Dr. Ruge this morning and he's had no [laughter] no patients suffering from AIDS or whatever it is.

Q: The President doesn't have gay plague, is that what you're saying or what?

Mr. Speakes: No, I didn't say that.

Q: Didn't say that?

Mr. Speakes: I thought I heard you on the State Department over there. Why didn't you stay there? [Laughter]

Q: Because I love you Larry, that's why. [Laughter]

Mr. Speakes: Oh I see. Just don't put it in those terms, Lester. [Laughter]

Q: Oh, I retract that.

Mr. Speakes: I hope so.

Q: It's too late.

While the government tried their best to ignore the problem, grassroots efforts began working quickly to find research funding and to protect the rights of those with the new disease. One of those pioneering grassroots groups was the Gay Men's Health Crisis (GMHC). The group began with 80 men meeting at the home of author Larry Kramer to discuss the gay community's health crisis. Staffed entirely by volunteers, GMHC set up an AIDS hotline in the basement of its future director, Rodger McFarlane. In the first night of operation, the hotline received over 100 calls. It was obvious that that AIDS had reached epidemic proportions. The CDC agreed. By the end of 1982 they officially declared AIDS to be an epidemic.

A Cause Is Found … But by Whom?

Over the next two years, work continued at a feverish pace in an effort to find the cause of AIDS. Public concern rose when the CDC announced that, given the blood borne nature of AIDS, the donated blood supply might be unsafe. If true, AIDS could no longer be considered a disease limited to the gay community. This fact was reinforced with the announcement of a major outbreak of AIDS in Africa. But unlike the outbreak in the U.S., the African outbreak was found to be spread primarily by heterosexual contact. This marked the beginning of the AIDS crisis in Africa, as well as the safer sex movement in the western world. The sexual revolution was officially coming to an abrupt and tragic end.

A major breakthrough occurred in 1983 when a lab in Bethesda, Maryland, headed by Dr. Robert Gallo cultured HIV cell lines from a lymph node tissue sample of a patient with KS, tissue samples sent to him from the lab of Dr. Luc Montagnier and Françoise Barré-Sinoussi of the Institut Pasteur in France. According to a piece jointly authored by Montagnier and Gallo that appeared in the *New England Journal of Medicine* in 2003, the tissue sample was actually a very aggressive cell line that contaminated a less aggressive strain of another sample. The aggressive strain overtook the less aggressive strain in the culture, resulting in the HIV cell line. Following the initial culture of the HIV, both labs and a third lab in California run by Dr. Jay Levy were able to repeat the culturing of HIV from samples of tissue obtained from AIDS patients with both KS and PCP. The new cell lines also led to a dependable HIV blood test and the conclusion that HIV was indeed the cause of AIDS.

Experts were hopeful that the discovery of a cause would pave the way to a treatment and possibly a cure. But the discovery was not without its share of controversy. A year after Institut Pasteur announced its discovery, Dr. Robert Gallo announced he too had discovered the virus responsible for AIDS. The two groups continued to dispute each other's claim until 1985 when they agreed to share credit for the discovery, Montagnier for first isolating the virus and Gallo for conclusively linking it to AIDS. Today, consensus among scientists is that Montagnier first discovered HIV and it was Gallo who provided further evidence that the virus did indeed cause AIDS. In fact, Montagnier and Barré-Sinoussi were awarded the Nobel Prize in Physiology or Medicine in 2008, and no mention of Gallo was made.

Soon after the discovery of HIV, the Food and Drug Administration (FDA) approved an HIV test. The test detects antibodies to HIV, antibodies produced by the body when a person is infected with the virus. In other words, the presence of antibodies confirms HIV infection. A test for HIV meant earlier detection of the infection, detection before the deadly infections like PCP and KS threatened the life of the infected. Blood banks could test their supplies to assure donated blood was HIV free. And finally, identifying a cause was the first step toward developing a treatment, a vaccine, or even a cure.

A cause had been determined, and a test to detect that cause had been developed. The final step was to find an effective treatment. While the world waited for such a breakthrough, people continued to die in alarming numbers. AIDS became a household word in 1985 when actor Rock Hudson was diagnosed with the deadly illness. When it was announced he was going to France for an experimental AIDS treatment the world could now associate a familiar face with the deadly epidemic. His death later that year made the list of the *Wall Street Journal's* most significant stories in its 100-year history.

Finally, a Treatment

Despite an annual investment in HIV research of $1.3 billion, a cure was nowhere to be found. The development of an effective HIV vaccine was as remote as a cure, so in an effort to improve prognosis and to lengthen lives, prevention methods and treatment options for the disease became a life and death priority. By executive order in 1985, the United States closed its borders to HIV infected immigrants and travelers. While President Reagan finally discussed the AIDS crisis publicly, negative public opinion regarding the Administration's handling of the AIDS epidemic was substantial. Vice President George Bush suggested mandatory HIV testing of its citizens in hopes of putting a halt to the illness's rapid spread. Prejudice, ignorance and fear had reached an unprecedented level when a Florida home was burned to the ground in an attempt to drive the family and their two HIV-infected sons from the neighborhood. Both sons had contracted HIV after receiving tainted blood products during their treatment for hemophilia. To their neighbors, the route of infection was not important. In the minds of their neighbors the fact that the boys were infected with HIV made them a threat to those who weren't—an all too common and very dangerous way of thinking in the United States during the age of HIV and AIDS.

The first glimmer of hope came in 1987 when drug manufacturer GlaxoSmithKline (known as Glaxo Wellcome at the time) gained FDA approval for the world's first medication to treat HIV. Retrovir (zidovudine) or AZT, as it became known, was to be given as a 400mg dose taken every four hours around the clock. Twenty years earlier, AZT was studied as an anti-cancer drug, but trials were halted because the drug showed little promise due to high rates of toxicity and significant side effects. Yet, short-term studies in HIV patients showed dramatic results. While side effects such as low blood count (anemia), headache, and fatigue were common, patient prognosis improved significantly. So, despite side effects, issues of toxicity, and because people were dying in large numbers, Glaxo stopped trials early and sought FDA approval for the use of AZT as an HIV medication.

While the development of an effective HIV medication was a wonderful step forward, the approval of AZT was not without its difficulties. First, Glaxo Wellcome was publicly blasted for what the HIV community called "price gouging," with its $7000-per-year AZT price tag ($14,500 in 2015 dollars). It took two years and intense pressure by HIV activist groups for Glaxo to reduce the price of AZT by 20 percent in 1989. The second controversy called into question the effectiveness and safety of AZT therapy. Some groups claimed that it was AZT itself that caused AIDS, not HIV. Stories of toxic side effects and birth defects were common, adding fuel to the AZT controversy. Even today, certain groups continue to insist AZT was the killer, not HIV or AIDS. But despite the controversy, AZT became widely prescribed and did show promising results, at least in the short term.

Given the positive results among those taking AZT, a new emphasis on HIV drug development was born. The FDA process for approving new drugs normally took years, but in the case of people infected with HIV, most didn't have years to wait. Pressured by AIDS activist groups like Act Up, the FDA announced a rapid drug approval system for HIV medications, shaving at least two years off the approval process.

Does Anyone Notice?

As the epidemic raged on, those in the HIV community struggled to get the world to notice what AIDS was doing to their friends, families and loved ones. The AIDS Memorial Quilt was started as a tribute to those who lost their struggle against HIV/AIDS. Authors and playwrights tried to explain HIV and AIDS through such works as *And the Band Played On* and *The Normal Heart.* Those dying from HIV were no longer faceless strangers. Pianist and song writer Liberace, actress Amanda Blake, and Michael Bennett, director of the Broadway play *Chorus Line,* all fell victim to AIDS.

Politicians of the time, while being slow to react to the epidemic, finally did realize the dangerous prejudice and discrimination that was occurring against those living with HIV. In response, a law was passed in 1988 making it illegal to discriminate against anyone infected with HIV. It was a small step in the right direction, but, unfortunately, discrimination and prejudice appeared to be here to stay.

In 1988, C. Everett Koop, Surgeon General of the United States, released a report emphasizing the need for sex education in order to slow the spread of HIV. To that end, the U.S. Department of Health and Human Services mailed out 107 million copies of its booklet *Understanding AIDS* in hopes that a better understanding of HIV and AIDS would slow the spread of the disease through safer sex practices (e.g., using condoms). At the same time politicians hoped a better understanding of the disease and how its spread could be prevented would quell the prejudice, discrimination and fear directed at those living with HIV. But, unfortunately, like previous attempts, it had little effect on the public's opinion of people living with HIV.

The Courage of Ryan White

The 1990s began with a public apology from Ronald Reagan for his neglect of HIV and AIDS during his presidency. In a public service announcement to benefit the Pediatric AIDS Foundation, Reagan called for compassion and understanding for those living with HIV and AIDS. One person living with HIV that Reagan was referring to was Ryan White. A teenage boy who contracted HIV/AIDS through blood products he received to treat his hemophilia, Ryan White experienced AIDS prejudice and hatred first hand. He and his family fought the Kokomo, Indiana, school board to allow Ryan to attend public school. Because of ignorance and fear, the people of Kokomo showed little support for Ryan's cause. Students vandalized his locker, townspeople vandalized the White home, and local restaurants threw away the dishes from which he and his family ate. After a gunshot was fired into their living room, the Whites moved to Cicero, Indiana, where, unlike Kokomo, they were welcomed with open arms. Ryan attended public school, got his driver's permit, and became an example of hope and courage for the entire HIV community. Ryan White lost his brave battle with HIV in 1990, but his struggle was not forgotten. Later that year, the United States Congress passed the Ryan White Care Act, a congressional act that continues to provide millions of dollars for HIV care and prevention. Today the act known as the Ryan White HIV/AIDS Program is arguably the most important source of HIV care funding in the world.

A Change of Course

The year 1991 saw the re-emergence of an old public health nemesis. Tuberculosis, or TB, as it is called, resurfaced after years of being controlled through organized testing and the development of antibiotics such as streptomycin. At one time, hospitals had TB wards, isolating the infected. TB sanitariums were commonplace in large urban areas. In fact, TB was once the leading cause of death in the U.S. But with the development of antibiotics, the deaths decreased dramatically, and new infections were all but eliminated. But with the emergence of AIDS, people whose immune systems were weakened by HIV became a high risk for TB. New cases started to emerge, especially in urban centers, among the homeless and throughout the U.S. prison system. Today, yearly TB screenings are standard of care for people living with HIV.

President George Bush continued the policies of his predecessor. Despite a recommendation to the contrary from his Secretary of Health and Human Services Louis Sullivan, Bush continued the ban on the immigration of HIV positive people. And while the Ryan White Care Act authorized $881 million of emergency relief for those cities hit hardest by HIV and AIDS, the administration eventually allocated only $350 million. But change was in the wind. Presidential candidate Bill Clinton promised full funding of the Ryan White Care Act, a lifting of the immigration ban, and the naming of an HIV "Czar" whose sole purpose was to address the problem of AIDS. Clinton's election in 1992 was seen by many as a positive step in the fight against HIV and AIDS.

On the treatment front, the choices of HIV medications were increasing. In a 204-month period between 1991 and 1994, the drugs Videx (didanosine), Hivid (zalcitabine), and Zerit (stavudine) were all approved by the FDA. Hivid was the first to be approved for use in combination with AZT. Study data made it clear that multiple drug therapy was superior to single drug therapy. Using multiple drugs, each attacking a different spot on the HIV life cycle, provided the best treatment results and durability of therapy. By 1993, experts reported that patients were beginning to show resistance to the drug AZT, especially among those first patients who used AZT alone. The consensus among HIV experts was that multiple drug therapy would be stronger and more effective, and would delay resistance to the medications. Their hypothesis was supported when, later that year, study results determined that AZT taken alone early in the course of infection did nothing to improve long-term prognosis or slow the progression to AIDS. In fact, that year's IX International Conference on AIDS made it clear that neither AZT nor any of the available antiretroviral drugs were useful for early treatment. The announcement couldn't come at a worse time. The statistics were quite sobering. By the end of 1993, almost 400,000 people had been infected since the epidemic began, and almost 200,000 of those had died.

AIDS was quickly garnering the attention of Hollywood. In response to the deaths of entertainers such as Rock Hudson, Amanda Blake, and Rudolph Nureyev, Hollywood producers, writers, and entertainers rallied to raise money and awareness. In September 1993, HBO premiered its film adaptation of the Randy Shilts novel *And the Band Played On*. In December, Tom Hanks starred in the movie *Philadelphia*, a story of an attorney fired by his firm because of HIV. Hanks won the Best Actor Oscar for his role as the attorney, yet some critics in the gay and HIV community claimed that his character fell short because the film lacked outward signs of affection normally found in gay relationships. Regardless, the Hollywood support was beginning to pay off in terms of money and awareness.

Bring Out the Big Guns: The Protease Inhibitor

HIV medications are classed according to where in the life cycle the medication has its intended effect. Prior to 1995, only one drug class was available, the nucleoside reverse transcriptase inhibitors (NRTI). That meant only one place in the life cycle could be attacked. When HIV enters a healthy cell it attempts to make copies of itself in part by using the enzyme reverse transcriptase. By blocking reverse transcriptase NRTIs prevent HIV from making more copies. Early regimens consisting of two NRTIs were used occasionally, but most often treatment consisted of only one NRTI medication. Unfortunately, studies soon revealed that one-drug treatment, or *monotherapy*, as it was called, was not strong enough to suppress HIV reproduction for very long. In addition, drug resistance developed quickly, eventually making the medications in that class ineffective. The most worrisome problem associated with monotherapy was that resistance to one NRTI medication usually meant resistance to all drugs in that class. That being the case, it was clearly evident that patients would run out of drug choices very quickly. A new and stronger class of drug was desperately needed. As the world waited for this new class, AIDS had become the leading cause of death in Americans 25 to 44 years of age.

Fortunately, the FDA recognized the urgent need for new treatments. In a record 97 days, the drug manufacturer Roche received FDA approval for a new class of HIV medication, the protease inhibitor (PI). Once HIV has entered the healthy cell and has made a copy of itself, the enzyme protease prepares the new HIV copy to leave the cell in order to infect other healthy cells. By blocking protease, the new HIV copy can't leave the cell and therefore can't infect other cells. The first medication in this class was the drug Invirase (Saquinavir). By attacking HIV at an entirely different place in the life cycle compared to existing drugs HIV could now be attacked on two fronts, meaning treatments would be more effective and their effect would last longer. Protease inhibitors like saquinavir made more powerful medication combinations or "drug cocktails" possible. The downside to PI-containing cocktails was the large pill burden and severe side effects, both of which made adherence to therapy more difficult. Still, the advent of the protease inhibitor prompted some media sources to report that the PI was the AIDS breakthrough that could spell the end of the epidemic.

More Meds, but Testing and Prevention Become Key

While preliminary results of combination therapy looked promising, experts agreed that the key to controlling the epidemic was testing and prevention. Prevention education, once generalized to target the public as a whole, was being retooled to address specific populations. Educators found that prevention messages were better received if they "spoke" to the intended population. For example, a prevention message targeted to gay white men might not be well received by bisexual black men unwilling to admit they had sex with other men. Many felt this small change was a very important step forward in HIV/AIDS education.

From the beginning of the epidemic, experts realized the importance of early diagnosis through HIV testing. Unfortunately, because of the stigma and prejudices associated with AIDS, a large share of the population was reluctant to get tested. People feared being diagnosed and feared that just being tested would bring on the same discrimination and prejudices faced by those people living with the infection. In response, HIV test manufacturers worked to develop a test that would alleviate some of those fears. In 1996 the FDA approved the first home test kit for HIV. Experts hoped that the anonymity of home testing would encourage people to get tested and learn their status. Unfortunately, it was discovered many years later that not all home test kits were created equal. Doubts about accuracy and reliability surfaced, and the home test kit idea suffered. While still available, home tests never became a primary mode of HIV testing.

Advances in HIV science continued in 1996. A third class of HIV medication, the non-nucleoside reverse transcriptase inhibitors (NNRTI), gained FDA approval, providing one more weapon against HIV. In order for HIV to infect healthy cells, the viral ribonucleic acid (RNA) must be converted to deoxyribonucleic acid (DNA). NNRTIs block that conversion, meaning the RNA can't be changed to DNA and therefore HIV can't infect the healthy cell. This third angle of attack meant regimens were even more powerful and lasted even longer than one and two drug regimens. The timing was perfect. Studies showed that more than 14 percent of all people taking existing HIV medications were exhibiting signs of medication resistance. Experts began to worry that if the trend continued there would eventually be no means to treat HIV. Fear of an out of control epidemic similar to what was happening in Africa at the time sent chills through the HIV scientific community. The addition of Roxanne Laboratories' new NNRTI, Viramune (nevirapine), was reason for hope. The drug added a new layer to HIV treatment, making regimens even more powerful and more effective. At about the same time, a new technology made it possible for doctors to monitor the fight against the virus. By the end of 1996, the FDA had approved for use the world's first HIV viral load test, allowing doctors to quantify and measure how many copies of the virus were active in the bloodstream—a perfect way to measure the effectiveness of HIV treatment regimens.

Since the epidemic began, most people, scientific and the general public alike, considered the Holy Grail of HIV research to be an effective and preventative HIV vaccine. Like the polio vaccine decades before, people envisioned an HIV vaccine that would offer permanent protection against AIDS. What many felt could be the realization of that dream was the announcement of the first human tests of an HIV vaccine in 1996. Over 5000 people from across the U.S. took that first courageous step by volunteering to receive the new vaccine. While hopes were high, researchers cautioned that a usable, effective HIV vaccine could still be decades away. And they were right. As of the printing of this text no effective vaccine is yet available.

More Sobering Statistics

As the end of the twentieth century neared, HIV/AIDS statistics from around the world did little to instill hope in those fighting the disease. By the year 2000, women and minorities were bearing the brunt of the HIV epidemic. AIDS had become the leading cause of death in women 25 to 44 years old, and African Americans accounted for 49 percent of AIDS deaths in the United States while only making up 12 percent of the U.S. population. And even with the emphasis on testing, New York City officials estimated that nearly 70,000 people were unaware they were HIV infected, a large percentage of those minorities. Public health experts feared that this fact would eventually translate into a geometric increase in new HIV infection numbers among minorities, a potential disaster that would eventually repeat itself in every large urban area in the United States.

While not all the news was bad, even the good news was problematic in some respects. From 1998 through 2001, deaths related to AIDS steadily declined from a peak of almost 18,000 to a low of just under 9000 per year. The consensus was that the declining death rate was the result of more powerful and effective HIV medication combinations. On the surface, this would appear to be very good news. Yet new HIV infections were on the rise, and there was a theory that explained the increased numbers. The success of multidrug HIV medication regimens meant HIV was becoming a long-term, manageable condition, not the death sentence it had been up to that time. However, experts feared the successes were beginning to diminish the public's appreciation of just how detrimental and potentially deadly HIV and AIDS truly were. Complacency was leading to an increase in high risk sexual behavior, namely sex without condoms. In turn, high risk sexual behavior resulted in more new infections. It became obvious that as medication regimens were saving lives, prevention efforts and risk reduction activities needed to be stepped up and targeted to those groups most at risk.

The New Century Arrives

As the new century arrived, scientists from around the world gathered in Durban, South Africa, epicenter of the HIV epidemic, for the XIII International AIDS Conference. Over

12,000 participants witnessed the devastation of AIDS first hand, prompting 5000 doctors to sign the *Durban Declaration*, a document of overwhelming affirmation that HIV was the cause of AIDS.

On the medication front, the age-old problem of medication adherence was being addressed with the development of many once-a-day therapies with diminishing pill burden. Experts had found that HIV drugs were very effective at controlling the virus but only if there was strict adherence to the prescribed regimen. Poor adherence eventually leads to medication resistance and in turn virologic failure. Experts learned very quickly that the major cause of an ineffective medication regimen was poor adherence. Medications not taken consistently, missed medication doses, or taking only a portion of a multidrug regimen all result in HIV mutating and adapting to the medication regimen rendering the combination ineffective. In an effort to improve adherence and thereby reducing the incidence of mutation and resistance, drug manufacturers began combining existing medications to create new combination drugs. For instance, Combivir, the combination of Retrovir (zidovudine, AZT) and Epivir (lamivudine), reduced a two-drug therapy from four pills each day to two. Trizivir, the combination of Retrovir, Epivir, and Ziagen (abacavir), reduced a three-drug regimen from six pills each day to two. The theory was that by decreasing the number of pills required each day, adherence would improve, the incidence of mutation and resistance would decrease, and therapies would be more effective for longer periods.

Medication improvements were not limited to NRTIs and NNRTIs. Protease inhibitors (PI), notorious for very large pill burdens that needed to be taken several times each day, were being improved as well. For instance, the drugs Norvir (ritonavir) and Lopinavir were combined into the drug Kaletra, a twice a day medication that diminished the amount of Norvir taken each day thereby decreasing side effects that negatively impacted medication adherence in the past. The 2003 FDA approval of the PI Reyataz (atazanavir) made it possible for doctors to prescribe the most powerful class of HIV drug as two pills once each day (one Reyataz capsule and one Norvir capsule to boost the effect of Reyataz. An excellent example of PI improvement came in 2003 with the release of Lexiva (fosamprenavir). By changing the formulation of the existing drug amprenavir to create the new drug Lexiva, the pill burden was decreased from sixteen pills each day to only four.

Despite all the success decreasing pill burden, drug manufacturers realized that decreasing the number of pills alone was not enough to significantly improve adherence. Some drugs, while very effective, were difficult to take because of side effects. Something had to be done to make drugs more palatable. A perfect example of advances made in drug formulation was the medication Videx EC (didanosine EC). The drug Videx (didanosine) had been part of drug regimens for several years. Consisting of four wafers that had to be chewed or dissolved in liquid to be effective, Videx was almost impossible to take consistently due to the horrid taste, so bad it caused some people to vomit immediately after taking. To address the problem, the manufacturer reformulated the drug into Videx EC, a one capsule once daily medication that could be swallowed whole instead of being chewed. This change in formulation, decreased pill burden and significantly increase in palatability made the drug much easier to take each day. This greatly improved adherence, so much so that Videx EC-containing regimens became one of the most popular regimens of 2004.

Another drug notorious for its severe side effects was Norvir. Originally taken as six capsules twice each day, Norvir caused severe gastrointestinal side effects, making adherence very difficult. However, researchers found that in small doses, Norvir improved the effect of other medications and was much more tolerable. In response to this finding, doctors began to prescribe Norvir as a *boosting* agent for other PIs, most often in doses as small as one capsule per day. But the softgel capsule required refrigeration and even in the smaller dose caused diarrhea in a majority of people. So again, a formulation changed to a tablet meant the medication no longer needed refrigeration and the incidence of diarrhea decreased. These changes to Norvir improved adherence while at the same time strengthening regimens.

Overseas, the effects of HIV were daunting; some parts of Africa were in financial ruins from a shrinking workforce due to a growing number of infected people. The number of orphaned children as a result of HIV and AIDS was staggering. In 2003 in response to the growing problem of HIV outside of the U.S., the 108th Congress passed the *United States Leadership Against HIV/AIDS, Tuberculosis, and Malaria Act of 2003*, also known as the *President's Emergency Plan for AIDS Relief (PEPFAR)*, which allocated $15 billion in part to combat the HIV/AIDS problem around the world. However, the funding came with political overtones, namely the conservative Congress mandated that one-third of prevention funds be dedicated to *abstinence until marriage* prevention measures, measures that had never been proven to be as effective as risk reduction education. In addition, any agency funded under the act could not be forced to endorse or teach any method(s) of prevention that they found morally or religiously objectionable, meaning condom education and condom distribution would, most likely, decrease or not occur at all.

2005–2006: The Epidemic Turns 25

After twenty-five years, and despite advances in treatment access, medication development, adherence tools, and education and prevention, the HIV epidemic was not running out of steam. The number of new infections in the United States continued at a rate of about 50,000 each year. In other parts of the world, such as Asia, India, and Russia, the rates of new infection were much higher. In Africa, the HIV epidemic was causing financial hardship, was orphaning millions of children, and brought about negative population growth in many areas. The main transmission routes were different in Africa than the U.S. While the majority of new infections were the result of men having sex with men (MSM), the majority of infections in Africa were by way of heterosexual sex and transmission from pregnant woman to unborn child or newborn via breast feeding.

It became more and more evident that the key to slowing the spread of HIV was easy and early access to health care and medications. Unfortunately, many countries lacked the resources to treat their population. Since the emergence of the epidemic the United States had pledged more than $50 billion globally for treatment, education, and prevention, but many felt this was not nearly enough. At the same time, drug manufacturers were beginning to ease their strict policies regarding generic formulations of HIV medications in an attempt to improve medication access outside the U.S. For instance, drug manufacturer Boehringer Ingelheim took an important first step, allowing a South African drug company to make a generic version of the drug Viramune (nevirapine), while Barr Laboratories gained FDA approval for its generic form of Videx EC (didanosine EC).

A constant concern within the HIV community and for HIV caregivers was adequate funding. The Ryan White CARE Act was reauthorized in 2000 and again in 2006, but not without significant cuts in funding, especially in those cities hardest hit by the epidemic. Ironically, the CARE Act title that provided funds for projects in the hardest hit cities had a decrease in funds, a cut that was passed on to the AIDS organizations in the cities. In addition, those programs not experiencing funding cuts were being *flat funded*. Simply put, each program received a predetermined amount of money to operate. While the costs of running their program increased, the amount of funding remained the same. Eventually, to maintain their program, budget cuts became necessary.

Debate continued on how best to fight the spread of HIV. While federal funding was slowly being shifted from prevention programs to treatment programs, prevention education had taken on political tones. Some lawmakers made HIV education a morality issue. The Bush Administration made it clear that prevention should be abstinence-based, and allocated almost one third of its prevention budget to abstinence training. Despite studies confirming abstinence education was not the most effective way to slow the spread of HIV, the CDC was ordered to remove condom educational material from its website, and replace it with abstinence educational material. After public and scientific outcry, the CDC returned the condom information to their government-sponsored website but in a watered down format, deemphasizing the effectiveness of condom use in preventing pregnancy and sexually transmitted diseases.

The benefit and morality of condoms was not the only source of controversy. Sharing needles and syringes among injection drug users was a well known HIV transmission route. Studies had shown that providing clean needles and syringes through needle exchange programs did decrease HIV transmission significantly. Yet, who should provide funding for such needle exchange programs was a constant source of controversy. Laws at that time prohibited federal funding of such programs, so agencies were left to find private funding, a task made much more difficult in times of economic troubles.

In 2003 a new drug class was added, the *Fusion Inhibitors*. This class was the first that attacked HIV before it entered a healthy cell. To make new HIV copies, the virus has to fuse with and enter a healthy host cell. Fusion inhibitors block HIV from fusing with the healthy cell. Without fusing with the cell, HIV can't enter the cell and make a new viral copy. With the addition of fusion inhibitors there were now four points of attack in the HIV life cycle. The first and only fusion inhibitor at the time was a medication known as Fuzeon (enfuviritide, T-20, a twice a day injectable medication. Each dose had to be reconstituted from a powder by the patient and given just under the skin (subcutaneously). If that wasn't difficult enough, almost everyone who used Fuzeon was left with swollen "lumps" at the injection sites. Because it was the first drug to act before HIV entered the cell, excitement for the drug was high among experts and patients alike. That excitement soon faded when people realized just how difficult it was to mix and inject the drug, take the oral HIV medications that completed the regimen, and deal with the unsightly and uncomfortable injection site reactions from the Fuzeon. At a time when manufacturers were trying to make taking HIV medications easier, Fuzeon did just the opposite and as a result the popularity of the drug peaked and crashed very quickly.

Just prior to 2005, two new combination medications hit the market. Epzicom, a combination of two existing medications, Ziagen (abacavir) and Epivir (lamivudine), was used primarily to further ease pill burden. The idea was sound, but Ziagen caused a potentially life-threatening hypersensitivity reaction in a very small portion of those people taking the medication so Epzicom's use had to be closely monitored. The other new combination, a drug called Truvada, was a mix of Emtriva (emtricitabine) and Viread (tenofovir) and like Epzicom decreased pill burden as a one tablet once a day medication. Because Truvada didn't have the concern over hypersensitivity that Epzicom did, Truvada became a very popular drug that is still being prescribed more than ten years after its approval.

As new medication classes and combinations were introduced into clinical trials the FDA created and initiated the *accelerated track system* in an effort to get new, improved HIV meds to the public in much less time. Getting new and improved HIV medications to the public quickly was certainly a benefit but not without risk, the risk that some side effects were not identified during the shortened clinical trial period. But for many that was a trade-off they were willing to make.

Meanwhile, vaccine research continued, but significant progress was still nowhere in sight. In fact, HIV vaccine researcher VaxGen announced that its trial vaccine, *AIDSVax*, proved ineffective in its initial testing of 5400 participants, a major blow to the worldwide vaccine effort. But on a positive note, the prevention world saw the CDC's first medication recommendations for Post Exposure Prophylaxis (PEP), a medication regimen that could be prescribed to HIV negative people to decrease their risk of infection after a possible HIV exposure. The triple-drug combination typically prescribed for 28 days was most effective if prescribed within 72 hours of the exposure. The idea was that PEP would be used after needle sticks, occupational exposures, and for those exposed while engaging in high risk sexual behaviors.

More Medications, More Classes, and More Money

As the first decade of the 2000s approached its conclusion, HIV and AIDS continued to be a serious public health issue, in the U.S. and abroad. The CDC found that their estimate of 50,000 new infections each year was a bit off, changing the estimate to 56,000 a year in 2008. On the medication front, the combination drug Atripla (efavirenz/emtricitabine/tenofovir) became the first one pill once a day HIV regimen—an entire multidrug therapy in one easy to take pill. Atripla became a very popular regimen, offering a very effective combination that also improved adherence dramatically. Isentress (raltegravir) became the first of a new class of drug called Integrase Inhibitors. Integrase is an enzyme necessary for HIV to make copies of itself. Integrase inhibitors block the enzyme and in turn prevent HIV replication. Another drug, Selzentry (maraviroc), was the first of another class of drug that works on HIV before it enters the healthy cell. *Entry Inhibitors* block proteins on the surface of the healthy immune system cell and in doing so prevents HIV from attaching and entering that cell. Unfortunately, Selzentry can only be taken by people with a specific type of protein on the surface of the cell, a protein known as CCR5. Regardless, it is another good option in the constant battle to fight HIV, especially those patients who have lived with HIV for several years and have developed resistance to many existing medications and classes.

While the number of people living with HIV worldwide continued to climb, the cost of caring for those people also soared to record amounts. In response to that rise in costs, President George Bush asked Congress to reauthorize PEPFAR for another five years and double the funding amount to $30 billion, which they did, and still some parts of the world said that the U.S. contribution wasn't enough. A year later, new U.S. President Barack Obama helped develop the first National HIV/AIDS Strategy, rolling out the strategy in 2010. Congress also voted to end two outdated laws, the HIV immigration and travel ban and the law against using government funding to support needle exchange programs.

The Berlin Patient: Could This Be the Cure?

Since the emergence of the epidemic, in the back of everyone's mind—researchers, patients, and physician alike—was the hope a cure could be found to stop this nightmare called HIV. In 2010 a vaccine was still years away if possible at all. The treatments were better but a cure was still a pipe dream. Then, quite by accident, the HIV world stumbled upon the "Berlin Patient." The Berlin Patient was a 40-year-old HIV positive man who had been taking Atripla to maintain his undetectable HIV viral load. Unfortunately, he was diagnosed with leukemia, a cancer that affects the blood. To treat his leukemia, the patient received an HIV-resistant stem cell transplant. Despite complications from leukemia and two stem cell transplants, the Berlin patient appeared to be HIV-free. Even biopsies of his brain, intestinal tract, and a variety of other bodily tissue were free of HIV or HIV genetic material. So for all practical purposes, the Berlin Patient was cured of his HIV. Without HIV medication his HIV viral load (the amount of active virus he has in his blood) has been undetectable ever since the stem cell transplant. While stem cell transplant is not a safe, reliable, or even feasible cure for HIV, the Berlin Patient gave new hope to patients and researchers alike, hope that an HIV cure may not be as far away as once believed.

One Pill Once a Day: Treatment and Prevention

Researchers continue to make treatment regimens as easy as possible to take and to tolerate. With the addition of Complera (rilpivirine/emtricitabine/tenofovir) and Stribild (elvitegravir/cobicistat/emtricitabine/tenofovir), patients had the option of three different one pill once a day regimens, bringing the total medication choices to 23 individual and 8 combination medications. Regimens were becoming easier to take with fewer pills each day and fewer uncomfortable and inconvenient side effects. While treatment was getting easier, a new prevention method was also added that could help decrease the spread of HIV. In 2012 the FDA approved the medication Truvada (tenofovir/emtricitabine) to be used as a prevention medication for high risk HIV negative people. Taken as one pill once a day, Truvada could now be used as an adjunct to condoms in order to further decrease the risk of spreading HIV from positive people to their negative partners. While this sounds like a very positive advance on the surface, the concept has created a few additional issues for providers.

1. Once prescribed by the HIV specialist, would primary care physicians be willing to prescribe the drug for the individual? Would the family physician feel comfortable enough not only to prescribe the drug but to monitor the necessary lab work? Would the family physician feel comfortable with performing sexual behavior risk assessments?

2. The drug Truvada contains the medication tenofovir. Tenofovir has been associated with kidney and renal issues when used as part of an HIV treatment regimen. Some of these renal issues can be serious, even life-threatening. Would that sort of risk be acceptable for some physicians to prescribe Truvada when condoms are a simple, effective, and safe alternative?

3. In the event that infection does occur despite taking Truvada and using condoms, would taking only Truvada for prevention lead to resistant virus, making initial treatment more difficult? In other words, by taking only Truvada to prevent HIV, is the person creating resistance that will complicate his HIV treatment in the future?

4. Will insurance companies be willing to pay for a medication used to treat HIV for a person who is HIV negative? Again, wouldn't it just be easier and cheaper to use a condom, a proven effective and inexpensive alternative to Truvada?

5. Will patients forgo condoms believing that Truvada alone is an effective prevention tool? Unfortunately, without condoms the effectiveness of Truvada is only 70 percent if taken each and every day without a missed dose. Not to mention, without condoms, the risk of sexually transmitted infections like chlamydia, gonorrhea, and syphilis rises dramatically.

Despite all these unanswered questions, people request Truvada and see it as an easy, and in some cases, a condom-free way to protect oneself from HIV without the inconvenience of condoms.

Where Are We Now?

With each passing year new advances in the treatment of HIV and AIDS become available for those living with the disease. Treatment guidelines are reviewed annually and now recommend that treatment be offered to all patients regardless of the strength of their immune system or the amount of virus they have circulating in the blood. That is a change from past guidelines that said treat but only when the virus has depleted the CD4 cells to a certain level. There are a couple reasons that philosophy is no longer recommended.

First, research has found that even in patients with undetectable virus, whether from medication or by being one of the rare few who can control the virus without medication, very low level viral replication can cause a persistent inflammatory reaction which can have long term effects on a person's health. In other words, if a person has a very low viral count, even an undetectable viral load, damage to organs, tissues, and the immune system nonetheless occurs. Medication regimens continue to decrease viral load even after it drops below the level of detectability. Continuing to decrease the number of active circulating virus will help diminish damage done by low level viral replication.

Another reason to treat HIV early is a concept know as *treatment as prevention.* Treating the HIV to continually suppress the virus in the blood and genital fluids decreases the risk of spreading HIV from person to person. The concept is not a new one, however. Treating pregnant women before and during delivery dramatically decreases the risk of *vertical transmission,* transmission of HIV from a positive pregnant woman to her newborn child. Studies have shown that treatment as prevention has decreased the incidence of vertical transmission by 90 percent. In fact, women who received at least 14 days of HIV medication have decreased the risk of transmission of the virus to their baby to less than one percent.

The new treatment philosophy means more people than ever are taking medications. More medications mean more money needed to care for those living with HIV. Thanks to the Ryan White Care Act, each state has a drug assistance program to help pay for HIV medications. That plus private and governmental sponsored insurance like Medicaid have helped get medications to those who need them. Since 2014, the Affordable Care Act, commonly referred to as "Obamacare" after President Barack Obama, has also helped defer some of the cost of HIV care and medications.

Thanks to improved treatment and medication, some populations living with HIV have a life expectancy on the rise. In fact, in some populations life expectancy for someone HIV positive and on HIV treatment is as long as or even exceeds that of people without HIV. A disease that was once a death sentence for anyone who contracted the infection is now a chronic illness much like asthma or diabetes, a disease that can be controlled so that those infected can live as long as or even longer than those without the infection. But with the good comes the bad. Among injection drug users and minority men and women, the life expectancy is much less than someone without HIV infection. So obviously work still needs to be done, especially among those populations.

Work continues on an HIV vaccine, and there is some progress to report. A new injectable HIV vaccine is beginning a National Institute of Health (NIH) sponsored trial in South Africa. There is another vaccine in capsule form that is created from a flu-like adenovirus that is very rare and doesn't cause illness in humans. The adenovirus is being used to carry an HIV protein in the bloodstream where the body recognizes the protein and forms antibodies to HIV. Finally, there is a new HIV medication that is so potent that it could be part of an HIV vaccine. The medication actually blocks two HIV attachment sites, making it impossible for HIV to enter the cell. It has been found to work on HIV-1, HIV-2 and SIV (simian immunodeficiency virus). Having such a broad effect makes it a good candidate for an HIV vaccine.

So as you see the learning process continues for those treating the disease, as well as for those living with HIV and AIDS. Now you know the history of the disease you're fighting. You know where we've been, and you've had a glimpse of where we're going. But that's just the beginning.

2

HIV Prevention and Testing

The first step in slowing the HIV epidemic is prevention. In fact, HIV is a preventable disease—if the proper precautions are taken. Since the onset of the epidemic, prevention efforts have significantly affected the spread of HIV. We need only to look at Africa to see what would be if not for prevention education. In 2002, David Holtgrave, a health policy educator at Emory University, published a report that discussed the impact prevention has had on the epidemic in the United States. By looking at infection rates in Africa, Holtgrave was able to calculate how the HIV picture would look today in the U.S. if not for the prevention efforts that have been in place for the last two decades. The numbers are frightening. Holtgrave has estimated that as many as 1.5 million more people in the United States would be infected today if not for HIV prevention.

Effective prevention starts with education. The public needs to know how HIV is transmitted, what behaviors increase the risk of transmission, and what steps can be taken to reduce the risk of acquiring HIV infection. Let's start by reviewing how HIV is spread from person to person.

Conditions Needed for HIV Transmission

Three conditions must be met for HIV transmission to occur. First, HIV must be present in the blood or bodily fluids involved in the exposure. Second, HIV must be in sufficient quantities to cause infection. In blood, HIV is very concentrated, so a very small amount of blood can infect. In other bodily fluids, such has semen, HIV is less concentrated, and so the amount needed for transmission is greater. Finally, HIV must make its way into the bloodstream. HIV on the surface of unbroken skin is not going to infect because the virus can't make it to the bloodstream. On the other hand, mucous membranes or open wounds give HIV access to the bloodstream, making transmission more likely.

Where in the Body Is HIV Located?

All bodily fluids contain HIV, but only some in concentrations great enough to cause HIV transmission. Table 1 illustrates which fluids do and do not transmit HIV.

TABLE 1

Fluids That Transmit HIV	*Fluids That Don't Transmit HIV**
Blood (Including Menstrual Blood)	Saliva
Semen	Tears
Vaginal and Rectal Secretions	Sweat
Breast Milk	Urine
Pre-cum	Feces

*Keep in mind that while these fluids do not cause HIV infection, they can transmit other diseases, such as Hepatitis B and Hepatitis C.

Transmission Routes

SEXUAL TRANSMISSION

The most common means of transmitting HIV is through sexual contact between two men, two women, or a man and a woman. Studies confirm that the transmission of HIV between men who have sex with other men (MSM) is most frequently due to unprotected anal intercourse. The receptive partner ("the bottom") is at higher risk than the inserting partner ("the top"). The mucous membranes that make up the lining of the rectum provide a large surface area for exposure to infected bodily fluids, namely semen. Rectal trauma from anal intercourse results in tears and tissue damage that make it easier for HIV to enter the bloodstream. The inserting partner can also be infected by exposure to rectal secretions and blood from rectal trauma via small tears in the skin of the penis and through the mucous membranes of the urethra (opening where urine and semen exit the penis).

The same mechanisms of infection hold true for vaginal intercourse. The mucous membranes of the vagina and cervix provide a large surface area where transmission can occur. Trauma to vaginal tissue or the presence of a sexually transmitted disease increases the risk of transmission. The risk of HIV being transmitted from a positive man to a negative female is about two times more likely to occur than transmission from a positive female to a negative male. However, the presence of special circumstances, such as IV drug use, male circumcision, or infection with a sexually transmitted disease, can make female to male transmission more likely to occur. There is also evidence that transmission from female to female can occur, but at a very low incidence. The most common means of transmission between two women is through the sharing of sex toys or through oral contact with infected bodily fluids. However, transmission during oral sexual contact is considered a very low risk by the CDC. Oral exposure to infected semen, vaginal secretions or rectal secretions has been known to transmit HIV; however, the risk is much lower than with vaginal or anal intercourse.

NEEDLES

The accidental injection of infected blood is a more effective means of HIV transmission than even sexual intercourse. In such places as Africa, sex between a man and woman is the most common means of HIV transmission. But outside of Africa, sharing needles among injection drug users plays a major role in the spread of HIV. As part of the process of injecting drugs, users pull infected blood into their needle and syringe. That needle and syringe is then used by another person, who injects the infected blood, along with the drug being injected, into his or her bloodstream. This process repeats itself over and over, leaving new HIV infections in its wake.

Another source of HIV transmission seen primarily in the healthcare industry is accidental needle sticks. The CDC estimates that approximately 384,000 needle sticks occur in hospital settings each year. Add to that needle sticks that occur in nursing homes, outpatient clinics, and home-based nursing care and that number approaches 800,000. Of these needle sticks the World Health Organization (WHO) reports that approximately 1000 infections occur each year; the majority of those infections are Hepatitis B, Hepatitis C, and HIV. A CDC study associated four factors with an increased risk of HIV infection from a needle stick.

- The needle stick injury is deep in the tissue
- There is visible blood on the needle
- The needle that caused the injury had been in the artery or vein of the source patient.
- The HIV-infected patient is not on HIV medications and has a high HIV viral load

While the Centers for Disease Control (CDC) reports less than 100 known cases of HIV transmission by accidental needle stick, the WHO estimates that 2.5 percent of health care workers who have HIV got infected through an accidental needle stick. Hollow-bore needles used to draw blood or give injections carry the highest degree of risk. In an attempt to decrease the number of accidental needle sticks, the 106th United States Congress in November 2000 passed the Needlestick Safety and Prevention Act, the only national-level legislation to mandate hospitals and medical practices to use safety-engineered devices and systems to protect healthcare workers from accidental needlestick injuries.

FROM MOTHER TO BABY

Vertical transmission, or transmission from an infected pregnant woman to her unborn child, can occur during pregnancy or during delivery. Exposure to infected blood or amniotic fluids while in the uterus or during a vaginal delivery provides the route by which HIV enters the baby's bloodstream. HIV transmission in this manner is very efficient, affecting about one in four births in pregnant women without proper treatment before, during and after delivery. With the right treatment before, the risk of vertical transmission decreases to less than 1 percent. To further reduce the risk of transmission, surgical delivery (cesarean section, C-section) of the newborn may be necessary. To decrease the newborn's exposure to HIV-infected bodily fluids from the mother a C-section may be scheduled for the 38th week of pregnancy if the mother's HIV viral load is greater than 1000 copies/ml, if the mother did not take HIV medications throughout her pregnancy, or if the viral load of the mother is not known at the time of delivery. If the mother has a viral load less than 1000 copies/ml and took an HIV regimen during her pregnancy a vaginal birth should be done unless contraindicated for other medical reasons. Unfortunately, the methods used to achieve this low rate of infection are not readily available to women and babies in such places as Sub-Saharan Africa, making vertical transmission a major source of new infections in that region.

Another way in which newborns are exposed to HIV is from breast milk during breast feeding. In fact, breast feeding carries an extremely high risk of transmission—somewhere between 24 and 42 percent. Because of the high risk, HIV positive mothers are cautioned not to breast feed or manually express breast milk to feed their baby. In parts of the world where resources provide clean water and baby formula, avoiding breast-feeding is not difficult. But in parts of the world where there is no clean water and no access to formula, breast feeding is the only option. This is an important reason why the African epidemic has been so devastating, because breast milk is the primary source of nourishment for newborn children in that country.

HIV–Infected Blood Products

Since 1985, blood products have been thoroughly screened for HIV, virtually eliminating transmission of HIV through infected blood products. While the chance of infection from blood products is remote, one in 1.5 million according to a 2008 study, the risk still exists. For instance, a person infected with HIV immediately prior to donating blood could donate blood that tests HIV-antibody negative but still carries the virus. During the "window" between HIV infection and HIV antibody production by the immune system, the blood donor would test negative but would still be infectious. Keep in mind that this scenario is extremely rare, and infection in this manner virtually never happens.

There is, however, a large segment of the HIV population that acquired the disease through infected blood products. Hemophilia is a genetic disorder characterized by the absence of blood clotting factors. Daily infusion of donated clotting factor is the treatment for the disease. Prior to testing of donated blood, thousands of people with hemophilia were infected with HIV by the very blood products they infused to save their lives. A scandal resulted in 6,000 to 10,000 hemophilia patients being infected by blood that was known to be contaminated with HIV. The blood was ordered to be destroyed but instead it was sold to a European blood product distributor which in turn sold it back to the U.S. blood product market. As a result, thousands of unsuspecting hemophilia patients were given the contaminated blood products all because someone wanted to line their pockets at the expense of hemophilia patients across the U.S. Today, however, the transmission of HIV infection through infused blood products has been all but eliminated due to strict testing of donated blood and blood donors. Table 2 summarizes the HIV transmission routes.

TABLE 2

Sexual Transmission	*Needle/Needle Sticks*	*Mother to Baby*	*Blood Products*
Anal (Male-Male & Male-Female)	Sharing needles while injecting drugs	During pregnancy	Via blood transfusion (prior to testing blood supply in 1985)
Vaginal (Male-Female)	Accidental needle sticks (occupational)	During delivery	Hemophilia Scandal (6,000 to 10,000 infected)
Oral		Breast Feeding	

Now we know how HIV spreads from person to person. Let's take a look at how the spread of HIV can be prevented.

HIV Prevention Basics

HIV prevention addresses all three primary modes of transmission: sexual, needle sharing, and vertical transmission. Before discussing specific prevention techniques, let's take a look at a major theory in prevention education—the theory of *risk and harm reduction*.

RISK REDUCTION

Early in the epidemic, prevention messages concentrated on teaching individuals how to avoid behaviors that lead to negative consequences. For instance, counselors instructed their clients to stop having sex with prostitutes in order to eliminate the risk of acquiring HIV. This prevention message ignores the effect certain personality traits have on a person's ability to do what's in their own best interest. Such educational approaches have proved ineffective for people fighting drug and alcohol addiction, as well as for those engaging in risky sexual behavior. Despite the risks, these people knowingly continue to engage in high-risk behavior. In order for prevention efforts to be effective, prevention specialists must consider these personality traits when developing their prevention tools and plans.

Risk reduction is a concept that considers personality traits when developing a holistic approach to HIV prevention. It takes into consideration the reality of human behavior. For example, teaching sexual abstinence as the only HIV prevention technique ignores the reality that a high percentage of teens will have sex despite the risks. Using risk reduction, teens are taught about abstinence as well as the proper way to use condoms in the event they do decide to have sex.

Risk reduction requires education, self-assessment and behavior modification. The risk reduction model consists of four stages:

- **Labeling**—an individual must be able to assess and recognize his or her at-risk behavior. For instance, a person at this stage would say, "I know unprotected sex is unsafe."
- **Commitment**—an individual makes a commitment to certain goals that will diminish his or her risk of HIV. For instance, a person at this stage would say, "I will use a condom each time I have sex."
- **Enactment**—an individual has achieved behavioral change by removing barriers to behavioral changes. A person at this stage would say, "I have discussed with my partner the importance of condoms, and we agree that we will use them each time we have sex."
- **Maintenance**—an individual sustains risk-reducing behavior. An individual at this stage would say, "Condoms are second nature to me now."

The term *safer sex* is a product of the risk reduction concept. Any sexual behavior can be unsafe. Safer sex refers to adjusting sexual behaviors in order to reduce risks associated with sexual activity. Other than complete abstinence there are no 100 percent safe sex techniques; therefore the outdated term safe sex may be misleading to some and, in fact, may lead to high-risk behaviors. For instance, at one time oral sex was thought to be "safe." Many engaged in what they thought was low risk oral sex, unaware that it carried the risk of sexually transmitted infections other than HIV. On the other hand, safer sex education assumes oral sex can be unsafe and teaches techniques to minimize the risk—thus, "safer sex."

SAFER SEX METHODS

There are several methods couples can employ to decrease the risk of HIV transmission. The most important thing is for couples to discuss safer sex prior to sexual activity. Trying to discuss safer sex in the "heat of the moment" is very difficult and most often not very effective. Discussions should be honest and frank. Being sexually intimate with a partner for the first time can be scary. Discussing the emotional and physical risks of sex and how to prevent those risks can be empowering and actually makes sex a more intense, enjoyable experience by creating an emotional understanding between the two partners. Remember, practicing safer sex does not mean eliminating sex from your life. It means being smart, minimizing risk, and staying healthy.

Abstinence

Abstinence is the voluntary choice to refrain from sexual activity and is the only safer sex method that is 100 percent effective in preventing HIV. Abstinence does not mean the absence of sexual intimacy, however. Non-coital (no sexual penetration, no intercourse) forms of sexual intimacy include holding hands, hugging, and kissing, as well as petting, mutual masturbation, and the use of stimulating devices such as vibrators, which can be enjoyable alternatives to intercourse. Keep in mind that while abstinence is an effective means of safer sex, if may be impractical for some and very difficult to maintain over the course of a long-term intimate relationship.

Condoms

Condoms are sheaths of thin latex or plastic that are placed on an erect penis prior to sexual intercourse. To be effective, condoms must be worn during sex and removed immediately after ejaculation. Condoms must be used during any oral, vaginal, or anal sexual contact. While using condoms, some very important points must be kept in mind.

- Condoms can break due to friction during sex, resulting in leakage of semen and possible exposure to infected bodily fluids. To reduce the risk of this occurring, a generous amount of water soluble lubricant should be used. Oil-based lubricants such as petroleum jelly will weaken a condom and should never be used. Some condoms are prelubricated so an additional water-soluble lubricant would not be necessary.
- Because it increases friction and therefore the risk of breakage, two condoms should never be worn at the same time.
- An erect penis can leak pre-seminal fluid ("precum") before ejaculation. This fluid can contain enough HIV to cause infection. For this reason, condoms must be applied prior to any sexual intercourse or oral sex.
- Condoms must be removed and discarded immediately after ejaculation. Never reuse a condom.
- For those people with latex allergies, non-latex, polyurethane condoms can be used. Keep in mind that sheepskin condoms have micro pores larger than HIV, allowing the virus to penetrate the condom. Consequently, they do not protect against HIV transmission and should never be used.
- Spermacides, such as *nonoxynol-9*, actually increase the risk of HIV transmission by irri-

tating mucous membranes, allowing HIV to enter the bloodstream through the irritated mucosa. For this reason, spermacides should never be considered as protection against HIV.

The Female Condom

The *female condom* is a polyurethane pouch about seven inches in length worn by a woman during sex. It has a flexible ring on each end—one ring holds the condom against the cervix, and one ring holds the condom outside of the vagina. There is silicone lubricant on the inside of the condom to reduce friction, decreasing the risk of breakage during sex. The female condom is the only female-controlled device that offers protection against HIV. There are a few important points to keep in mind when using the female condom.

- Used correctly and all of the time, the female condom is 95 percent effective in preventing HIV.
- The female condom can be put in place up to eight hours prior to sexual activity.
- Because friction can break condoms, a female condom and male condom should not be used at the same time.
- The female condom must be held in place during intercourse to prevent accidental displacement.
- After ejaculation, carefully remove the female condom and discard. Never reuse a female condom.

Dental Dams

Dental dams are rectangular squares of latex that are used during oral-vaginal and oral-anal sex. During sex, dams are stretched across the genitals to prevent bodily secretions from coming in direct contact with the mucous membranes of the mouth. While their effectiveness has not been studied, dental dams are probably as impermeable to sexually transmitted organisms as are condoms. However, dental dams can be a bit cumbersome and difficult to hold in place. A small amount of water soluble lubricant applied to the genital side of the dam can help keep them in place. Once used they should never be flipped over to use the opposite side or to use a second time. Dental dams are a one use only device and should be discarded immediately after the sexual encounter.

PREVENTING PREGNANCY DOESN'T MEAN SAFER SEX

Regardless of their effectiveness in preventing pregnancy, there are several birth control methods that do nothing to prevent HIV transmission and therefore should not be used as a prevention method.

- Diaphragms
- Intrauterine devices (IUDs)
- Birth control pills
- Hormonal implants and injections
- Hormonal patches
- Contraceptive sponges

- Spermacides (actually increase the risk of HIV transmission)
- Withdrawal
- Surgical sterilization of men or women

PREVENTING MOTHER TO BABY TRANSMISSION

Vertical Transmission

The HIV epidemic rages out of control in much of Africa in part due to the high incidence of infected pregnant women passing HIV to their unborn children. In the absence of medical care, this mode of transmission occurs in about one out of every four pregnancies. However, in the western world, advances in HIV treatment and abundant financial resources have nearly eliminated vertical transmission, decreasing the incidence to less than 1 percent. The keys to this success include early diagnosis through aggressive screening programs, regular obstetrical care, and HIV treatment for the mother during pregnancy and delivery, and treatment for the newborn baby after delivery. Let's look at the three parts of HIV treatment for pregnant women: throughout pregnancy, during delivery and after delivery.

In accordance with the latest treatment guidelines, most pregnant women in HIV care should already be on an HIV medication regimen. However, a woman may have to change her HIV regimen once she is pregnant. Certain medications are not recommended in pregnancy due to the increase risk of side effects and possible damage to the unborn fetus. During pregnancy the current guidelines recommend the mother's HIV regimen include two NRTIs plus an integrase inhibitor (INSTI), an NNRTI, or a PI with low dose Norvir as a boosting agent. Because the NRTIs abacavir, emtricitabine, lamivudine, tenofovir, and zidovudine all cross the placenta to the unborn baby, the mother's regimen should contain at least one of these medications. Once in the baby's system, the medication protects the unborn baby from mom's HIV.

When it is time to deliver, the answers to two questions will determine how the baby will be delivered. First, has the mother been taking an HIV regimen throughout her pregnancy? Second, is mom's HIV under good control? Any mom that has been taking HIV medications throughout her pregnancy and has less than 1000 copies of circulating HIV (HIV viral load) can deliver vaginally, provided there are no other medical reasons that would necessitate a C-section. If there has been no medication regimen during the pregnancy, mom's viral load is not known, or the viral load is greater than 1000 copies, a C-section delivery should be done and mom should be given a dose of intravenous (into the vein) zidovudine during delivery.

The final step in preventing HIV vertical transmission occurs after delivery. After delivery the newborn receives a 6-week course of zidovudine and has HIV testing at 14 to 21 days, 1 to 2 months, and 4 to 6 months. If baby has two negative HIV tests that include one at 1 month and one at 4 months after delivery than the baby is presumed HIV-negative.

Breast Feeding

The *Breastfeeding and HIV International Transmission Study* reports that 24 to 42 percent of all children breast fed by an HIV infected woman will acquire the disease. The study also estimates that between one-third and one-half of vertical transmission is a result of breast-feeding. However, this incidence does vary greatly depending on the population being studied.

So in order to eliminate this transmission route, HIV infected women who have alternatives to breast-feeding, namely commercial formula, should not breast feed. Unfortunately, there are parts of the world where bottle feeding is not available. In regions that lack financial resources, clean water, and commercial formula, bottle feeding is not an option. In this situation, breast-feeding should be done exclusively and both mother and child should be taking an HIV medication regimen.

SHARING NEEDLES AND INJECTING DRUGS

Outside of sexual contact, needle sharing among injection drug users is the most common means of HIV transmission. Therefore, in order to significantly slow the spread of HIV, needle sharing must be eliminated, ideally by halting injection drug use. However, as our discussion of risk reduction revealed, human behavior and certain personality traits make eliminating substance use unrealistic. A more realistic approach is to treat those who want treatment for their substance use and to reduce the risk for those who feel they need to continue injecting drugs or are unable to stop.

RISK REDUCTION—NEEDLE EXCHANGE

Risk reduction takes a realistic approach to preventing the spread of HIV among drug users. One type of risk reduction is needle exchange. The process of needle exchange is simple: intravenous drug users bring their used needle and syringe to a collection point somewhere in the community and a sterile needle and syringe is given to the drug user in return. Needle exchange is a proven method of decreasing not only HIV transmission but Hepatitis C transmission as well. Unfortunately, needle exchange is a politically controversial subject. Opponents of needle exchange fear that making clean needles available to intravenous drug users promotes and facilitates further drug use. Political opponents have also made needle exchange a morality issue, refusing to fund a program that would supply the tools that support illegal drug habits. In the U.S. it is illegal to fund a needle exchange program with federal monies; however, some states have passed bills appropriating funds for needle exchange. Faith-based groups, HIV agencies, and private donors also provide needle exchange dollars. At the time of this printing Texas was the only state to outlaw needle exchange programs entirely.

Where needle exchange programs aren't available, injection drug users must take steps to minimize exposure to blood borne illnesses like HIV. The equipment of drug use, commonly known as "works," includes needles, syringes, cotton balls, bowls, filters, spoons ("cooker"), citric acid, and water. While using a new needle and syringe is preferable, properly cleaning the "works" prior to injecting drugs can help reduce the risk of HIV infection. Cleaning the needle and syringe must be done after each use and should never encourage the sharing of needles. Its importance can't be overstated: drug users should NEVER share their needles and syringes. These cleaning steps will help reduce exposure to blood borne illnesses:

- Draw cold, clean water into the syringe and needle, and flush. Repeat two more times for a total of three.
- Draw household bleach into the syringe and needle. Let the bleach stand in the syringe

at least 30 seconds, then flush. Repeat this procedure two more times for a total of three.

- Draw cold, clean water into the syringe and needle, and flush. Repeat two more times for a total of three.

Keep in mind that cleaning your "works" in this manner will kill HIV but it does little to prevent the transmission of Hepatitis C, another epidemic fueled by needle sharing.

TREATMENT AS PREVENTION

Treatment as prevention is a concept that began as more and more people were achieving undetectable viral loads due to their HIV medication regimens. The concept is that by treating HIV and decreasing the HIV viral load to an undetectable level (less than 40 copies), HIV transmission can be decreased significantly. In August 2011, the *New England Journal of Medicine* published the results of a study called the *HPTN 052* trial. The trial showed that HIV-infected people taking HIV medications were less likely to spread their HIV than those people not taking medications. In fact, the National AIDS Treatment Advocacy Policy (NATAP) pooled the results of six different studies including HPTN 052 and found there was a 96 percent reduction of risk when the positive partner was taking an HIV medication regimen. Stated a little differently, if there were a thousand couples with one HIV positive partner and one negative partner (serodiscordant) and they had sex for one year, only one or two of the negative partners would become HIV positive. Even more promising, in couples with one partner taking HIV medications and the couple is using condoms, the risk of transmission decreases to essentially zero if the positive partner has an undetectable viral load. Simply put, another important way to decrease the risk of HIV transmission is for positive partners to take their medications religiously and maintain an undetectable HIV viral load. Do that and add condoms, and the risk of transmission is just about zero.

POSITIVE PREVENTION

A common misconception is that HIV prevention stops once a person becomes HIV infected. Nothing could be further from the truth. Obviously, prevention techniques such as condoms must be used to prevent HIV exposure to those not infected. But what precautions need to be taken in relationships with two positive partners? Simply put, the same precautions that are taken in HIV negative couples. The concept of *positive prevention* refers to safer sex precautions taken in HIV positive couples to prevent *HIV reinfection.*

HIV REINFECTION

For many years, experts suspected that HIV-infected partners could infect one another with their specific strain of HIV, including any mutations and drug resistance. Initially, the proof of reinfection was scarce. But according to three studies presented at the 19th Conference on Retroviruses and Opportunistic Infections (CROI) in 2012, the risk of being reinfected with HIV is similar to the initial risk of HIV infection. These studies confirm what scientists have suspected for years: reinfection can and does occur, it could have many public health ramifications, and it will affect future work on HIV vaccines.

HIV reinfection occurs when HIV-positive partners expose one another to their specific HIV virus. Because of natural changes or mutations that occur, HIV varies slightly from person to person. When HIV infected people expose one another to their own specific HIV types, a mixing of two HIV types can occur, resulting in one or both partners having multiple types of virus to treat.

HIV reinfection complicates an already complicated illness. For example, person "A" has a type of HIV that is effectively treated by Drug #1. His partner, person "B," has a type of HIV that is not treated effectively by Drug #1. If person "A" is reinfected by person "B," there is a new HIV variant introduced to person "A"; one that is not treated effectively by Drug #1, a drug that is working well in person "A." The resulting mix of HIV types means person "A" must find a new drug regimen to treat his HIV. Reinfection has made his old drug regimen ineffective, allowing his HIV to multiply and damage his immune system, which eventually will lead to infection and illness. Because of the potential harm caused by reinfection, precautions to prevent HIV transmission must be employed—especially safer sex methods, condoms with each oral, vaginal, or anal sexual encounter, and adherence to HIV treatment regimens.

HIV Testing Basics

Another important aspect of HIV prevention is testing. The Centers for Disease Control estimates that by the end of 2012 approximately 1.2 million people 13 years and older were living with HIV in the United States. Incredibly, that number includes more than 156,000 people who are unaware of their HIV infection. In addition, the CDC estimates approximately 50,000 new infections each year. Imagine the potential for infection those 156,000 people have. One only has to look to Africa to see the public health disaster that exists when people are not aware of their infection.

THE PRICE OF NOT KNOWING

Knowing one's status is paramount to staying healthy and slowing the HIV epidemic. What are the advantages of early diagnosis? What are the consequences of not knowing?

Early Intervention and Care

HIV testing and diagnosis allows for earlier access to medical care, which greatly improves the prognosis of people infected with HIV. Experts universally agree that early HIV medical care keeps a person healthier for a longer period of time. A 2010 study in Argentina showed that diagnosing an HIV infection before symptoms of the illness occur increases life expectancy by almost 11 years. The availability of effective HIV medications allows the HIV specialist to treat the disease sooner, thereby preserving the immune system and health of the infected individual. In addition, early HIV treatment is also an effective means of preventing its spread from person to person. Being aware of an HIV infection and maintaining an undetectable HIV viral load are key components to slowing or even stopping the epidemic. But to access care, a person needs to take that first step and get HIV tested.

HIV Prevention

Being unaware of HIV infection greatly impacts HIV prevention efforts. While the presence of an HIV infection is no guarantee, individuals have a greater incentive and are more likely to use safer sex methods after their HIV infection has been diagnosed. With knowledge of an HIV infection, mothers who would otherwise choose to breast feed would bottle feed, thereby protecting their children from HIV exposure and infection. Imagine this very real scenario: A woman is unknowingly infected with HIV by her husband, who also is not aware of his infection. She gets pregnant but still is not aware of her infection so there is no prevention of vertical transmission. The baby is born and mom decides to breast-feed; as a result, the baby gets infected as well. In this scenario, had the husband been tested and made aware of his infection, two other infections—that of his wife and his newborn—could have been avoided. Simply put, one test could have avoided two additional infections. If this scenario plays over multiple times across the U.S. and the world, the numbers are staggering.

In the over-fifty population, many believe that condoms are used only to prevent pregnancy. Even health care providers neglect to perform sexual histories and safer sex education in their over-50 and post-menopausal patients, thinking that since they are not of child bearing age and presumed monogamous why should they need safer sex education. Since becoming pregnant is not a concern for the over 50 population and healthcare providers are not encouraging safer sex, condoms are not used. And the numbers show us that HIV testing and condom use is needed. In 2013 there were approximately 7,500 new infections in people older than 50. The fact of the matter is that being aware of an HIV infection increases the probability that condoms will be used; important in all populations, including the over 50 crowd.

Knowing your HIV status is an important part of HIV prevention. Knowing you are infected motivates you to make lifestyle changes that will decrease your risk of infection or infecting others. If you are positive, knowing so allows you to get medical care sooner rather than later, decreasing the risk of spreading HIV to others. Knowing your status answers the question "Can I infect others?" And if you are negative, being aware of that will relieve the anxiety and stress of not knowing.

HIV TESTING METHODS

Testing for HIV can be accomplished in many ways. Testing can be confidential or anonymous, free or for a fee, at home or in a testing facility, and by drawing blood from a vein, taking cells from inside the cheek, or taking a sample of oral fluid. Let's explore each of these testing options.

Confidential vs. Anonymous

For many, HIV testing can be a very threatening and frightening experience. Prejudices and stereotypes surrounding HIV are well known. There are people who avoid testing because they fear the social backlash of a positive test. Some are even fearful that the very test itself will label them, regardless of the result. For this reason, two methods of HIV testing exist: confidential and anonymous. Table 3 illustrates the differences.

- *Confidential*: These tests are usually done through commercial laboratories, hospitals, or medical practices. The person being tested provides his or her name, address, and other vital information prior to testing. The results of the test, positive or negative, are stored indefinitely in the person's medical record, readily available to anyone permitted to access medical records kept at the testing facility. All medical practices and hospitals have a strict policy of confidentiality in accordance with the *Health Insurance Portability and Accountability* Act (HIPAA). But unfortunately there are no guarantees that the results will remain confidential at all times.

- *Anonymous*: This type of testing is done by community agencies, in-home test kits and free-standing testing facilities. No name is ever associated with the test, and no connection can be made between the person being tested and the random code assigned to him or her. Results are kept for a brief period, usually several weeks, and then destroyed. Anonymous testing provides the privacy and safety that people need in order to alleviate their fear of HIV testing.

TABLE 3

Confidential Testing
- Typically done through commercial labs, hospitals, or medical practices.
- There will be identifiers attached to the test and results (e.g., name, address, telephone, etc.).
- The results are stored indefinitely and are forever attached to the identifiers.
- Typically, these tests are done for a fee and may or may not be covered by medical insurance.
- Regulations try and assure confidentiality, but, unfortunately, there are no guarantees.
- Results are readily available to anyone permitted to view the facility's medical records.

Anonymous Testing
- Typically done in community agencies, free-standing testing and HIV facilities, and as part of home test kits.
- No name is ever associated with the test or the results.
- While unique identifiers (random numeric codes) are used, there is no way to connect test results to a specific person.
- Results are kept for a brief period of time and then destroyed.
- These tests are typically free of charge.

Free vs. Fee

HIV testing can be very expensive for those without financial means or medical insurance. The inability to pay deters people from being tested. To assure testing is readily accessible for everyone regardless of his ability to pay, two types are available.

- *For a Fee*: These tests are usually provided by medical practices, hospitals and laboratories. Coincidentally, these tests are usually confidential, as opposed to anonymous. Testing fees vary in amount but are paid for by most types of medical insurance, private and government sponsored (e.g., Medicaid).

- *Free*: As the name implies, these tests are free of charge. Most often these tests are provided by HIV testing organizations and are usually anonymous. Government-funded testing programs also provide free tests through state and local agencies, and county health departments.

Home vs. Community Testing

The majority of tests, both confidential and anonymous, are done in the community in testing agencies, medical practices, laboratories, and hospitals. But, as mentioned earlier, HIV testing can be a very scary and threatening experience to many people. In an effort to engage those people reluctant to be tested because of anxiety and fear, the FDA has approved home testing as an alternative to community testing.

- *Home Testing*: Home test kits are available without a prescription at local pharmacies. Currently there are two types of home tests approved by the FDA. One uses a dried drop of blood applied to a special card. The other home test uses oral fluid collected by swabbing the inside of the mouth. The swab or the card are packaged according to instructions provided as part of the kit and mailed to a testing laboratory. Much like anonymous testing, a random code is assigned to each kit. With this code, the user can retrieve test results by telephone; typically, the results are available 24 hours per day. While the home test kit does provide the privacy people want, test accuracy has come into question; specifically, user error can affect the results. There are two other factors to consider when thinking about using a home test kit. First, some kits require you wait up to three months after a potential exposure to get an accurate test result. Second, because you have to send the sample to a lab for processing, it may be up to a week to ten days before a test result is available. Testing at a lab or a community agency will decrease the time after exposure a test can be done and the time it takes for the results to be available. Finally, keep in mind that any positive result or a negative result in the presence of HIV risk factors should be confirmed by a blood test provided by a community agency or medical lab.

- *Community Testing*: Community testing is done in testing agencies, hospitals, laboratories, and medical practices. Community agencies usually use the cheek swab method, collecting oral fluid that is tested for the presence of HIV antibodies. Laboratories, hospitals, and medical practices, on the other hand, use blood samples drawn from a vein. Unlike home test kits, community testing is considered more reliable and accurate, and can be done sooner after a possible exposure. A big advantage the community testing has over home test kits is the results are available sooner, sometimes in less than 30 minutes depending on the test being used. Depending on the testing site, community testing can be free and anonymous, or for a fee and confidential.

How Do HIV Tests Work?

To understand HIV testing, you first must understand what occurs in the body when HIV enters the bloodstream. The *immune system* is the body's natural defense against foreign organisms and infectious agents, such as HIV. When the immune system senses a foreign invader like HIV, the immune system produces substances known as *antibodies* that attempt to fight off the infectious agent. Antibodies are specific to the organism they are fighting. For instance, the body produces hepatitis B antibodies to fight off hepatitis B, and flu antibodies to fight off the flu. Likewise, when your body is exposed to HIV, antibodies are produced that are specific to HIV. It's these specific HIV antibodies that are detected by HIV tests. When HIV enters the bloodstream, HIV antibodies are produced, which are then detected by HIV testing. If antibodies are detected, the HIV test is positive and the person is said to be HIV-infected.

In addition to antibody testing, there are ways to test for HIV by looking for actual viral copies. While antibody testing looks for the body's response to the HIV infection, there are tests that look for evidence of the actual virus. These tests are known as *antigen tests*. Specifically, antigen tests look for viral proteins or genetic material to confirm infection with HIV. Let's look at the different antibody and antigen tests.

Antibody Tests

- *ELISA*: The ELISA test is actually a laboratory technique used to detect HIV antibodies. It is most often used on blood, but can be used to test oral fluid (as in the cheek swab tests) and urine. The ELISA is the first testing technique used on a blood sample because it's very sensitive and rarely provides "false negative" results (negative results in the presence of HIV antibodies). "False positive" results, or positive test results in the absence of HIV antibodies, are much more common. Because of this, ELISA testing alone can't diagnose an HIV infection. If the ELISA test results are negative, the testing process ends and the person is considered not to be HIV-infected at that time. If the ELISA test is positive, the testing process moves to the next step, the Western Blot Assay.

- *Western Blot Assay (WB)*: The Western Blot Assay is another technique that is only used after the ELISA test is positive. Because of the very rare incidence of "false positive" results, this test is used to confirm the results of the ELISA. The test looks for the presence of HIV *protein bands* in the blood being tested. Proteins are organic compounds that make up living organisms. HIV is made up of HIV proteins. If three or more of these HIV protein bands are detected, the sample is said to be Western Blot positive, confirming the positive ELISA. While the ELISA has two possible results, "positive" or "negative," the Western Blot has three:
  - *Positive*: Three or more proteins are present, confirming an HIV-positive result.
  - *Negative*: No HIV protein bands are present, confirming an HIV-negative result.
  - *Indeterminate*: One or two protein bands are present. This result is neither positive nor negative. If a sample is indeterminate, and if the person being tested has HIV risk factors or has a known HIV exposure, another antibody test should be performed in six to twelve weeks. An *antigen test* could also be done to help confirm a negative or positive result.

- *Indirect Immunofluorescence Assay (IFA)*: The IFA testing method is seldom used but acts as a confirmatory test, much like the Western Blot. A reaction occurs between HIV antibodies in the blood sample and HIV antigen fixed to a microscope slide; the reaction glows (fluorescence), confirming the presence of HIV antibodies in the blood sample. If there are no antibodies in the blood, there is not reaction on the slide and thus no glowing. Faster than a Western Blot, labs sometimes use the IFA when the speed in which results are obtained is an issue.

- *Oral Mucosal Transudate (OMT)*: This test is an alternative to blood testing. A specially treated pad on the end of a wooden stick is swabbed between the lower cheek and gum, picking up a substance called *oral mucosal transudate (OMT)*. This substance is then tested for the presence of HIV antibodies. Keep in mind that OMT is *not* saliva.

- *Urine HIV Antibody Test:* An alternative to the blood test, the urine Elisa and Western Blot test detects HIV antibodies while protecting the tester from potential needle sticks. The FDA does approve this test as an alternative to a blood test.
- *Rapid HIV Antibody Test:* Faster than conventional blood tests, the rapid test uses a drop of blood mixed with a vial of developer and a test stick to identify the presence of HIV antibodies. Test results are available in 5 to 60 minutes. This test is perfect for those situations where getting the person into care may be difficult. Using this test allows for quick results and a rapid referral process to an HIV provider. Again, this test requires a conventional serum test to confirm a positive result.

Antigen Tests

- *p24 Antigen:* The protein p24 is an HIV viral protein that makes up most of the viral core or central part of the virus. In the first few weeks after infection, p24 can be detected in high levels in the blood. Because the amounts of p24 rise very quickly after infection, the p24 antigen test can be used very early after being infected when HIV antibodies are too low to be detected by HIV antibody tests.
- *HIV RNA:* As we know from our brief discussions of HIV medications, HIV is comprised of genetic material called *ribonucleic acid* (RNA). The HIV RNA test detects HIV RNA sequences in the blood of an infected person by using *nucleic acid testing* (NAT). Until recently, HIV RNA testing was not generally used for HIV testing but rather to quantify the amount of active virus in the blood (viral load) of someone already confirmed as HIV-infected. But with new 4th Generation antibody testing (HIV-1 and HIV-2 are tested for in one antibody test) HIV RNA testing is required to confirm a negative HIV-1 and HIV-2 test result.

WHEN NEGATIVE ISN'T NEGATIVE

At first glance, a negative Western Blot test means that there is no HIV infection. A majority of the time this is true, but there is a circumstance when the ELISA and Western Blot tests can be negative, yet the person can still be HIV-infected. How is that possible?

The body has a built-in defense mechanism that detects infectious organisms and produces specific antibodies that help fight the organism. If HIV antibodies are present, the person is HIV positive; if not, they are HIV negative. The problem is that the body needs time to manufacture these HIV antibodies, meaning the test has some degree of inaccuracy.

There is a "window period" defined as the time between HIV entering the bloodstream and the time when the body has made enough HIV antibodies to be detected by an HIV test. Depending on the sensitivity of the test that period could be anywhere from four to six weeks after the initial infection. It's during this "window period" that a person will have a negative HIV antibody test despite having HIV in their blood. Simply put, in this case, negative doesn't necessarily mean negative. More importantly, despite having a negative test, the person is infectious and can transmit HIV to other people.

In order for an HIV antibody test to be considered accurate, the body must be given ample time to produce antibodies in quantities great enough to be detected by HIV testing. To assure an accurate result and to make certain sufficient quantities of antibodies have been manufactured by the body, a series of HIV antibody tests—one at six weeks, three months and finally six months after a potential exposure is required. If after the six-month test there are still no HIV antibodies detected, a person can feel confident that he or she is not HIV-infected.

An alternative to early antibody testing is the HIV antigen tests which, as we have discussed, detect actual HIV proteins. These tests can detect HIV infection much earlier and can be used to determine infection soon after the HIV exposure. In fact, some of the new 4th Generation antibody tests use HIV antigen tests to confirm HIV antibody results.

So what if the test is positive? What happens next? Where do we go from here?

3

HIV 101 ... THE BASICS

Understanding HIV and AIDS starts with a good foundation of knowledge, understanding the basics. "HIV 101," as it is called among HIV educators, is an essential first step to building the strong foundation needed to live with the disease. Someone once said that the best place to start is the beginning. It all begins with a virus. Before we can understand HIV, we must first understand viruses and why they need us to survive.

What Is a Virus?

As the name implies, Human Immunodeficiency Virus (HIV) is a virus. But what exactly is a virus? By definition, a virus is a microscopic living organism that makes copies of itself by using genetic material from the cells of a living host. In the case of HIV, we are the living host and it is our genetic material HIV uses to make more HIV. Specifically, there are two types of genetic material needed for a virus to replicate (make copies of itself): *Ribonucleic Acid (RNA)* and *Deoxyribonucleic Acid (DNA)*. Big words, but what do they mean?

The human body is made up of many substances and compounds that all work together to make us who we are. One such substance is called a *protein*. Proteins are the building blocks of the human body. Proteins come together to form tissues, muscles, and organs. *DNA* is a double strand protein that contains the genetic information needed during the manufacture of new proteins. *RNA*, on the other hand, is a single strand protein which transports DNA instructions that control the synthesis of new proteins. It's that genetic information that makes a virus a virus, a monkey a monkey, or a human a human. Through chemical reactions, DNA is changed to RNA. The RNA then transports the genetic code of the DNA to the sites of protein manufacturing. On a car assembly line, parts for the car must be brought to the line so they can be assembled. RNA brings the genetic parts to the protein assembly line.

In most living organisms, including viruses, DNA is converted to RNA in order to replicate. HIV, on the other hand, is a *retrovirus,* meaning it converts RNA to DNA in order to replicate. Regardless of whether DNA is converted to RNA or vice versa the key point to remember is that viruses and retroviruses need genetic material from a living host in order to survive and multiply. In the case of HIV, we are the living host and our cellular RNA is changed into viral DNA in order to make more HIV copies.

The HIV Life Cycle

What happens after HIV enters the bloodstream? How does HIV make copies of itself? The HIV life cycle is comprised of several complex physiologic steps, each with a very specific and important role in the replication of HIV. The life cycle is a very difficult concept to understand but a necessary one to discuss as a foundation for our upcoming discussion of HIV medication regimens. Keep in mind that the theory behind HIV medications is that multiple medications in the regimen attack multiple steps in the life cycle. Understanding that one concept is essential to a good foundation for the discussion of medications in upcoming chapters.

INTRODUCTION OF HIV INTO THE BODY

Before HIV can replicate, it must enter the body. As we learned earlier, exposure to infected bodily fluids during sexual contact or by sharing needles are the primary means by which HIV enters the body. While less common, HIV can also enter the body during pregnancy, child birth or by ingesting HIV-infected breast milk.

VIRAL ATTACHMENT

Once in the body, HIV needs a *host cell* in order to replicate. In the case of HIV, the host is a specialized cell from the immune system known as the *T-cell* or *CD4 cell*. The CD4 cell is considered a "helper cell" because it triggers the body's response to infection. Ironically, it's the CD4 cell, the very cell that triggers the defense against HIV, that the virus seeks out in order to replicate. Once in the bloodstream, HIV attaches to the CD4 cell in a "lock and key" system. Proteins on the surface of HIV attach to complementary proteins on the CD4 cell much the way a key fits into a lock. Once attached to the CD4 cell, HIV can move on to the next step in the life cycle.

VIRAL FUSION

Once attached to the cell, HIV injects proteins of its own into the cellular fluids (cytoplasm) of the CD4 cell. This causes a *fusion* or joining of the host cell membrane to the outer envelope of HIV. As part of this fusing, a fusion pore develops, creating a "tunnel" between the virus and the CD4 cell. It's through this "tunnel" that the HIV genetic material enters the healthy CD4 cell.

THE UNCOATING

In order for HIV to use its genetic material (RNA) for reproduction, the protective coating (capsid) surrounding the RNA strand must be disassembled. The capsid organizes and contains the viral RNA for optimal delivery to the target cell, in this case the CD4 cell. Once the capsid's coating is disassembled the two RNA strands are exposed, triggering the next step in the life cycle.

REVERSE TRANSCRIPTION

Once in the cell, the single-stranded HIV RNA must be converted to double-stranded DNA. This takes place with the help of the enzyme *reverse transcriptase*. Reverse transcriptase uses proteins from the CD4 cell to help change the HIV RNA to HIV DNA. Reverse transcriptase allows genetic information to flow from RNA to DNA, opposite of the typical virus in which the genetic material flows from DNA to RNA. The resulting DNA contains the HIV's genetic information that's required for HIV replication to continue to the next step.

INTEGRATION

Once inside the nucleus of the CD4 cell, HIV releases an *enzyme* called *retroviral integrase*. Enzymes are special proteins that start or help a chemical reaction to occur. Retroviral integrase fuels the chemical reaction that facilitates the transfer of viral DNA into the CD4 cell. HIV uses the integrase to insert the HIV DNA into the CD4 cell DNA. Once inserted, the HIV DNA initiates the next phase in the HIV life cycle.

VIRAL LATENCY

Webster's Dictionary defines *latency* as an incubation period or a period of waiting. After successful integration of viral DNA into the host CD4 cell, the cell is said to be "latently infected." At that point the viral DNA is called a *provirus*. During viral latency, the provirus is waiting to be activated. Once activated the provirus instructs the cell to manufacture the proteins and components of HIV. Simply put, the HIV must wait for additional proteins to be manufactured before replication can be completed.

FINAL ASSEMBLY

Once the viral proteins are manufactured, they must be cut in pieces and assembled into new HIV particles. This *cleavage* or cutting is accomplished with the help of another protein enzyme called *protease*. The enzyme cuts the proteins into smaller pieces, allowing those pieces to reassemble into new HIV proteins. Some of the protein segments form HIV structures and others are used to create enzymes like reverse transcriptase. The new HIV proteins and viral RNA move to the surface of the CD4 cell and assemble into immature and non-infectious copies of HIV.

BUDDING/MATURATION

Budding is the final step in the HIV life cycle. The newly formed HIV, complete with viral genetic material and a new outer coat made from the cell membrane of the host CD4 cell, "pinches off" of the host cell and enters the body's circulation. After a period of maturation—an HIV "growing up," so to speak—the newly formed HIV is ready to attach to another CD4 cell and start the process all over again. Unfortunately, the HIV life cycle, the process of HIV replication, destroys the host CD4 cells while producing new and infectious HIV copies. Now that HIV has started replication and destruction of CD4 cells, what effect does this have on the human body?

The Immune System

The body's defense against parasites, bacteria, viruses and other sources of infection is the *immune system*. The immune system is composed of specialized cells, organs, and a circulatory system all working together to detect foreign substances and organisms that can cause infection and illness. Once an infectious agent is detected, an *immune response* is initiated that protects the body by killing the foreign invader and systematically eradicates the infection from the body. For example, when a cold virus enters the body, the immune system detects the virus and produces a response that fights the cold. While the virus is able to produce cold symptoms, the immune system limits the severity and duration of those symptoms.

How Does the Immune System Work?

Foreign organisms that enter the body are called *antigens*. Once in the body, these antigens are detected by the immune system, triggering a sequence of events that allow the body to fight off the foreign invader. During step one the body transports the antigen to a specialized part of the body called the *lymph system*. Once in the lymph system specialized cells called *macrophages* ingest the antigen and display it on the exterior surface of the macrophage. The antigen on the exterior of the macrophage causes *helper T-cells* (CD4 cells) to signal the rest of the immune system to respond to the foreign invader. *B-cells*, another type of specialized immune system cell, produce millions of antibodies in response to the T-cell signals. These antibodies attach to the antigen in a manner very similar to the lock and key method that HIV uses to attach to the CD4 cell. Antibodies are specific to the antigen they attach to— the way a key is specific to the lock it opens. Once attached, the antibody "tags" the antigen, allowing other cells of the immune system to recognize, engulf, and destroy it before it causes illness or disease. Finally, when the number of antigen cells in the body drops below a certain level, *suppressor T-cells* signal the immune system to rest, essentially shutting off the immune response to the foreign invader. This is important because if left unchecked the immune response could start damaging healthy cells.

Once antibodies are produced to fight a specific antigen, they remain in the body, standing guard in case the antigen that triggered their production enters the body some other time. For instance, when the chickenpox virus enters the body, our immune system produces antibodies that help rid the body of the virus. Once the virus has been eliminated, the antibody remains, providing us with *immunity*, or protection, from future exposures to chickenpox. Because of this, once you've had chickenpox, you have lifelong protection, meaning you will not get chickenpox again even if you are exposed.

What Occurs After HIV Enters the Body?

Remember from the discussion about the HIV life cycle that the virus needs our genetic material to make more viral copies. The virus gets the genetic material it needs by attaching and fusing to CD4 cells. Specifically, HIV attaches to highly specialized cells in our immune system called T-cells or CD4 cells. When a foreign antigen is detected, CD4 cells instruct other immune system cells to start making antibodies. CD4 cells also activate specialized cells that attack and destroy host cells that have been infected by the foreign antigen. It's obvious that CD4 cells play a very important role in the immune response.

Unfortunately, the process of HIV replication destroys the CD4 cell, interfering with its role as the body's defense against infection. As HIV attaches to more and more CD4 cells, the number of healthy, functioning CD4 cells decreases. Imagine an army of CD4 soldiers guarding the body from enemy viruses—in this case, HIV. The enemy sneaks into the body, catching the soldiers off guard. HIV attacks the soldiers, destroying them one by one. Eventually, so many CD4 soldiers are destroyed that those remaining are unable to protect the body from the HIV enemy. With a weakened immune system, HIV replication goes unchecked, like the enemy pouring over the walls of a fort because the soldiers protecting the walls have been weakened and destroyed. As the example illustrates, HIV replication damages so many CD4 cells that the immune system becomes weak and unable to protect the body from foreign antigens. Simply put, the fort (your body) is overrun by the enemy (HIV).

Does HIV Make You Sick?

Over thirty years ago when the epidemic started, people died shortly after being diagnosed with AIDS, after the immune system had already been ravaged by HIV. Today that's no longer true, but after being infected, people do get sick on occasion. Is it HIV that makes us sick? Indirectly, the answer is yes, but HIV itself doesn't cause illness or infection. If that's the case, why do people get sick after being infected with HIV? Why did people die in such large numbers thirty years ago?

During the replication process, HIV destroys CD4 cells and in doing so weakens our immune system. By fighting off infections and other illnesses, a strong immune system keeps us healthy. On the other hand, a weak immune system places the body at risk for infections caused by foreign antigens. As the immune system grows weaker the body is unable to fight off any infectious organism, resulting in serious illness and, in some cases, death. Keep in mind that this is the natural course of an HIV infection without medical intervention. Medications and regular health care alter this scenario significantly. To better understand the process, let's look at it step by step.

Step 1: HIV enters the bloodstream and begins to replicate, using CD4 cells as its source of genetic material.

Step 2: As more copies of HIV are made, more and more CD4 cells are destroyed, gradually weakening the immune system.

Step 3: As HIV replication continues, the immune system eventually becomes unable to fight off infection.

Step 4: With little or no functioning immune system, infectious organisms find minimal resistance when they enter the body. Soon, serious infections overrun what's left of the immune system resulting in serious illness and death.

Infectious organisms take advantage of weak immune systems, seizing the opportunity to cause sickness. It's the *opportunistic infections* that make people sick, not HIV.

HIV vs. AIDS

The mainstream media, lay people, and even some health care providers use the terms HIV and AIDS interchangeably. For many, HIV and AIDS are one and the same. Actually, they're not the same at all.

Acquired Immune Deficiency Syndrome, or AIDS for short, is actually the name given to a collection of the most serious opportunistic infections that strike when the immune system is at its weakest. These AIDS-defining illnesses include:

- Bacterial infections, multiple or recurrent (in people over the age of 13 years)
- Candidiasis, esophageal
- Cervical cancer, invasive
- Coccidioidomycosis, disseminated or extrapulmonary
- Cryptococcosis, extrapulmonary
- Cryptosporidiosis, chronic intestinal (greater than 1 month's duration)
- Cytomegalovirus disease (other than liver, spleen, or nodes)
- Cytomegalovirus retinitis (with loss of vision)
- Encephalopathy, HIV-related
- Herpes simplex: chronic ulcer(s) (greater than 1 month's duration), or bronchitis, pneumonitis, or esophagitis (onset at age older than 1 month)
- Histoplasmosis, disseminated or extrapulmonary
- Isosporiasis, chronic intestinal (greater than 1 month's duration)
- Kaposi's sarcoma (KS)
- Lymphoma, Burkitt's (or equivalent term)
- Lymphoma, immunoblastic (or equivalent term)
- Lymphoma, primary, of brain
- Lymphoid interstitial pneumonia or pulmonary lymphoid hyperplasia complex
- *Mycobacterium avium* complex or *Mycobacterium kansasii*, disseminated or extrapulmonary
- *Mycobacterium* tuberculosis, any site (pulmonary or extrapulmonary)
- *Mycobacterium*, other species or unidentified species, disseminated or extrapulmonary
- *Pneumocystis jirovecii* pneumonia (PJP) (formally known as *Pneumocystis carinii* pneumonia, or PCP)
- Pneumonia, recurrent
- Progressive multifocal leukoencephalopathy (PML)
- *Salmonella* septicemia, recurrent
- Toxoplasmosis of brain
- Wasting syndrome due to HIV

It's not important to remember the complex medical names of all the AIDS-defining illnesses. Just remember that if a person has ever been diagnosed with one of them, he or she is said to have AIDS. AIDS is a result of severe immune system damage caused by HIV replication.

Being diagnosed with one of the AIDS-defining opportunistic infections is not the only way to be diagnosed as having AIDS. An AIDS diagnosis can also be made according to the total CD4 count. The number of CD4 cells is measured by a simple blood test. The normal value ranges between 500 and 1,500 CD4 cells per cubic millimeter of blood (1 drop of blood equals about 50 cubic millimeters). When the CD4 level falls below 200 CD4 cells per cubic millimeter of blood, the person is said to have AIDS.

As you can see, HIV and AIDS are definitely connected, but they are certainly not the same thing. But what does it mean if a person has been given an AIDS diagnosis? In the minds of many patients, an AIDS diagnosis is a signal that their health is failing and HIV is winning the battle. Does AIDS change the way the HIV specialist treats a patient? Does the patient have to change the way he or she approaches day-to-day life? What is the true significance of an AIDS diagnosis?

The Significance of an AIDS Diagnosis

When the epidemic emerged over thirty years ago, an AIDS diagnosis signaled that the end of life was near. Prior to the development of an HIV antibody test, people were diagnosed after they were diagnosed with AIDS-defining infections such as pneumocystis pneumonia (PCP) or Kaposi's sarcoma (KS). By the time the most serious opportunistic infections appeared, the HIV was in an advanced stage, already having done irreparable damage to the immune system. Most often people died within months of an AIDS diagnosis. Obviously, being diagnosed with AIDS thirty years ago was very significant.

Since the development of the HIV antibody test, people are diagnosed much earlier in the course of the disease. The advent of HIV medications has delayed the progression to AIDS in some cases indefinitely. Even after an AIDS diagnosis is made, medications keep people healthy and alive for a very long time. AIDS is no longer the death sentence it was three decades ago and having an AIDS diagnosis is nowhere near as significant today as it was then.

Tracking the epidemic is an important part of HIV prevention and care. Federal funds are allocated based on the epidemic patterns among populations and geographic areas. Prevention messages and prevention education must be targeted to specific populations to be affected, those hardest hit by the epidemic. At the beginning of the epidemic, the only way to track the epidemic was to count the number of AIDS cases. Because people were diagnosed only after they acquired AIDS-defining infections, the number of AIDS cases was an accurate representation of the number of HIV-infected people.

Today, counting the number of AIDS cases is not an accurate method of tracking the epidemic. HIV testing makes it possible to diagnose people long before they have AIDS-defining infections. Counting only AIDS cases would be inaccurate because the method omits a large number of people with HIV that have yet to progress to AIDS, and may not for several years if ever. While many of those infected with HIV place great significance to an AIDS diagnosis, the fact is that AIDS is in many ways an outdated classification that has outlived its usefulness.

The Natural Course of HIV

Without medications or medical intervention, HIV is free to follow its natural course and, in the process, destroy the body's immune system. Soon after infection, HIV begins replicating at a very rapid pace, damaging CD4 cells along the way. Soon after infection, the amount of circulating virus is very high, and the number of functioning CD4 cells declines dramatically. Simply put, HIV has caught the immune system off guard. Three to six weeks after being infected, many people experience a flu-like illness known as *acute HIV infection*. Symptoms include fever, diarrhea, rash, fatigue, malaise, and weight loss. Quite often, the symptoms are attributed to the flu or some other benign viral illness. Because the body has not had ample time to develop antibodies, an HIV test done at this time can be negative, despite the presence of HIV in the blood. Many times, the opportunity for early diagnosis is missed because of the negative HIV test and symptoms that are attributed to other illnesses.

About six weeks after infection, most people will have developed enough HIV antibodies to be detected by the HIV antibody test. In fact, there are newer fourth generation antibody tests that can detect HIV antibodies much sooner than the older generation tests, in some cases, 14 to 21 days earlier than the traditional western blot antibody test. Once antibodies are formed, the body begins to fight the new infection. The symptoms of the acute infection resolve and the person begins to feel much better, reaffirming the belief that what they experienced was nothing more than a typical viral illness.

As the body begins to realize what is happening, the remaining healthy CD4 cells begin to fight HIV. About six months into the infection the immune system is successful in stabilizing the number of circulating HIV at a level known as the viral load *set point*. The set point varies from person to person and can be a predictor of how fast HIV will progress to AIDS in the future.

Once the set point is reached, the virus begins a chronic phase during which the body's immune system is able to suppress viral replication enough to maintain the strength of the immune system. The duration of this chronic phase can vary greatly from person to person, ranging from a year to ten years or more. During this time, the infected person feels well and has few, if any, symptoms. Because a fairly stable CD4 count can be maintained, the immune system is able to protect the body from opportunistic infections, and the person's overall health remains good.

Years after the initial infection, HIV replication continues, slowly chipping away at the number of healthy CD4 cells. On average an untreated HIV infection will diminish the typical CD4 count by about 100 cells per cubic millimeter of blood per year. Eventually, sometimes after many years, so many CD4 cells have been destroyed by HIV that the immune system is significantly weakened and the body becomes at risk for opportunistic infections. Remember the normal CD4 count ranges from 500 to 1500 cells per cubic millimeter of blood. When the level falls below 200 cells per cubic millimeter of blood the person is at significant risk for the most serious opportunistic infections, and is diagnosed as having AIDS. Thirty years ago it was not until this point in the infection that a person was diagnosed with AIDS.

Still, HIV replication continues, and opportunistic infections become more common as the number of functioning CD4 cells continue to decline. Once the level falls below 100 CD4 cells per cubic millimeter of blood, HIV becomes stronger than the immune system, and the most serious, potentially fatal opportunistic infections become commonplace. Without some sort of medical intervention, the body will soon be unable to fight any infection, eventually leading to the person's death.

Typically, people will live on average about 10 to 15 years without any type of treatment. Some people with more aggressive strains of HIV survive as little as a couple of years, while others with less aggressive strains of HIV can live twenty years or more. But as an unpredictable infection people will progress at varying rates. Based on the rate of progression HIV infection can be divided into three categories.

- *Rapid Progression:* HIV infection will progress to AIDS in three years or less
- *Intermediate Progression:* HIV infection will progress to AIDS in three to ten years
- *Long-term Non-progressor (Elite Controllers):* People maintain high CD4 counts while being treatment naïve, while not being on a medication regimen

The advent of HIV medication regimens has significantly altered the progression of HIV to AIDS. The newest guidelines recommend treatment be offered to everyone, but what about long-term non-progressors? They maintain high CD4 counts without being medicated; should they be treated too? Let's take a closer look at the elite controller/long-term non-progressor.

The Long-Term Non-Progressor/Elite Controller

The natural progression of HIV infection slowly destroys the immune system, lowering the CD4 count over the course of several years. Some people infected with HIV are *long term non-progressor* also known as *elite controllers,* maintaining stable CD4 counts for ten years or more without any medical intervention or HIV medications. Actually, long-term non-progressors can be divided into two categories: those that persist with a low level of circulating virus, around 5,000 copies or less, and those that maintain an undetectable amount of virus, less than 50 copies of circulating HIV. Research is being conducted to determine why some people progress slower than others. Understanding long term non-progressors could result in new and better HIV treatments that may extend the lives of HIV-infected people even further.

While about one percent of people infected with HIV are elite controllers, 98 percent of those have circulating virus at a detectable level. That circulating virus, even at a very low level can slowly erode the CD4 count until the immune system is weak enough to make the body vulnerable to opportunistic infections. For that reason, even elite controllers/long-term non-progressors should be treated with an HIV medication regimen.

Now that we understand the basics of HIV and AIDS, the discussion turns to those first days and weeks after diagnosis. If the HIV test result is positive, what comes next?

4

THE TEST IS POSITIVE .... NOW WHAT?

Many people are reluctant to be HIV tested because they're afraid of what it would do to their lives if they were indeed HIV positive. Being diagnosed with any chronic and potentially fatal disease is frightening, but a diagnosis of HIV gives a new meaning to the word fear. So what if the unthinkable does occur? What if that HIV test is positive? The first few days and weeks can be the most important and the most difficult. Making the right choices from the beginning can mean the difference between you taking control of your disease or your disease taking control of you.

Informed Consent/Test Counseling

Getting HIV tested entails a lot more than just holding out your arm and having blood drawn. HIV testing is more than just finding out if you are positive or negative. It's an opportunity to educate and an opportunity to learn. Testing policy and procedure varies from state to state. In the past, because of the sensitive nature of HIV information and the stigma surrounding HIV, there needed to be signed consent from the person being tested. In 2006 the CDC revised their HIV testing and counseling guidelines. Since that time, every state except Nebraska has passed a testing law that aligns with CDC guidelines. However, while those guidelines recommend routine testing, they do differ from previous informed consent requirements, and pre- and post-test counseling requirements. The new requirements state:

- Separate written consent for HIV testing is not necessary. General consent for medical care should state HIV testing may be performed unless the person declines at the time of testing ("opt-out"). The provider should document that the HIV test procedure was discussed prior to the testing.
- Prevention counseling that assesses the risk of HIV infection, identifies at-risk behavior, and develops a plan to reduce risk, while very useful, should not be required for HIV testing to be done.

If pre and post-test counseling is done the United States Department of Health and Human Services recommends that counseling include an explanation of the HIV test itself, basic HIV and AIDS information, methods to diminish the risk of spreading HIV from person to person, the importance of test confidentiality, the possible social impact of being HIV tested, and finally, the people in your life that legally must be notified of your positive HIV test. Post-test counseling provides an opportunity for medical and psychosocial referrals in the event of a positive test. If the test is negative, post-test counseling provides an opportunity to share information that will diminish the risk of HIV exposure.

What Happens During Pre-Test Counseling?

Again, due to changes in the law, pre-test counseling is no longer a required part of getting an HIV test, but it still is done in many circumstances. If your test includes pre-test counseling, you will meet with a state trained and certified test counselor. Because of the complexities inherent to HIV testing, most states have some sort of counselor training or certification. A test counselor needs to wear many hats, being part medical professional, part mental health professional, and part supportive friend. The counselor will discuss your medical and sexual history in an effort to identify behaviors that put you at additional risk for HIV exposure. Some of those at-risk behaviors include unprotected sex, trading sex for drugs, having sex with multiple anonymous partners, having sex while under the influence of drugs or alcohol, or having unprotected sex with a known HIV-infected partner. The counselor will also ask about any history of recreational drug use or sharing needles while injecting drugs because those behaviors increase the risk of HIV exposure and high risk sexual encounters. The purpose of these intimate questions is to assess your HIV risk and to counsel you on ways to reduce or avoid risky behaviors in the future.

As part of your pre-test counseling, the HIV counselor will explain the basics of HIV and AIDS, including transmission routes, methods of safer sex and ways to reduce your risk of infection. He or she will discuss the social impact HIV testing can sometimes have on the person being tested. Finally, you will have an opportunity to ask questions of the test counselor. When all your questions have been answered, the counselor will make certain you are still interested in being tested and if so the test will be done. The test counselor will arrange an appointment for you to return to get your results. Results, positive or negative, should never be given over the telephone.

What Happens During Post-Test Counseling?

While pre-test counseling is not always done, a majority of test results are given as part of post-test counseling. Depending on the type of HIV test you have and where you have it done, your test results will be ready anywhere from a few minutes to several days. Your test counselor will have you come into the test center for your results. Test results, either negative or positive, will never be given over the telephone. Receiving your results is more than just learning if you're positive or negative. If your test is negative, your counselor will review safer sex methods, discuss ways to reduce your risk of HIV exposure, and stress the importance of not sharing needles. Your counselor will also discuss the importance of repeating your test several weeks later to confirm your negative results. Finally, depending on the testing site, condoms are typically available free of charge in order to encourage their use during each and every oral, vaginal, or anal sexual encounter.

Receiving positive test results is a very stressful and emotional event. Shock, fear, anger, and disbelief are all common emotions after learning you are HIV-infected. Your test counselor is specially trained to help deal with the sudden onslaught of emotions that occur after receiving positive results. The counselor will assist with medical referrals and, if needed, mental health referrals. Finally, the counselor will discuss disclosure of your positive status, whom you legally must tell, and whom you want to tell in search of support. Remember, the only people you are required to tell are those you may have sexual contact with after diagnosis. While it is highly recommended that you tell your physicians, dentists, and nursing staff, legally it is not required. Keep in mind, however, that medical professionals can take better care of you if they are familiar with your entire medical history, especially conditions that affect the entire body like HIV. Finally, before telling friends, family, or employers make certain telling them will help you and provide you with much needed support. Telling someone just to tell them could bring you undue stress and difficulties you don't need at this time. If you can't think of a good reason to tell someone your status, then you probably shouldn't tell them. If you aren't sure whom to tell, discuss this with the test counselor or your HIV care provider.

TABLE 4

Pre-Test Counseling (if you get counseling with your test)

- The purpose of pre-test counseling is to assess HIV risk.
- Trained and certified test counselors will take a medical and sexual history.
- Sexual history will include the number of partners; questions regarding trading sex for drugs; and any history of having sex with anonymous partners.
- The counselor will ask about any history of recreational drug use or sharing needles.
- Part of your pre-test counseling is an explanation of basic HIV/AIDS information.
- Some pre-test counseling involves a discussion of the possible social impact of HIV and being tested.
- Finally, you will be given the option of being tested now that you have all the information.

Post-Test Counseling (typically will receive when getting test results)

- Keep in mind, test results, either positive or negative, will never be given by telephone.
- If your test is negative, your counselor will discuss safer sex methods and ways to reduce your HIV risk.
- The counselor will discuss ways to decrease your risk of HIV when injecting drugs, including offering to refer you to substance abuse treatment.
- The counselor will instruct you on the importance of being retested several weeks later to confirm the results.
- If your results are positive, your counselor will assist with medical referrals, mental health referrals, and will help with the initial shock of a positive diagnosis.
- Often, condoms will be available to take with you after post-test counseling.

A Positive Test: Taking the First Steps

Being diagnosed with HIV can be an incredible shock, filling a person with fear, desperation, and confusion. The initial reaction may be to throw in the towel, to give up and let the disease take control. Like any medical diagnosis, learning you are HIV-infected is not the news anyone wants to hear. Every person will handle the news differently. For many, the initial reaction may be to give up and let HIV take control. Others choose to cope by using alcohol or drugs. Still others will deny they have any illness at all and give in to the "out of sight out of mind" mentality. People who ignore their diagnosis and do not take steps to fight their disease will eventually have to face their disease, but by then they may be very sick.

Initially, most people will feel helpless, but the truth is it's possible to take control of your life while living with HIV. To do so requires preparation, determination, and the will to move forward. There are several things that must be done in order to move forward with an HIV diagnosis. They include:

- deciding whom if anyone you should tell of your diagnosis;
- finding a qualified HIV specialist to assume your medical care, and
- taking control of your healthcare and your life by learning as much as you can about your disease.

Each is an essential step when preparing for a life with HIV. The sooner you get a handle on the emotions that have you afraid, depressed, and uncertain about your future, the sooner you can get into HIV care and as a result the longer, healthier life you will live. Let's look at each of these three things a little closer.

Whom Do You Tell About Your HIV?

As is true with all medical information, HIV test results are strictly confidential. For the most part, it's the individual's decision whom to tell, if anyone, about their HIV status. However, there are circumstances when the law requires HIV-infected people to disclose their status.

DISCLOSURE IS MANDATORY

HIV disclosure laws vary from state to state but most require a person to disclose their HIV status to any potential sexual partner prior to sexual contact or intimacy. Knowingly exposing a sexual partner to HIV without their knowledge is, in most cases, a criminal act, punishable as a felony. In fact, over the last several years more and more cases of knowingly exposing a sexual partner to HIV without their knowledge are being prosecuted and jail time is being handed out. Also, any past sexual partners should be made aware that they may have been exposed to HIV. In fact, your local health department will contact you to assure that partner notification has been done. While these discussions will be very difficult, speak with any potential sexual partner before intimacy and any past sexual partners that may have been exposed.

DISCLOSURE IS RECOMMENDED

While it's not required, it is recommended that you disclose your HIV status to other doctors, dentists, and medical providers that care for you. The purpose of disclosure is not to protect your medical providers from potential HIV infection. Medical professionals employ the same universal precautions for all patients, regardless of their HIV status. The fact is that disclosing your HIV status benefits you. All medical providers need a complete picture of your health and medical history to care for you properly. Having HIV can impact the way other conditions are treated and how certain symptoms are interpreted. Most experts agree that disclosing your HIV status to all of your health care providers is a good idea.

THE CHOICE IS YOURS

Disclosing your HIV status to anyone else other than those people in the previous examples is strictly your decision. Before disclosing, ask yourself why you are doing so and what will be gained. For instance, telling your family of your diagnosis may provide you with a support system to help you cope with your new diagnosis. On the other hand, disclosing your status to coworkers or casual acquaintances may not benefit you at all. Keep in mind that disclosing your status is not something to take lightly and should be thought out carefully before doing so. Before disclosing your status to anyone, especially an employer, consult with your provider, nurse, or case manager/social worker. He or she can guide you through the process of disclosure. Other resources that will help you when it's time to disclose your status include local HIV agencies and HIV advocacy groups. Remember, nobody has the right to disclose your status. If you feel that has happened, seek legal advice from an attorney.

TABLE 5

Mandatory Disclosure
- Past sexual partners.
- Potential sexual partners prior to any sexual contact.

Recommended Disclosure
- Doctors, dentists, and any medical professionals that will be caring for you.

The Choice is Yours
- Friends, family, acquaintances, and employers.

How to Disclose Your HIV Status

Telling someone you have HIV, be it a loved one or your best friend, can be one of the hardest things you will ever have to do. You may feel awkward, afraid, or embarrassed. The person you are telling may react in any number of ways. Some may be angry; others will be sad. Some will be frightened and still others won't know exactly how they feel. While the task of disclosure is a difficult one, there are steps you can take to prepare for the task.

- Learn as much as you can about HIV before discussing your HIV status. Knowledge is power. Having an understanding of HIV and AIDS will allow you to answer questions and ease the fears of the person you are telling.
- Know why you want to tell the people you are telling. What do you want from them? Are they at risk for infection? Have you unknowingly exposed them to your HIV? Will they be a source of support? Have an idea why you are disclosing before you disclose.
- Before disclosing think about what the person knows about HIV. Do they have preconceived opinions or feelings surrounding HIV? Does the person have attitudes or issues that may affect their ability to support you or deal with the news of your diagnosis?
- Anticipate their reaction. What's the best you can hope for? What's the worst you can expect? Often, the person you tell will experience emotions much like you did when you were told of the diagnosis. Be prepared for a variety of emotions ranging from anger to fear. Ironically, you may have to be their support before they can be yours.
- To promote an understanding of HIV and AIDS, have educational materials on hand to help answer questions that may arise. Provide educational resources and places to get more information if needed.

- For each person you want to tell, ask yourself if that person needs to know now or if it can wait until things settle down a bit. For instance, current or past sexual partners need to know soon so they can get tested while "Uncle Bob" can wait until you are settled and in HIV treatment.

- If you have someone who already knows your status, bring them along for support, both for you and the person you are telling. Along with that person, come up with a disclosure plan. While it may not always be appropriate to bring along another person, a support person can help come up with a plan of action prior to disclosure, making the process much less stressful.

- Be prepared for any reaction and allow the person you are telling to express their emotions freely. Often the person being told will need as much support as the person who is disclosing their HIV status. Remember, you can't control the fears and feelings of others, and it may take time for the person to adjust to and accept what you have told them.

- Be patient. It may take some time for those you tell to process the information and be supportive of you. Everyone deals with difficult news in their own way and in their own time.

- Understand your rights if you choose to disclose to your employer. Don't sign anything from your employer until discussing it with a legal advocate. There are lawyers who specialize in the rights of those living with HIV. Typically, HIV community based organizations will have lists of attorneys who offer such services. First and foremost, don't assume your employer will be supportive.

Partner Notification

One type of HIV disclosure is partner notification. HIV can remain undiagnosed for several years. During that time an HIV infected person can unknowingly expose their sexual partners to the virus. Because early diagnosis is so important, an infected person must notify their past sexual partners that they have been exposed to HIV. This allows their sexual partner(s) to get tested and into medical care if they are found to be HIV-infected. Partner notification also provides a means by which HIV exposure between sexual partners can be reduced, which in turn will slow the spread of HIV. There are three ways to notify a partner.

NOTIFICATION BY THE INFECTED PERSON

Partner notification can be done by the HIV-infected person. Hearing about a potential exposure can sometimes be easier if the news is delivered by a partner, loved one or friend. However, it can also be a very awkward encounter. In some cases, being told your partner has HIV will create stress in the relationship, both in the short-term and long-term. But it doesn't necessarily mean the relationship is over. Being honest and understanding will go a long way in saving and even improving the relationship.

Many times disclosing your HIV status may also mean disclosing a sexual behavior or substance abuse problem that was kept secret before diagnosis. For instance, a husband who secretly has sex with men or shares needles while injecting drugs must disclose his new HIV status to his wife and in doing so his other secrets—having sex with men or using recreational drugs—are disclosed as well. Many infected people would rather not be the one to pass on such troubling news. Doctors, counselors or social workers can offer support to those people who wish to notify their partners themselves.

Notification by the Local Health Department

In all fifty states, new HIV infections are reported to the local health department. In fact, in many states each CD4 count and HIV viral load is reported electronically directly from the lab to the local health department. And part of the health department's role is to assist and assure partner notification is done. Even in circumstances where little is known about past sexual encounters, the health department can assist in partner notification. For instance, people meeting for anonymous sexual encounters may know little about one another. The local health department can take any little bit of information, such as a first name or where the sexual encounter took place, and track down the person or persons potentially exposed.

The involvement of local health departments is not limited to anonymous encounters. Health department staff can assist in notifying known partners as well. Despite their diligence in finding and notifying sexual partners, they take great care not to compromise the confidentiality of the HIV-infected person. Notification is vague, making the person aware that they may have been in contact with someone HIV-infected without giving specifics about the person who exposed them.

Notification by the Physician

Physicians caring for newly diagnosed HIV-infected people can do partner notification as well. In fact, many states require physicians to perform partner notification, or, at the very least, make sure the infected person or the health department notifies those people exposed. Most times physicians have neither the resources nor the time to do a thorough and complete partner notification. Usually the task is delegated to social workers, nurses, the HIV-infected person or the local health department. Regardless of who does the notification, it's the physician's responsibility to make certain it's documented.

Take Control

Regardless of your personality, an HIV diagnosis can wreak havoc with your level of confidence. Before you were diagnosed, if you were one to take control of difficult situations, then you can do so now that you're HIV-infected. If taking charge came easy to you before, with hard work, support and time, it should again.

On the other hand, if you were one to let things happen around you or take a passive approach to life, needing to "step up" and take control may be intimidating. The tendency would be to sit back and let others take control of your health care. Taking a passive approach to your disease will shut you out of the healthcare process. Once you give others control over your medical issues, it's very difficult to get it back. Without having a say in your healthcare you become a powerless outsider. Taking control from the start assures that you will be included in every aspect of your healthcare, from planning medication regimens to expressing concerns. Many would argue that taking control and being empowered is the key to staying healthy.

Fortunately, being in control of your own healthcare and being part of the healthcare team can be achieved by understanding your disease. It requires very hard work and determination. At times the urge will be to quit and assume a passive role. At times you will want to quit, to throw in the towel. It won't always be easy but it is worth the effort and the hard work. Pushing forward, despite these urges, will help you resume your life after your diagnosis. In order to move take control of your life and disease, there are a few things you must first learn.

You Are Number One

Now that you have been diagnosed with HIV, your health and quality of life must become your priority. Depending on your personality, it may be difficult for you to put yourself first. You may feel guilty or selfish, or have mixed feelings about putting your health first. If your relationship is one where your partner is in control, he or she may have trouble with you taking the lead in some aspects of life. It will take time for them to adjust to the "new you." Resist the tendency to revert back to the "old you." The work you and your partner will invest in your health will be worth it. Your health and well-being is much too important to leave solely in the hands of others.

Putting yourself first doesn't mean becoming isolated or abandoning your responsibilities. It does mean that it's okay and necessary to sometimes say "no." It's necessary to make your needs known to your doctor and the people around you. Learning to say no and expressing your needs is simply becoming empowered.

Women living with HIV tend to abandon their own needs in order to care for their family and children. When a woman takes care of herself, she is doing something good for her family as well. Doing what is needed to stay healthy allows a woman to care for others and teaches her children an important lesson—how to love yourself.

Finally, taking control also means resisting the temptation to think of yourself as "helpless" or as a "victim." Don't identify yourself or allow others to identify you by your diagnosis. You are not an "AIDS patient", you are a person with a chronic disease. That fact can never diminish the person you are or the respect you deserve. If you feel someone is treating you in a disrespectful manner, tell them. Demand their respect; you deserve nothing less.

Believe in Yourself

Nobody knows what's best for you except you. Who better to understand how you're feeling physically and emotionally than yourself. If you feel something is not right, even if you don't know why, then it's probably not. If something doesn't feel right, let your doctor know about your concerns sooner rather than later. Know your body and trust your instincts. Survival is a very strong instinct that you should not ignore.

There is no doubt that a chronic illness makes life more difficult. But keep in mind that more difficult does not mean impossible. Certainly there will need to be adjustments and changes in your routine. Learning to live with your chronic illness will take a lot of work and some getting used to for certain. But believe in yourself. Believe that you can make those lifestyle adjustments and that you are up to the task; after all, your health hangs in the balance.

GIVE YOURSELF SOME TIME

While finding an HIV specialist is very important. You don't have to rush into any rash decisions now that you have HIV. Decisions that impact your health and your life should not be made on a whim but should be made with good facts and a good knowledge base. Make sure you give yourself all the time you need. Decisions should be made according to *your* time frame, not that of the doctor, the nurse or anyone else. No one can tell you how long it should take to adapt to your new diagnosis. Keep your expectations realistic and don't try to do too much too soon. Especially during those first days and weeks after receiving your diagnosis, don't expect too much of yourself too soon. A lot of changes are taking place in a very short period of time. Give yourself all the time you need; after all you have a very long life in front of you. That being said, keep in mind that getting into quality HIV care as soon as you can will improve your quality of life for a long time to come. Simply put, don't rush into any decisions but be proactive and get into HIV care as soon as you feel you are ready for the next step.

TABLE 6. TAKE CONTROL OF YOUR LIFE

You Are Number 1

- Your health and quality of life must become your highest priority.
- Feeling guilty or selfish, or having mixed feelings is common.
- Your partner or spouse may have trouble adjusting to you "taking the lead."
- If being the priority is new to you, resist reverting back to the "old you."
- Being first doesn't mean you need to isolate yourself.
- It is ok and sometimes necessary to say "no."
- It is necessary to make your wishes and needs known to your doctor.
- Women must not abandon their own needs for the needs of their children and family.

Believe in Yourself

- Nobody knows how you feel emotionally or physically better than you.
- If you feel something is not right, then it probably is not, even if you don't know why.
- The survival instinct is very strong and should not be ignored … in other words, trust your instincts.
- Difficult adjustments in your life will have to be made, but believe in yourself…. YOU CAN DO IT!
- You are up to the task.

Give Yourself Some Time

- Finding an HIV specialist is important but take a deep breath … you have time to make the right choices.
- Do not rush into any rash decisions regarding your medical care or to whom you disclose your diagnosis.
- Decisions should be made on *your* timeframe, not your doctor's.
- Have realistic expectations … don't try to do too much too soon.
- Change takes time, so leave yourself plenty.

Choosing a Doctor That's Right for You

The most important decision you will make in those first few days after learning you have HIV is choosing a doctor to handle your HIV care. It's a decision that will impact your health as well as your quality of life for many years. Obviously it's not a decision you should take lightly. Take a systematic approach to finding the right doctor for you. Here are several things you should consider when choosing your HIV specialist.

- *Find a Doctor:* To find a doctor you have to know where to look. If you live in or near a large urban area, large medical centers or university-based hospitals are a good place to start. Not only do they have the very qualified HIV specialists needed to manage the complex medication regimens and treatment protocols common to HIV but those providers have access to essential specialty services such as gastroenterology (stomach issues), pulmonology (lung/breathing issues), endocrinology (diabetes), and cardiology (heart diseases). In addition, large university based medical centers typically have access to clinical trial medication and HIV treatment studies, keeping your HIV care on the cutting edge of HIV therapy and treatment protocols. In large cities such as Detroit, Chicago, or New York, which have been hard hit by the HIV epidemic, free-standing medical practices or clinics are a good source of quality HIV care. Keep in mind, however, that if you choose a free standing clinic or medical practice, you may need to use a local hospital for such services as radiology, blood draw, and specialty services typically not available at free standing community clinics. In rural areas it may be necessary to travel several miles to the nearest city to get your HIV care. To minimize travel, a local family physician can be retained for illnesses and issues not related to HIV such as colds, sinus infections, and high blood pressure. But whether you choose the large medical center or the stand alone clinic, the most important thing is that you have your HIV managed by an HIV specialist. If your search for an HIV specialist comes up empty, you can call the National AIDS Hotline at 1-800-CDC-INFO (1-800-232-4636). By providing your ZIP code, the hotline will provide the names and contact information for HIV specialists in your area. You can find a provider online as well at the website AIDS.gov (https://www.aids.gov/locator/).

- *Find an HIV Specialist:* HIV is a very complex disease requiring an expertise in HIV and infectious diseases in order to be managed properly. HIV specialists are infectious disease doctors that further specialize in the treatment of patients with HIV and AIDS. However, being an infectious disease specialist is not enough. HIV is so complex, and treatment guidelines change so often, that doctors need to devote their full-time attention to HIV medicine. In 2010, the HIV Medicine Association (HIVMA) a subgroup of the Infectious Diseases Society of America (IDSA), released their qualifications for an HIV specialist. According to HIVMA, an HIV specialist should have at least 40 hours of HIV continuing medical education every three years and manage the HIV care of at least 25 patients per year. The doctor you choose should keep up to date on the most current advances in HIV medicine by attending continuing education conferences, and through extensive journal review. The importance of choosing an HIV specialist to manage your care can't be stressed enough.

- *Choose a Full Service Medical Practice:* HIV and AIDS affect the whole person, physically as well as emotionally. For that reason, it is important to choose a doctor whose clinic offers more than just medical care. Does the clinic employ social workers, nutritionists, and nurses who specialize in HIV? Does the practice have access to specialty care such as ophthalmology, gynecology, substance abuse treatment and psychiatry? Because HIV impacts the entire person both physically and mentally, people living with HIV need more than just medical care. Choose a doctor that treats the entire person.

- *For Women: Choose a Doctor That Understands the Special Needs of HIV–Infected Women:* Women living with HIV have special needs that must be addressed by their doctor. Choosing a clinic that offers a special emphasis on women's issues insures that the needs of HIV-infected women will be addressed. Are there processes in place that assure women will get yearly Pap exams, breast exams, and the proper reproductive health counseling? Does the doctor understand the importance of HIV care for the pregnant women? To remain healthy, a woman living with HIV needs a doctor who understands their special needs.

- *Access to Clinical Trials and Studies:* The science of HIV medicine is always advancing and new improved medication regimens are being developed every day. New medicines and treatments have helped people live longer and healthier lives with HIV. It's important for people living with the disease to have access to the most advanced treatments and medications. Choose a doctor that participates in or has access to clinical trials and studies. As the years pass, having access to clinical trials and cutting edge drugs can mean the difference between chronic illness and long-term health.

- *Choose a Doctor That Encourages Patient Participation:* Insist on a doctor that includes you in all medical decisions and care planning. Studies have shown that patients fare much better if they are participants in their own care. Doctors who empower their patients by allowing them to help make health related decisions, better understand the needs of their patients. Avoid doctors or medical practices that exclude patients from medical decision making and treatment planning.

The importance of choosing the right doctor can't be overstated. The decisions you and your doctor make together will impact your health and quality of life for a very long time. But remember, the doctor you choose today may not necessarily be your doctor for life. If you find the doctor you have chosen is just not working out, don't hesitate to look for another. It is absolutely imperative that you and your doctor have a good patient-doctor relationship. Without a good relationship, you are less likely to attend appointments, report problems that arise, and adhere to medication regimens. Without adherence to medication regimens and scheduled appointments and without a comfortable relationship with your HIV specialist, your health will ultimately suffer. Keep in mind that since you are infected with HIV, the relationship you have with your doctor may be one of the most important relationships you will ever have.

Who Will Manage Your Care?

Chances are you had a family doctor or a primary doctor prior to your HIV diagnosis. That doctor cared for you when you had the flu, a cold, or a fever. Now that you have HIV, you have chosen a doctor to monitor your immune system. What becomes of the doctor that has been caring for you perhaps since you were a child? There are three ways to manage your HIV.

- *Care Managed by Your Family Doctor:* After years of seeing the same family doctor, a trusting doctor-patient relationship develops. After being diagnosed with HIV, the tendency may be to stay with your family doctor and allow him or her to manage your HIV. As discussed earlier, HIV is a very complex disease that requires the expertise only an HIV specialist can provide. For this reason, experts adamantly recommend that HIV not be managed by primary care physicians or family doctors. Fortunately, fewer and fewer primary care physicians are comfortable managing HIV, realizing the complexities of HIV care requires an HIV specialist for the best care possible.
- *Care Managed by Your Family Doctor and an HIV Specialist:* An acceptable way to manage your HIV care is to maintain a relationship with your family doctor, leaving him or her to manage your basic healthcare needs, and an HIV specialist to manage your HIV and immune system. If you choose this method, make certain that your family doctor and HIV specialist communicate with one another in order to assure continuity of care.
- *Care Managed by an HIV Specialist:* The preferred method of managing your healthcare needs, both HIV-related and basic health care, is to employ an HIV specialist that is willing to manage both. HIV specialists are typically internal medicine (primary care, family medicine) doctors that go through two to three years of additional training to specialize in infectious disease and HIV care. With the internal medicine background, he or she is able to manage the basic health needs of their patient while managing the HIV and immune system, possible because of the additional training in infectious disease. With one physician managing the whole person, continuity is assured. Having an HIV specialist manage your care does not mean he or she won't refer you to other specialists if needed. If you want to keep your family doctor apprised of your care and condition, make it known to your HIV doctor and he or she can arrange to have regular updates sent to your primary care physician.

Before Your First Visit to the Doctor

Once you have chosen a doctor to manage your HIV, it's time to prepare for that first visit. There are a number of preparations you should make prior to your first visit to the doctor.

- *Get Your Insurance in Order:* To make sure you aren't saddled with a large medical bill, talk to your insurance provider to determine if any referrals are required prior to your first visit. Many times, especially if your insurance is a Health Maintenance Organization (HMO), you will need a referral from your primary care physician (PCP) in order to see a specialist, in this case an HIV specialist. If you don't have insurance coverage, don't let that prevent you from getting into the HIV care you need. There are many resources available, especially for those living with HIV, to help defer the cost of medical care and medication costs. Prior to your visit assemble past tax returns, old pay stubs, and a list of your monthly expenses. This information will be needed for you to apply for community resources, plans available through the Affordable Care Act ("Obamacare"), Medicaid, and state run drug assistance programs. Provided the clinic you choose has social worker support, contact them prior to your first visit so they can assist you in getting the insurance coverage and the medication coverage you will need. If there is no social work support, contact the local HIV case management agency in your area and make an appointment with one of the case managers. They will help you get insurance and medication coverage before incurring any bills. Again, if you don't have insurance DO NOT allow that to prevent you from seeking out medical care. There are resources that will help.

- *Find Your Old Medical Records:* Assemble any old medical records you have, either at home or by asking your family doctor for copies of your past medical record. Get a copy of your positive HIV test result along with any other labs results from blood tests done at the time of your HIV test. This will give your new HIV doctor a more complete picture of your medical history and your HIV test history. If possible, find the date of your last negative HIV test. It can help the doctor estimate how long you have been infected. Finally, bring a list of any prescription and over-the-counter medications you are taking along with a list of any medication or food allergies you may have. It's very helpful for the doctor to know what type of reaction you have with each of your medication allergies.

- *Find a Family Member or Friend to Come with You:* If possible, arrange to have someone attend your first doctor's appointment with you. Obviously it should be someone you trust knowing your diagnosis. That first visit will seem very confusing and overwhelming. This may be the first time since you received your test results that you have had to discuss your HIV infection, your treatment, and your prognosis. It will be extremely helpful to have someone alongside you to help make sense of the large amount of information you are about to receive. Having a friend or family member at your side is not required but the support during your visit may be more helpful than you think.

- *Be on Time:* Make certain to arrive to your appointment on time. In fact, arriving a few minutes early is advisable. There will be paperwork that needs to be completed prior to seeing the doctor. Filling out forms before you see the doctor allows for more time with the physician. Every minute of your appointment is important, especially at your first visit. Arriving on time or early makes the best use of the time allotted for your appointment.

- *Bring Plenty of Questions:* Assemble a list of questions for your doctor. Write the questions down as they occur to you. It's common to forget questions and concerns the minute you walk into the doctor's office. How many times have all of us had a burning question for our doctor, only to forget it the minute we walk into the office? Then, like clockwork, it occurs to us the minute we pull out of the doctor's parking lot. Writing your questions down will insure that they will not be forgotten and will get answered. Remember, you are new to this diagnosis and disease so there are no dumb questions. If you don't know the answer, ask the question. The worst thing you can do is not ask the question or assume you know the answer. Again, if you don't know the answer ask the question and don't leave without an answer.

Ask the Right Questions

The first thing to keep in mind is that there are no trivial or silly questions; if you don't know the answer then absolutely ask the question. It's essential that you fully understand your HIV treatment plan and how it is developed by your HIV doctor. So never hesitate to ask questions, and don't leave your doctor's office without the answers you seek.

There are a few questions that you should ask during that very first visit to the doctor. It's important to develop a good doctor-patient relationship. Just as the doctor asks questions to get to know you better, the answers to your questions will teach you a lot about your doctor and how he or she plans on approaching your HIV care. Asking the right questions not only educates you but also tells your doctor that you have a vested interest in your HIV care and expect to be an active participant from the start. Some important questions to ask your doctor include:

- *Will I be able to play an active role in planning my care and structuring my treatment?*
- *How much time will I have to ask questions at my appointments?*
- *Will I be seen by the same doctor at each visit?*
- *Will I see an attending physician, or will there be resident physicians involved in my doctor visits?*
- *Are walk-in appointments available?*
- *Is there a nurse line I can call if I have an issue that can't wait until my next visit?*
- *Is there a number to call if I have problems after hours and on weekends?*
- *How do you decide what medication regimen is right for me?*
- *Will I have access to clinical trials?*
- *Can I bring a family member, a loved one, or a friend to my visits?*

These are just a few of the most important questions. But, obviously, the questions you ask are specific to your needs. Again, there are no right and wrong questions. In order for you to make sound judgments and decisions regarding your HIV care, you must have the right answers to your questions.

Ryan White HIV/AIDS Treatment Extension Act of 2009 (Formerly Ryan White CARE Act)

It became evident very early in the epidemic that getting quality medical care soon after diagnosis is the key to living a healthy, productive life with HIV. Unfortunately, the specialty care necessary does not come cheap. While many have the good fortune of medical insurance, a number of HIV-infected people lack medical insurance or the monetary resources to get necessary medical care. In 1990, the United States government passed the Ryan White Comprehensive AIDS Resources Emergency (CARE) Act, providing funds that assure each and every HIV-infected person has access to HIV care.

When the act was initially put into law, it was comprised of several titles, each providing funding for specific services. But because the act was never designed to be a static piece of legislation, changes have been made over the years to adapt to the changing HIV epidemic. In 2000, the act was reauthorized but with some significant changes addressing the following issues:

- access to care
- quality of care
- capacity development
- targeting of resources
- early intervention services
- administrative issues

With each reauthorization the U.S. Senate and House of Representatives examine trends in HIV care and prevention to make certain the act is addressing the needs of those particular aspects of the epidemic. Surveillance data is also examined to see where the new infections are coming from and where education is needed. Finally, before reauthorization, programs funded by the act are examined to make certain they are making good use of the funds they receive: Are the programs providing quality care in a fiscally responsible way, or should funds be reallocated to other areas that are lacking the resources they need?

In 2006 the name of the act was changed to the Ryan White HIV/AIDS Treatment Modernization Act and as the new name suggested, changes were made that improved and modernized how treatment funds were allocated. The changes in 2006 were important in emphasizing the act had always been geared toward the health care needs of those living with HIV. With that in mind, new stipulations added to the grant mandated 75 percent of awarded funds had to be used for core medical services. This change assured that funds were used in a way that directly impacted the health of Ryan White consumers, those living with HIV. When President Barack Obama took office in 2009 there was some concern among providers that the act would not be renewed. Luckily, however, in 2009 Congress voted to extend the act, changing the name to the Ryan White HIV/AIDS Treatment Extension Act of 2009. But the cost of delivering the needed care was and still is not cheap. In 1990, the first year of the CARE Act, $220 million was allocated to fund HIV care across the country. In 2010 that amount soared to $2.29 billion. Let's look at where all that money is going.

- *Part A (formerly Title I)—Grants to Emerging Metropolitan & Transitional Grant Areas:* This part provides funding to those metropolitan areas hardest hit by HIV and AIDS. The areas can be one city, one county, or an area that spreads across multiple cities or even multiple states. There are two ways areas can be eligible for these funds.
- Eligible Metropolitan Area (EMA)—an area has at least 2000 HIV cases in the previous five years and a population of at least 50,000.
- Transitional Grant Area (TGA)—an area that has 1000–1999 HIV cases in the previous five years and a population of at least 50,000.
  This part's funding provides such services as:
  - Outpatient and ambulatory health services, including substance abuse and mental health treatment;
  - Early intervention including outreach, counseling and testing, and referral services designed to identify HIV-positive individuals unaware of their HIV status;
  - Outpatient and ambulatory support services including case management and adherence services

- Home health care; nutrition services; hospice services; and drug assistance programs

- *Part B (formerly Title II)—Grants to States & Territories:* This title provides funding for all fifty states, the District of Columbia, Guam and Puerto Rico, Virgin Islands, and Pacific Territories. These funds are used for:
  - The AIDS Drug Assistance Program (ADAP);
  - Health insurance premiums including those purchased through the Affordable Care Act;
  - Adherence tools and services;
  - Drug treatments monitoring

- *Part C (formerly Title III)—Early Intervention & Capacity Building Services:* This part actually provides funds earmarked for two different purposes. A portion of these funds is used for Early Intervention Services, funds that provide core medical services and primary health care for HIV-infected people who receive their care in free-standing clinics, hospital-based clinics, community health centers, and family planning agencies. The funds provide:
  - Outpatient medical care;
  - Risk-reduction counseling and prevention, antibody testing, medical evaluation, and clinical care;
  - Antiretroviral therapies; protection against opportunistic infections; and ongoing medical, oral health, nutritional, psychosocial, and other care services for HIV-infected clients;
  - Case management to ensure access to services and continuity of care for HIV-infected clients; and
  - Attention to other health problems that occur frequently with HIV infection, including tuberculosis and substance abuse.

The remaining funds are used for Capacity Building Grants. As the name suggests the money is for the purpose of improving infrastructure so the agency's capacity to care for patients can increase. Because patients are living longer and there are always new infections, the demand for HIV services is always increasing, thus increasing the need for quality HIV care. Funded programs can use these grants to:

  - Improve program management and care delivery systems
  - Improve retention in care
  - Improve or initiate an electronic medical record system and telehealth program
  - Purchasing dental, anoscopy, or colposcopy equipment
  - Pay for staff training to maintain cultural competency
  - Fund Continuous Quality Management (CQM) activities within Part C programs

- *Part D—Services for Women, Infants, Children and Youth & Their Families:* This part provides funding for family centered care including women, children, and their families. While all parts of the CARE Act are required to care for these populations, Part D funding is specifically for them. This funding provides:
  - Primary and specialty medical care;

- Psychosocial services;
- Logistical support and coordination; and
- Outreach and case management.
- Continuous Quality Management (CQM) activities within Part D programs

- *Part F—Special Projects of National Significance (SPNS)*: This funding advances knowledge and skills in the delivery of HIV health care. Considered the research portion of the CARE Act, it provides funding for:
  - Assessing the effectiveness of particular models of care;
  - Supporting innovative program design; and
  - Promoting replication of effective modes of care.
- *Part F—Dental Reimbursement Program*: Also a Part F program provides funding that supports oral health and dental care for those HIV-infected people without the means or resources to maintain regular dental care.
- *Part F—Minority AIDS Initiative*: Another Part F program, supports a range of activities to address HIV/AIDS care needs unique to African-Americans.
- *Part F—AIDS Education and Training Centers (AETC)*: One more Part F program that supports a network of eleven regional centers (and more than 130 local associated sites) that conduct targeted, multidisciplinary education and training programs for health care providers treating people living with HIV/AIDS.

Experts agree that the Ryan White CARE Act of 1990 forever changed how HIV care would be funded and delivered. One could argue that if not for the act, tens of thousands more people would have died of HIV and AIDS because the care they desperately needed would not have been possible or available. However, there is a new player in town that may help people get the medical care and medications they need in order to stay healthy. Let's take a look at another act that will change the way we access medical care, The Affordable Care Act.

The Affordable Care Act ("Obamacare")

In March 2010, President Barack Obama signed into law the *Affordable Care Act (ACA)*, more commonly known as "Obamacare." The legislation's goal is to make medical insurance available and affordable for everyone. Partisan politics has debated the effectiveness and long-term impact of the ACA from day one, but regardless of your politics it has made some progress toward affordable insurance and medication coverage for everyone. Despite many issues with online sign-up and sudden unexpected insurance cancellations, people have gotten coverage for medical care and medications, including people living with HIV and AIDS. So far, the ACA does appear to have some positive implications for those living with HIV.

- *Improving Access to Coverage*—One important aspect of the ACA is that no one can be dropped from coverage or denied coverage for any pre-existing condition, including HIV/AIDS. In addition, there are no lifetime coverage caps, meaning there is no limit to the amount of claims a person can make to get medical care. This is very significant for people with chronic health care issues because with the numerous diagnostic tests, blood tests, medications, and regular visits to their doctor, lifetime caps in coverage are met very quickly. Finally, the ACA policy can't be cancelled or denied if honest mistakes are made on the application. All these provisions remove the fear of being denied coverage and in the process encourage them to seek care since patients don't have to worry about accumulating medical bills.

The ACA has made it possible for many states to expand their Medicaid coverage by raising the income limits and family size restrictions, which in turn allows more people in need to qualify for coverage. But most important for people living with HIV, because of Medicaid expansion an AIDS diagnosis or having children will no longer be required to qualify for Medicaid coverage. For those families with private insurance, the ACA now permits parents to keep their dependent children on the insurance policy until they turn 26 years of age. Finally, the ACA will provide affordable coverage options with lower out-of-pocket expenses for lower income individuals and families that already have financial challenges.

- *Ensure Quality Coverage*—The ACA requires insurance policies to cover a majority of preventative healthcare services including HIV testing for everyone 15 to 65 years old. Given the number of people who are infected and are not aware of their infection, this provision alone could have a significant impact on HIV care and prevention. The ACA legally provides for coverage of the "essential health benefits," those health services that we all need to remain healthy and to be cured of sickness when it occurs. For the HIV-infected person, this type of coverage is very important in order to remain healthy. Examples of essential health benefits include lab work, inpatient and outpatient care, prescription drug coverage, mental health service, and substance abuse services. Finally, quality coverage under the ACA includes coverage for care of the whole person, which assures not only medical care but support services like mental health and nutrition services as well.

- *Enhance the Capacity of the Healthcare Delivery System*—The ACA has made major investments in expanding the capacity of the current healthcare delivery system by providing funding for outpatient health centers, providing technical assistance to improve the healthcare infrastructure, providing care for underserved populations, and by providing support and training for culturally competent care. Because the HIV population is very culturally diverse and has a large number of people from underserved and at-risk populations (e.g., transgender, homeless, and minority populations) the ACA will have a profound impact on HIV care.

There is no question that the ACA has made great strides in providing insurance for millions of U.S. citizens and in doing so it has also provided another resource for those who are living with such a costly disease, financially, emotionally, and physically. In fact, many would argue that second to the Ryan White Care Act, the ACA is the most important piece of legislation in the fight against HIV and AIDS.

TABLE 7—HOW THE AFFORDABLE CARE ACT HELPS PEOPLE LIVING WITH HIV

- Ensures coverage for people with pre-existing conditions.
- Expands Medicaid

- Provides more affordable healthcare coverage
- Lower prescription drug coverage
- Provide preventative services, including HIV testing
- Expands coverage for dependent children of the insured
- Assure coverage for essential health benefits
- Provide resources for coordinated care for people with chronic health conditions.

5

YOUR FIRST VISIT TO THE DOCTOR

When it's finally time to meet your doctor for the first time, what can you expect? No doubt it will be a very confusing, stressful and frightening time. As you may know, fear is a product of not knowing what to expect. Fear of the unknown can also create stress and anxiety. Knowing what to expect that first visit can help minimize the stress, anxiety and fear. Let's look at the first visit, how to prepare, what to expect, and who you may see.

What You Need to Bring

Getting the most from your doctor's visit requires more than just showing up. You need to prepare for the visit as much as the physician does. As was mentioned in the previous chapter, there are a few items you should get together and bring with you to that first visit. They include:

- *Your HIV Test Results:* Your doctor will want to review your HIV test results. When you receive your results, make certain to ask for a copy and bring that copy to your first doctor's visit.

- *Insurance Cards:* If you have insurance coverage, be it private or government sponsored insurance, the clerical staff at the doctor's office is going to want to see your insurance cards. Most likely they will make copies of those cards, make the copies part of your electronic medical record (EMR), and return them to you by the end of your visit.

- *Insurance Referral:* In this day of Health Management Organizations (HMOs), the insurance referral is very important. HMOs employ a network of general medicine physicians from which you can choose to get your primary care. Every member of the HMO must choose a primary care physician from the network, and it is that physician who must refer you to other specialists, HIV specialists included. Be sure to get a referral prior to your first visit to the HIV specialist, and bring a copy of the referral with you for the clerical staff at the doctor's office. Some insurance systems employ an electronic referral system that will send the referral directly to the HIV provider from your primary care physician's office. Without a referral some practices will not schedule your first appointment, and at the very least *you* instead of your insurance company will be billed for your visit. If you are having issues securing a referral to an HIV specialist, most primary care physicians employ referral specialists that submit referrals for their patients. Call your primary doctor and ask to speak to the referral specialist to request the needed referral.

- *Appointment Information:* If you receive an appointment confirmation, reminder, or itinerary from your doctor prior to your appointment, bring it with you in case there is any confusion surrounding the date or time of your appointment once you arrive at the doctor's office.

- *Old Medical Records:* If you have time prior to your first visit, obtain copies of your past medical records from other physicians who have treated you before your HIV diagnosis. Even medical information not related to your HIV is important to your new doctor. Items of particular interest to your new HIV provider include immunization records, medication lists, medication allergies, and records of the past twelve months of medical care. The better he or she knows your past medical history, the better care you will receive now that you have HIV.

- *Questions for Your Doctor:* As was mentioned in a previous chapter, bring a list of any questions you have for your doctor. Because questions can be easily forgotten among all the stress and anxiety of your first visit, write them down as they occur to you and present that list to your doctor when you arrive. Leave plenty of room on your list for notes and answers to each question.

- *Friend or Loved One for Support:* As discussed earlier, bringing someone along to your first visit for emotional support will be a great help in digesting the large amount of information you will receive. Obviously, the person you choose should be someone who knows your diagnosis and can offer the assistance and support you need. While your doctor may ask for that person to leave the room during portions of your examination, HIV care providers are more than happy to include your support system during that first visit. If there are aspects of your visit you would prefer to be alone with the physician, just ask your support to step out so you can have the privacy you are looking for.

TABLE 8

Questions for Your Doctor at Your First Appointment

1. Will I be permitted to play an active role in planning and structuring my care?
2. How much time will I be allotted for my appointment and my questions?
3. Will I be seen by the same doctor each visit?
4. Will I see an attending physician or a resident/student?
5. What days are clinic appointments available?
6. Are "walk-in" appointments available?
7. Is there a nurse-line I can call if my issue can't wait until my next visit?
8. Is there an emergency number I call after office hours and on weekends and holidays?
9. Will I have access to any experimental treatments or clinical trials?
10. May I bring my partner/spouse/loved one to my visits?

What Should You Expect Upon Arrival?

Most likely, the first people you will encounter at your visit are the clerical staff responsible for registering you for that first visit. Usually, the clerical staff has limited medical training but is responsible for getting all the insurance paperwork out of the way before you see the doctor. Normally the staff will ask for your insurance information, any referrals that may be required of your insurance, your appointment time, and the name of the physician you are scheduled to see. While the staff is bound by the same confidentiality rules and regulations as the medical personnel, there's no need to provide the check-in staff with details of your diagnosis or medical history. In fact, it's best not to discuss those things in a public area such as the check-in desk or waiting room. If you feel the check-in staff are not observing your right to confidentiality—for instance, the staff are speaking loud enough to be heard by others waiting nearby—remind them of your right to privacy. Once they get you "checked in," your doctor will be notified that you are ready for your appointment. You'll be taken back to an exam room when a room becomes available.

What to Expect Once You're in the Exam Room

When an exam room becomes available, you will be escorted to the room by some member of the medical staff. Depending on the type of practice you choose, it may be a medical assistant or a nurse who accompanies you to the room. Once in the room, the nurse or medical assistant will take your blood pressure, heart rate, respiratory rate and temperature.

Many practices employ registered nurses who make the initial patient contact at each visit. The nurse will perform a basic assessment to see if there are any specific complaints, issues, or concerns (e.g., sore throat, anxiety, or a fever) you would like to pass on to your doctor. Often times the nurse will do a medical history, which includes assessing past and current illnesses, medication history, surgical history, and mental health history. This is a good time for you the patient to begin a relationship with the nurse. You will find that the nurse will be a very valuable part of your HIV care. Due to the doctor's busy schedule, most often it is the nurse who is available when issues or concerns arise. The nurse is a liaison between you and your doctor. Be upfront and forthright with your concerns and complaints. Many times the doctor relies heavily on what the nurse has learned in the initial assessment. If you leave items out, the doctor may not address them at all during your visit. A good relationship with the nurse will help your relationship with the doctor as well.

When the nurse has completed his or her focused assessment, the information gained will be forwarded to the physician. Depending on how busy the practice is that day, you may have a short wait in the exam room. Keep an eye out for any educational material available in the room. The time spent waiting can be a valuable learning period if the right educational materials are available. Soon, it will be your turn to see the doctor.

What Should You Expect from Your Doctor?

The first visit to your doctor will likely be a bit longer than subsequent visits after the doctor-patient relationship has been established. At that first visit the doctor is starting with a clean slate, knowing little about you. Much of the visit will be a discussion centering on your past medical history and your current medical condition. This discussion provides your doctor with very important information necessary to provide you the best and most complete medical care. It's important to be honest and forthcoming with facts and information. Some questions the doctor will ask may seem very personal and intrusive. Rest assured that every question has a purpose, so answer each honestly and as completely as possible. Without completely honest answers, pieces of your medical puzzle will be missing, preventing the doctor from providing the medical care you need. If confidentiality is what concerns you, rest assured that physicians and all medical personnel are bound by very strict rules of confidentiality. The information you share with the doctor, nurse or any other person in the medical office remains confidential.

A part of every medical visit is the physical examination. On your first visit, this exam will cover all the body's systems from head to toe. On subsequent visits your doctor will probably limit his physical exam to those systems giving you problems currently or at your last visit. For instance, if you are having a cough now or are recovering from a cough, the doctor will assess and examine your breathing and your lungs. If you are complaining of abdominal pain or nausea, the doctor will examine your stomach. The complete head-to-toe exam performed during the first visit will include:

- *The Head and Neck:* The doctor will examine your head, eyes, and ears. Are you having headaches, visual changes, ringing or pain in your ears? The doctor will palpate or feel your neck for any enlarged "glands" or lymph nodes. While enlarged lymph nodes can signal an acute (new) infection, they can be a common symptom with a chronic (old) infection like HIV. The doctor will also ask if you've recently had fevers, chills, or night sweats.

- *The Chest:* The doctor will use a stethoscope to listen through your chest and back to assess your lungs. Lung infections such as pneumonia can cause changes in the way your lungs sound when you breathe. Hearing that change through the stethoscope helps your doctor identify illnesses that have to be evaluated and treated. The doctor will also use the stethoscope to listen to your heart to identify any abnormal heart rhythms or heart sounds that signal illness or disease. Your doctor will also feel under your arms and around your chest for any enlarged lymph nodes. Female patients will get a breast exam to check for any breast lumps that would need to be evaluated further using more invasive tests (e.g., mammogram or biopsy). Finally, the doctor will ask if you've had any cough, shortness of breath, difficulty breathing, or chest pain. If so these symptoms could mean a heart or lung condition that would need to be evaluated much more closely using an electrocardiogram (EKG), chest X-ray, or various blood tests.

- *The Abdomen (stomach):* Using the stethoscope again, the doctor will listen to your abdomen for bowel sounds—the sounds your intestines make when working to digest your food. The doctor will palpate (press on) your abdomen and your groin, looking for enlarged lymph nodes. He or she will also press on your abdomen to assess for pain or enlargement of the liver and/or spleen. Finally, the doctor will ask about your bowel habits, specifically, are you having any constipation, nausea, vomiting or diarrhea. Your doctor will also ask about the presence of pain or burning with urination, low back pain, abdominal pain, foul smelling urine, or the presence of blood in your urine.

- *Rectal and Genital Areas:* The doctor will do a physical inspection of your genitals and rectal area, looking for any open sores, lumps or lesions that could indicate a sexually transmitted disease or underlying infection or illness. While women will be encouraged to have a complete pelvic exam and Pap test by a gynecologist, that exam probably will not be part of your first visit. Men will have a testicular exam to feel for any lumps or masses in the scrotum. The doctor will do a rectal exam by placing a gloved finger in the anus to feel for lumps or masses, and to assess for any blood that may be in the stool. In men, the prostate will be assessed during the rectal exam to see if there is any enlargement or tenderness when the prostate is palpated. Finally, the doctor will ask if you have had any abnormal pain or abnormal discharge from the vagina, penis, or anus. Female patients will be asked about any past pregnancies, abortions, and miscarriages, as well as questions about the menstrual cycle. While these questions and exams are very personal, intrusive, and invasive, it's important to be open and honest with your doctor. Remember, the doctor and his staff are not there to judge or be critical, they are there to take care of you. Your HIV provider's office is a safe place to be completely honest for the sake of your health. For instance, if you deny any penile discharge because you are embarrassed you may be hiding an infection that could be easily treated. By not being treated you are jeopardizing your health and that of your partner or spouse. Be honest and receive the treatment you need if there is an issue.

- *Leg, Arms, Hands and Feet:* The upper and lower extremities will be assessed for any swelling or open wounds. The doctor will ask if there is any history of numbness, tingling, or needle-like pain in the hands and feet. The doctor will also assess how well you move your extremities, the color and temperature of hands and feet, the condition of your toenails and fingernails, and the presence of palpable pulses in the feet and the wrists. Finally, the doctor will assess hand and foot strength by having you squeeze his or her hands, and pushing down on his or her hands with your feet.

- *Psychosocial/Mental Status:* The doctor will assess your mental health status by asking a variety of questions. Do you have a history of "passing out"? Do you use alcohol or tobacco? Have you ever abused prescription or recreational drugs? Do you feel depressed or are you having trouble sleeping? Have you ever thought about hurting yourself or hurting others? Depending on the provider, some will administer a short depression screening tool to identify any early signs of depression, common with a new HIV diagnosis. Remember, being honest and forthright with your answers no matter how difficult or embarrassing is in the best interest of your health and will benefit you in the long-term.

- *Sexual and Risk Factor History:* An important part of your first visit's assessment will be a discussion about your sexual risk factors and your sexual history. This allows the doctor to determine how you contracted HIV and to educate you regarding safer sexual practices. Information on the route of transmission is also an important part of tracking the epidemic. The doctor is required to report new infections to the state health department. The information is tabulated by health department staffers and used by prevention specialists in order to target their prevention messages to those populations most at risk. Once again, it's important to be forthright with your sexual history. Nobody is there to judge you only to take care of you, keeping you healthier longer. If you don't use condoms say so; if you have multiple anonymous partners tell your provider. Being upfront with your doctor is in your best interest and is the only way to keep you and all future sexual partners safe and healthy.

Who Else Will See You That Day?

Depending on the type of practice you choose, the doctor may not be the only person you will see that first visit. Because HIV affects the whole person, proper HIV care includes many medical and social disciplines. They include:

- *Registered Nurses:* The nurse could be considered the liaison between the doctor and the patient. All practices will have at least one nurse to handle such things as injections, patient teaching, patient telephone calls, and assisting with medical procedures. In larger practices, the nurse may have his or her own schedule of patients to address issues ranging from medication and adherence teaching to well care visits and immunizations. When a patient is sick, the nurse is typically the first person they will encounter, either by telephone or in the clinic.

- *Social Workers:* Depending on the practice, social workers play a huge role in the care of the HIV-infected patient. The social worker is primarily responsible for those things not physical in nature, including mental health counseling, accessing community resources, and negotiating the medical insurance maze, including the Affordable Care Act. In addition, social workers play a big role in medication and adherence teaching, HIV prevention, testing and counseling, and safer sex education. Finally, social workers play a very important role in those first few days after diagnosis when the patient is desperately trying to adjust to their new illness.

- *Nutritionists or Dieticians:* Proper diet and nutrition is an important part of staying healthy. If you are fortunate enough to choose a practice that employs a nutritionist, he or she will help you optimize your diet by choosing foods high in the calories and nutrients necessary to fight your illness and remain healthy. The nutritionist can assist with diet and menu planning, exercise programs and medication related-issues surrounding eating and food. Some HIV medications can increase your cholesterol and blood sugar. Dieticians can assist with menu planning in an effort to normalize cholesterol and blood sugar while maintaining adequate calories to maintain a proper body weight. Finally, because HIV medicines can cause side effects such as nausea and vomiting, the dietician plays an important role in medication teaching and adherence by instructing the patient in ways to deal with unpleasant medication side effects.

- *Medical Assistants:* Most practices employ medical assistants to handle such tasks as injections, vital signs, and clerical duties. Medical assistants are often responsible for the flow of patients through the clinic, from check-in, to seeing your doctor, to checking out and making the next appointment. Hospitals often employ medical assistants to work alongside the registered nurse performing tasks like checking and routing voice mail messages, initiating medication refills and prior authorizations, and administering immunizations.

- *Others:* Depending on the type and size of the practice you are part of and whether you are a patient in an HIV program funded by the Ryan White CARE Act, you may find that there are several other disciplines involved in your care. Pharmacists, psychiatrists, and dentists are often part of Ryan White programs so those important services are available to patients when they come to see their HIV provider. If you are being seen in a large hospital based program you will also encounter specialists from all branches of medicine—dermatologists to address issues with your skin, cardiologists to address issues with your heart, and gynecologists to address women's issues to name a few. It just goes to show you it takes a team approach comprised of many disciplines to care for the HIV patient because HIV affects the entire person.

Specialty Services

It's inevitable, despite the best medical care, there will be times of poor health. In certain practices, the HIV specialist can also act as the patient's primary care physician, handling such issues as high blood pressure, diabetes, asthma, and the common problems that we all face from time to time. However, there are times when specialists are needed to address illnesses other than HIV. For instance, patients will be referred to a hepatologist (liver specialist) if they have a hepatitis C coinfection or other conditions of the liver. Patients who have heart disease will be referred to a cardiologist (heart specialist) to manage their heart problems. Finally, if a woman with HIV is having problems specific to women, she will be referred to a gynecologist (women's issues specialist). Depending on your needs at the time of your first visit, your HIV specialist may refer you to another specialty physician to address concerns not related to HIV.

Now you know what to expect during your first visit to the doctor. Depending on your health status, most HIV specialists will see you once every month or two until you are stabilized on an effective HIV medication regimen. After that, the standards of HIV care recommend that a person living with HIV should see a doctor at least once every six months. Obviously, the number and frequency of visits will change according to your health status. For instance, certain illnesses or changes in medication regimens will require more frequent visits. Regardless of the frequency, the purpose of regular visits to your doctor is to keep you as healthy as possible for as long as possible. So in addition to regular visits to your HIV provider, there are many blood tests, diagnostic tests, and procedures that help monitor your HIV, immune system and overall health. In the next chapter, we will discuss each of these tools in detail.

6

Monitoring Your Health

Obviously, the goal of your HIV care is to stay as healthy as possible for as long as possible. And people in regular HIV care are definitely meeting that goal. Experts now agree that among some segments of the HIV population, people living with HIV have life expectancies equal to or even better than people living without HIV. Achieving those kinds of results requires consistent HIV care by an HIV specialist and strict adherence to HIV medication regimens. During regular visits to your doctor, your current state of health will be assessed using physical examination and a combination of lab tests, X-rays, and diagnostic procedures. The goal of your HIV care is to preserve the health of your immune system by controlling the replication of HIV. This chapter will review the most commonly used diagnostic and screening tools.

Blood Testing

Blood testing provides information that your doctor will use to interpret the health and functioning of your body, most notably your immune system. The results of these tests provide clues to your overall health, the functioning of your organs, the strength of your immune system, and the amount of viral activity in your body. During or before most visits your doctor will order an assortment of blood tests that will help him or her assess the health and functioning of various systems in your body. Let's look at each blood test in a little more detail.

Electrolytes (Lytes)

Serum electrolytes are a collection of salts and minerals circulating in the blood that control fluid balance, blood pH, energy generation, and muscle contraction. Electrolytes are an essential part of almost every major biochemical reaction in the body. While there are several electrolytes in the blood, this panel of tests measure four important electrolytes and two important indicators of normal kidney function.

- **Sodium (Na):** Sodium is primarily responsible for maintaining osmotic pressure (fluid pressure) within cells and the vascular system. In other words, it maintains a balance between intracellular (fluid inside the cell) and extracellular (fluid outside the cells) fluid levels in the body. Increased serum (blood) sodium is present in states of dehydration resulting from diarrhea or vomiting. Low sodium levels usually result from too much fluid within the cells resulting from excess free water intake or fluid retention due to a disturbance in the body's fluid balance system.

Normal values: 135–145 milliEquivalents/liter (mEq/L)

- **Potassium (K):** Potassium is the major electrolyte involved in heart and muscle function. Even small changes in potassium levels, either too much or too little potassium, can cause abnormal heart rates and rhythms, which in turn negatively impact cardiac (heart) function. Too much potassium in the blood is usually a result of poor kidney function and can adversely affect heart rhythm. Low potassium levels are usually the result of potassium loss through excessive urination or vomiting, and can cause serious changes in heart rhythm.

  Normal values: 3.5–5.0 (mEq/L)

- **Chloride (Cl):** In combination with sodium, chloride maintains fluid levels by regulating osmotic (fluid) pressure in the blood. An elevated chloride level usually results from excessive water loss from diarrhea or vomiting or low fluid volume (dehydration) in the blood. A chloride level below normal usually results from ongoing vomiting or excess fluid (free water) in the body.

  Normal values: 100–106 millimoles/liter (mmol/L)

- **Bicarbonate (HCO3):** Bicarbonate is a substance that helps maintain a proper blood pH. The pH is the measure of the blood's acidity. If the blood is too acidic the blood has a lower than normal pH (<7.35). If the blood is not acidic enough, it's said to be basic and has a higher than normal pH (>7.45). Keep in mind that the pH of water is 7.00. Bicarbonate is basic; it has a high pH. When the blood becomes too acidic, the body releases bicarbonate to raise the pH into the normal range. If the blood is too basic, the body decreases the bicarbonate, which lowers the pH, making the blood the proper acidity. Keep in mind that the body must have a pH between 7.35 and 7.45 to function properly. Any variation can be very serious, even deadly.

  *Normal HCO3 values: 35–45 mmol/L; **Normal pH:** 7.35–7.45 (low pH—acidic/high pH—basic)*

- **Blood Urea Nitrogen (BUN):** Urea is a waste product produced in the liver by the breakdown of protein during the production of energy in the body. Typically, the body uses glucose for energy, but if there is not enough glucose, as is the case in dieting or an abnormally low blood sugar, the body breaks down protein and urea is produced. Urea is transported via the bloodstream to the kidneys where it is excreted. An elevated BUN can be a result of poor kidney function or inadequate blood circulation to the kidneys. However, BUN is not a good indicator of kidney function because its level can be affected by many things, especially dieting and weight loss.

  Normal values: 8–25 milligrams/deciliter (mg/dl)

- **Creatinine (Cr):** Creatinine is a waste product formed when muscle tissue uses energy sources found in the body. Creatinine is transported to the kidneys via the bloodstream, is filtered from the blood by the kidneys, sent down the ureters into the bladder and then out of the body via the urethra. Unlike an elevated BUN that is affected by weight loss and dieting, elevated creatinine is a specific indicator of impaired kidney function. Damaged kidneys are unable to filter creatinine from the blood and it accumulates, elevating the serum creatinine. If too much creatinine accumulates in the body it must be filtered from the blood by the mechanical process known as dialysis.

Normal values: 0.5–1.1 mg/dl

- **Blood Sugar:** Glucose (blood sugar) is the main source of energy for the human body. The glucose is released from energy stores and makes its way to the bloodstream where it can be used by the body. The amount of sugar in the blood is kept within a normal range by a substance the body produces called insulin. If too much or too little sugar is in the blood the body will not work properly. There is a common lab test known as the blood sugar. The doctor will check the amount of sugar in your blood on a regular basis to make certain in never gets too high or too low.

  Normal values: 70–110 (varies depending on lab) **Hypoglycemia:** *<70mg/***Hyperglycemia:** *>110mg*

- **Hemoglobin A1C (HgbA1C):** The HgbA1C blood test is used by your physician to assess how well your blood sugar has been controlled over the past two to three months. Compare that to the blood sugar test that in essence is checking the blood sugar value for a specific moment in time, the time of the blood draw. Over time, some of the sugar circulating in the bloodstream adheres to the hemoglobin of red blood cells, remaining there for the life of the red blood cell. HgbA1C measures the percentage of red blood cells that have sugar adhered to its hemoglobin. The more sugar circulating in the blood over a period of time the greater number of red blood cells that have sugar attached to the hemoglobin. The HgbA1C is used to diagnose diabetes or to monitor blood sugar control of someone living with diabetes.

  Normal values: **Without diabetes**—*5.0–6.5 percent*
  With diabetes—*less than 7.0 percent*

COMPLETE BLOOD COUNT (CBC)

One of the most important blood tests that your doctor will order is the complete blood count (CBC). There are many different types of cells in your blood, and all of them can be grouped into one of three categories: red blood cells, white blood cells, and platelets. A complete blood count helps your doctor determine if your body is trying to fight infection, if your body is producing the cells necessary to fight that infection, and if your body is producing the specialized cells that carry oxygen to your organs and tissues.

- **White Blood Cells (WBC):** Also known as leukocytes, white blood cells are produced in the bone marrow and are part of the body's system of fighting infection. An elevated WBC count usually indicates that the body is fighting some type of infection. A count lower than normal suggests that too few white blood cells are being produced, possibly because of a medication (e.g., chemotherapy for cancer) or a disease process (e.g., HIV) that is interfering with the bone marrow's ability to produce white blood cells. As the WBC count declines, the body's natural defenses against infection grow weaker.

  Normal values: 5000–10000 cells per cubic millimeter of blood (reported as 5.0–10.0)

- **Red Blood Cells (RBC):** Also known as erythrocytes, red blood cells are produced by the bone marrow and are responsible for delivering oxygen to tissues and organs throughout the body. As the number of red blood cells declines, so does the body's ability to oxygenate organs and tissues. If the red blood cell count falls too low, organs will fail from lack of oxygen. A low red blood cell count (anemia) can be caused by poor diet, bleeding, or vitamin deficiency. In addition, there are certain medications, including some HIV medications (e.g., zidovudine, AZT) that suppress bone marrow, interfering with red blood cell production, eventually causing anemia. Fortunately, the newer HIV medications do not suppress bone marrow and are used more often than AZT. As a result, low red blood cell counts and anemia from HIV medications are less of a concern than they once were.

Normal values: 4.20–5.70 million red cells per microliter of blood

- **Hemoglobin (Hgb):** Hemoglobin is an iron containing protein located on the red blood cell. Oxygen molecules are able to attach to the hemoglobin because of the iron molecules. It's the hemoglobin that makes it possible for red blood cells to carry oxygen from the lungs to tissues and organs throughout the body. A lower than normal hemoglobin means the blood's ability to carry oxygen is diminished, impairing all bodily functions. Obviously, without enough oxygen the body begins to fail, causing symptoms such as shortness of breath, chest pain, muscle pain and fatigue. Conditions that cause lower than normal hemoglobin levels include bleeding, diminished red blood cell production by the bone marrow, iron deficiency, and poor diet. Because the human body does not make iron, it must be included in the diet or as dietary supplement. If the diet is deficient in iron, this will decrease hemoglobin and the red blood cell's ability to carry oxygen.

  Normal values: Male—14–17 grams of hemoglobin per deciliter of blood (g/dL); Female—12–15g/dL

- **Hematocrit (Hct):** Whole blood is composed of red blood cells, white blood cells, hemoglobin, platelets, and serum. Hematocrit is a calculated value that represents the ratio of red blood cells to the total blood volume. A higher than normal hematocrit is most often a result of dehydration that changes the ratio between red blood cells and the total blood volume. As the amount of blood volume decreases, as is the case when a person is dehydrated, the ratio of red blood cells goes up. A lower than normal hematocrit can be caused by bleeding, states of fluid overload, or conditions that diminish red blood cell production (e.g., diseases affecting the bone marrow).

  Normal values: Male—41–50 percent; Female—36–44 percent

- **Platelets (PLT):** Also known as thrombocytes, platelets are produced by the bone marrow and are involved in the blood clotting process. When an opening develops in the vascular system (the blood vessels), platelets are dispatched to the area and begin to clump together, forming a plug to seal the opening. Having too few platelets causes prolonged clotting time, which, in extreme cases, can result in severe bleeding. Some diseases, illnesses, and the side effects of certain medications can cause the platelet count to drop below normal, increasing the risk for prolonged bleeding.

  Normal values: 140,000–390,000 platelets per microliter of blood

LIVER FUNCTION TESTS (LFTS)

Liver function tests assess the functioning of the liver by examining the amounts of certain substances and enzymes in the blood. From these studies, your doctor can identify possible liver disease, medication stress on liver function, and infections of the liver (e.g., hepatitis). There are a variety of tests that comprise LFTs.

- **Albumin (ALB):** Albumin is a protein produced by the liver that helps maintain osmotic (fluid) pressure in the vascular space (blood vessels). Albumin helps maintain a pressure balance between the inside and outside of the vessels, assuring that fluid stays in the vascular system instead of leaking out into the tissues, causing swelling (edema). Albumin also carries certain essential minerals in the bloodstream and throughout the body. Elevated albumin levels usually indicate dehydration, while lower than normal albumin levels can indicate liver dysfunction or insufficient protein intake.
  Normal values: 4–6 grams per deciliter of blood (g/dl)

- **Alkaline Phosphatase (ALK PHOS):** Alkaline phosphatase is an enzyme found in many organs of the body, including the liver. This enzyme is released into the bloodstream when there has been damage to the liver caused by such things as infections, medications, and blockages within the liver's biliary ducts. While lower than normal alkaline phosphatase levels are not related to any health problems, elevated levels indicate liver dysfunction and/or damage to the liver.
  Normal values: 30–120 units per liter of liter (U/L)

- **Alanine Aminotransferase (ALT or SGPT):** This protein is found primarily in the liver. It is released into the blood when there has been some sort of liver tissue damage. While lower than normal levels are really insignificant, elevated levels result when there has been liver tissue damage caused by such things as infection, medications, chemicals, obstruction, cirrhosis (hardening), or injury to the liver.
  Normal values: Less than 35 U/L

- **Aspartate Aminotransferase (AST or SGOT):** This protein, unlike (ALT), is found in the liver as well as the brain, pancreas, heart, skeletal muscle, kidneys and lungs. Because of that fact, an elevated AST alone does not necessarily mean there has been damage to the liver. Physicians can use a ratio between the AST and ALT to get a clue about the cause of liver damage. Like ALT, lower than normal levels are not significant, but elevated levels accompanied by elevated ALT levels result when there has been liver tissue damage caused by things like infection, medicines, obstructions, cirrhosis, chemicals, or trauma to the liver.
  Normal values: less than 35 U/L

- **Total Bilirubin (TBILI):** Bilirubin is a yellow pigment found in red blood cells. When red blood cells break down, bilirubin is released into the bloodstream. Bilirubin is then carried to the liver, where it is broken down, metabolized, and excreted in the feces or stored in the gall bladder. When the liver is not functioning properly, bilirubin builds up in the body, and the yellow pigment causes dark urine and a yellowing of the sclera (white portion of the eye), mucous membranes, and the skin. Such an elevation can be caused by an obstruction, liver disease or liver failure. The HIV medication Reyataz (atazanavir) causes the same jaundice but not for the same reason. When taking Reyataz the jaundice occurs because the metabolic pathway for Reyataz and bilirubin are the same, causing the pathway to be overwhelmed resulting in the accumulation of bilirubin. In this scenario there is no damage or problem with the liver at all.
  Normal values: less than 1.0 milligrams/deciliter of blood (mg/dl)

- **Unconjugated (Indirect) Bilirubin (BU):** Also known as indirect bilirubin, unconjugated bilirubin is a type of bilirubin that is not water soluble. Bilirubin needs to be water soluble in order to be excreted through the urine. Unconjugated bilirubin is carried to the liver by albumin and is then transformed to a water soluble form with the help of special enzymes. Elevated BU can occur with many blood disorders, liver disease, or resolution of large blood clots. As mentioned earlier, an elevated BU can also be caused by the HIV medication Reyataz (atazanavir).
  Normal values: less than 1.0 mg/dl

- **Conjugated (Direct) Bilirubin (BC):** Conjugated or direct bilirubin is the water soluble form of bilirubin. Elevated conjugated bilirubin is indicative of impaired liver function, and can signal impending liver failure. As the amount of bilirubin in the blood rises, the skin and the whites of the eyes will yellow. Also, the urine will darken and mucus membranes under the tongue will yellow. This yellowing is typically a sign of poor and failing liver function. If you notice this type of yellowing contact your HIV specialist right away.
  Normal values: less than 1.0 mg/dl

THE CHOLESTEROL PROFILE

Cholesterol is a substance produced naturally in the body having many important roles in the body, most notably hormone production, proper immune function, and cell membrane integrity. However, many of the foods we eat are sources of cholesterol as well. While cholesterol is a necessary substance in the body, too much can actually be harmful. Cholesterol does not dissolve in the blood so excess cholesterol will deposit on the walls of blood vessels, causing narrowing and eventually blockage. The narrowing or blockage deprives important tissues and organs of oxygenated blood, causing damage and eventual death of the tissue or organ. For that reason, it is important to keep cholesterol levels normal, avoiding cholesterol deposits in the vessels.

- **Cholesterol:** There are two sources of cholesterol—the cholesterol your body produces naturally and the cholesterol present in animal products that you eat (fish, meats, eggs, and poultry). In addition, certain foods that don't contain cholesterol (e.g., saturated fats) do contain fatty acids that the body uses to produce more cholesterol. Certain disease processes (diabetes) as well as genetics can cause higher than normal cholesterol levels. Because elevated cholesterol has been associated with heart disease, it is important to monitor cholesterol levels on a regular basis, especially in people living with diseases that have been associated with increased risk of heart disease, such as HIV. There are many causes of increased cholesterol levels but the two primary causes are genetic (e.g., family history), meaning your body just makes too much cholesterol, and dietary (e.g., fatty foods and red meats), meaning a person is taking in too much cholesterol or fats that the body ultimately converts to cholesterol. Regardless of the cause, too much cholesterol is detrimental to the health of the person. Limiting the intake of fatty foods and red meats is the best way to keep your cholesterol at a healthy level.
  Normal values:
    - *Desirable—less than 200 mg/dl*

- *Borderline High Risk—201 to 239 mg/dl*
- *High Risk—greater than 240 mg/dl*

• **Triglycerides:** A triglyceride blood test measures the amount of the fatty substance circulating in your bloodstream. Fats that are taken into the body as part of the diet are used as an energy source. However, if more fat is taken in than is needed by the body for energy, the excess is stored in the blood as triglycerides. Excess triglycerides are deposited along the lining of blood vessels, most notably those vessels that supply the heart muscle. If those vessels become narrowed or clogged with triglycerides, the heart muscle doesn't get enough oxygen, causing heart muscle damage. Heart muscle damage caused by a lack of oxygenated blood is commonly known as a heart attack. Having elevated levels of triglycerides increase the risk of a heart attack. Therefore, it's important to keep the amount of triglycerides in your blood within normal limits to avoid heart muscle damage. Meals high in saturated fats (e.g., red meats and fried foods) and simple sugars (e.g., candy and sweetened soft drinks) raise the triglyceride level in the blood. Alcohol also raises triglycerides; even a small amount of alcohol can increase triglycerides dramatically. Finally, some HIV medications can dramatically elevate triglyceride levels, so much so that lipid-lowering medication is required to bring triglyceride levels down. Simply put, decreasing the intake of saturated fats, simple sugars, and alcohol is the best way to keep triglycerides within normal limits.

  Normal values: 90–150 mg/dl

• **High-density lipoprotein cholesterol (HDL):** This type of cholesterol is known as the "good cholesterol." Like cholesterol, the level of HDL is primarily related to diet. Higher levels of HDL have been shown to decrease the risk of heart disease. Some studies have shown that HDL slows the build-up of cholesterol in blood vessels. Without cholesterol build-up in the vessel, plenty of blood gets to the heart muscle and the heart stays healthy and strong. The ability of HDL to slow the build-up of cholesterol and in turn help keep the heart muscle healthy is why HDL is known as the good cholesterol.

  Normal values (Based on gender and age):

Male 20–39 years old >51mg/dl	*Female 20–39 years old >63mg/dl*
40–59 years old >52mg/dl	*40–59 years old >69mg/dl*
60+ years old >60mg/dl	*60+ years old >74mg/dl*

• **Low-density lipoprotein cholesterol (LDL):** This type of cholesterol is known as the "bad cholesterol" because excessive amounts will slowly build up along the inner walls of blood vessels. In combination with other substances present, LDL forms plaque, a semi-hard substance formed by the combination of LDL and white blood cells that build up on the vessel walls and eventually causes blockages that stop blood flow to the heart muscle. Like most cholesterol, LDL level is primarily dependent on diet.

  Normal values (Based on gender and age):

Male 20–39 years old 100–117mg/dl	*Female 20–39 years old 90–108mg/dl*
40–59 years old 118–140mg/dl	*40–59 years old 109–128mg/dl*
60+ years old 122–143mg/dl	*60+ years old 126–149mg/dl*

Monitoring Your Immune System…. Monitoring Your HIV

As mentioned in an earlier chapter, one of the keys to staying healthy is regular monitoring of your immune system. The HIV standards of care recommend that a CD4 count, the measure of immune system strength, should be measured at least twice in twelve months and those two checks should be at least 90 days apart. The presence of opportunistic infections, cancers, or other illnesses and diseases can signal a weakening immune system. But wouldn't it be better to know the immune system is weak before getting sick? Recognizing a weakened immune system or active HIV replication before a person gets sick is an important step in keeping a person healthy for a longer period of time. Let's look at blood tests used by your HIV provider to monitor your illness, your immune system, and your viral activity.

CD4 CELLS (T-CELLS)

White blood cells come in many specialized types that work together to protect the body from infection and illness. T-cells (or T-lymphocytes) are one type of specialized white blood cell that plays an important role in the immune system and the immune response. There are two types of T-lymphocytes but most impacted by an HIV infection are the CD4 cell and the CD8 cell. The CD4 cell is considered the immune system's "helper" cells, initiating the body's defensive response to microorganisms such as bacteria and viruses. The other type of T-cell is called CD8 and their job is to destroy infected cells by producing antiviral and antibacterial substances. Unfortunately, HIV is able to attach to CD4 cells, allowing the virus to enter and infect the CD4 cell, damaging it in the process. The more CD4 cells infected by HIV the fewer that are available to initiate the immune response. The CD4 count is a reflection of how many functioning CD4 T-cells are circulating in the blood. Your doctor can assess the health and strength of your immune system and its ability to fight off infection by monitoring the number of healthy CD4 cells. Your doctor will monitor your CD4 count at least every six months, more often if you are sick or have recently started a new HIV medication regimen.

Normal values:

- In the HIV-negative person:
  - 500 to 1500 CD4 cells per cubic millimeter of blood
- In the HIV-infected person:
  - less than 200 cells—Requires antibiotic protection (prophylaxis) against opportunistic infections
  - greater than 200 cells—Minimum goal
  - greater than 500 cells—Long-term goal

HIV VIRAL LOAD

The HIV viral load blood test measures the number of active HIV copies in a milliliter of blood. Scientific evidence has proven that keeping the HIV viral load as low as possible for as long as possible decreases the complications of HIV disease. It makes sense. HIV attacks CD4 cells, damaging them and weakening the immune system in the process. As the immune system weakens, the body becomes more at risk for infections and sickness. By keeping the HIV viral load low, fewer CD4 cells are damaged and the immune system stays strong and able to fight infection and illness. Your doctor will monitor your HIV viral load on a regular basis—at least every six months, and more often if you are sick or have recently begun a new medication regimen. By measuring the number of active HIV copies in circulation, your doctor can assess several things:

- *The status of your HIV disease:* Is your HIV under control? Is your current HIV regimen working? Are you at risk for disease progression and opportunistic infections?
- *The predicted course of your disease:* Will your disease progress rapidly or slowly? Will you be at risk for opportunistic infections in the future? Will your disease respond to your current or future regimens?
- *The effectiveness of your HIV medication regimen:* Is this regimen working? If not, which regimens will work? Is poor adherence causing this medication regimen to fail?

What Does the Viral Load Result Mean?

As mentioned above, the HIV viral load measures the number of HIV copies in a milliliter of blood. The greater the number, the more copies of active virus are present. As the number of active virus increases, so does the damage done to CD4 cells in the immune system. In addition, as the viral load value increases so does the risk of transmitting HIV to another person during unprotected sex.

Depending on where you get your viral load drawn, the range of sensitivity can vary. Typically, the upper value remains about the same but the lower part of the scale is a bit different. While there used to be two separate tests, one for normal sensitivity and the other for ultra-sensitivity, today that is no longer the case. Most tests used in the U.S. have a lower limit sensitivity of 40 copies but there are tests being used that go as low as 20 copies. Regardless of the sensitivity, the results are usually one of the following:

- **Viral Load > 10 million copies:** This viral load is so high that there are too many copies of HIV to be counted individually. With a viral load this large the patient is sustaining major damage to the immune system. In fact, like any virus, having this much HIV circulating in your blood is most likely going to cause the patient some significant symptoms including fever, fatigue, weight loss, and night sweats. A viral load this high requires treatment with an HIV regimen as soon as possible.
- **Viral Load from 10 million to 40 copies:** This range of viral load is really saying the same thing: it's time to get started on an HIV regimen. A viral load within this range can last several months after starting HIV medication regimens, depending on the level of the viral load when the regimen was started. The rate at which viral load declines once medication is started varies from person to person. That being said, the sooner the viral load gets below 40 the better it is for the health of the immune system.
- **Viral Load < 40 copies (*"undetectable"*):** This is the ultimate goal of treatment with an HIV medication regimen: to get the viral load less than 40 copies. Again, the time it takes to reach this goal can vary from person to person, depending on the virus starting point, the strength of the medication regimen, and the adherence to the medication regimen. Getting to a value of <40 copies means the immune system is now able to grow

stronger by rebuilding its complement of CD4 cells. In addition, a viral load of <40 makes it more difficult to transmit HIV to another person during sexual encounters. In fact, an undetectable viral load has become a very important part of HIV prevention and risk reduction.

Interpreting Results

There is no way to completely eradicate HIV from the body. HIV not only circulates in the blood but also "hides" in other areas of the body including the lymph system, cerebral spinal fluid, the brain, and in the genetic code of resting and dormant CD4 cells. In the latter, this genetic material waits for a break in HIV therapy and then restarts HIV replication without the protection of HIV medication. That is why adherence to medication regimens is so important, to maintain the fewest HIV copies possible. The success or failure of a medication regimen can be determined by the following results:

- *Undetectable Viral Load:* This is a viral load less than 40 copies (<40) or less than 20 copies (<20) if the lab uses the most sensitive viral load test. Undetectable means that the number of circulating HIV copies is less than the test's sensitivity or the test's ability to measure.
- *Detectable Viral Load:* This value is reported as the number of HIV copies per milliliter of blood. The values range from greater than 40 (or 20 using the most sensitive test) to greater than 10 million copies. The higher the viral load the more damage to the immune system and its complement of CD4 cells. Also, the higher the viral load the higher risk there is of transmitting HIV to sexual partners during unprotected sexual encounters.
- *Viral Load "Blips":* On occasion, a person who has had consistently undetectable viral loads (viral loads less than 40) will have an episode when the viral load jumps to just about the level of detectability (e.g., viral load of 45 copies) and then will return to undetectable at the very next viral load check. In HIV care this scenario is often called a viral load "blip." For a patient who has been undetectable and takes his or her medications religiously, even a small "blip" above detectability can be very stressful. Viral load "blips" do not mean that a person's medication regimen is no longer effective. Experts attribute such blips to things like differing lab technique or minor infections like a cold. If such blips are isolated there is no reason for concern. If you are having frequent "blips" or you have a detectable viral load in two consecutive tests your doctor may want to look at your regimen and adherence patterns to see if resistance to your medicines has occurred.

Your doctor uses the HIV viral load results to determine the activity of your HIV infection and the effectiveness of your current HIV medication regimen. Maintaining an undetectable viral load is the goal of every medication regimen. An undetectable viral load allows your immune system to rebuild and grow stronger despite your infection. Keeping the viral load undetectable not only keeps you healthier but it protects your sexual partner(s) as well. HIV medications work very well and will maintain an undetectable viral load when they are taken as prescribed. But what happens if we can't get the viral load to an undetectable level?

HIV Genotype Test

One of the characteristics that make HIV such a formidable disease is its ability to change and mutate in response to medications. After prolonged exposure to an HIV treatment regimen, the virus has the ability to change its genetic structure (mutate) in a way that makes it resistant to the medication regimen being taken. Eventually, the regimen must be changed in order to effectively control HIV replication. But how does your doctor know which regimen will be most effective given the virus type and mutation pattern? The HIV genotype test assists the doctor in choosing a new medication regimen that will be effective.

As the name suggests, a genotype study uses genetics and the genetic make-up of HIV to predict which medications will work and which medications will have little or no effect. A sample of blood containing HIV is examined and genetic markers that cause resistance to HIV medications are identified. The presence of certain markers (mutations) translates to resistance to a certain medication or in some cases an entire class of medications. Some mutations are more damaging to a drug's effectiveness than others. Sometimes a mutation will actually make the virus weaker; however, because multiple mutations are usually present, the weaker virus is typically overrun by a strong mutated HIV strain. Mutations and resistance makes the virus harder to treat. For that reason, HIV professionals stress adherence because poor adherence leads to mutations and in turn resistance to medication. And remember, there are only so many medications and medication regimens to choose from.

HIV Phenotype Testing

As mentioned earlier, HIV can change and mutate, making it difficult to choose an effective HIV medication regimen. Another blood test that can help your doctor choose an effective therapy is an HIV phenotype. Unlike the genotype test, which identifies resistance by looking at viral mutations, phenotype testing actually exposes the virus to individual drugs, identifying which have the greatest effect on viral replication. That information makes it possible for the doctor to choose a drug regimen containing medications proven by the phenotype test to be effective against the type of virus present.

Abacavir Hypersensitivity Test (B*5701)

In the next chapter we are going to discuss HIV medications and medication regimens in more detail. One of the medications we will be discussing is abacavir (Ziagen). A member of the drug class known as nucleoside reverse transcriptase inhibitors (NRTIs), abacavir is a commonly used medication in treatment regimens and combination drugs (e.g., Triumeq). Since its FDA approval, five to eight percent of patients who take the medication experience hypersensitivity reactions to abacavir. In some cases, these reactions can be life threatening and even fatal. The risk of hypersensitivity is increased by stopping and restarting abacavir, as patients often do when they have poor adherence. So in response to that potential catastrophic occurrence the U.S. Department of Health and Human Services (DHHS) Panel on Antiretroviral Guidelines for Adults and Adolescents now recommends an abacavir hypersensitivity screening prior to starting the medication.

The abacavir hypersensitivity test, also known as a B*5701, is a blood test that examines a specific gene on a specific chromosome of the person being tested. Those patients that have experienced hypersensitivity reactions were found to have a specific *allele* or subtype of the gene in question. That type of gene is called B*5701. If that gene type is present on the chromosome of the patient, then the chances are greater that the person will have a hypersensitivity reaction to abacavir. If the B*5701 is not present on the chromosome, then the risk of a hypersensitivity reaction is very low, even a zero percent chance according to some studies.

Because of the popularity of abacavir containing regimens and combination drugs, the abacavir hypersensitivity test has become the standard of care for patients who will be started on abacavir-containing HIV medication regimens. If the test indicates that B*5701 is present, then abacavir or abacavir-containing regimens and combination drugs should not be prescribed.

INTEGRASE GENOTYPE

The class of HIV medications called the integrase inhibitors do what the name implies; they interfere with the integration of viral DNA into the genetic structure of human CD4 cells. These medications are very effective components of HIV medication regimens. However, as with all HIV medications, poor adherence, mutations, and resistance can make them ineffective. HIV specialists are now using a special kind of genotype test to identify resistance to integrase inhibitors. The Integrase Genotype is able to identify gene mutations that confer resistance to the integrase inhibitors; the regular genotype test mentioned earlier is unable to identify those mutations. In many HIV practices, if the regular genotype study is ordered the provider will order the integrase genotype as well, assuring he or she gets a complete picture of HIV mutations and resistance.

TROFILE ASSAY

HIV attaches to the CD4 cell by first attaching to the CD4 molecule. After attaching to the CD4 molecule HIV uses a second attachment point, with one of two co-receptors called the CCR5 (R5) or the CXCR4 (X4). The virus's "tropism" is classified according to the co-receptor the virus uses: R5, X4, or Dual if the virus uses both R5 and X4. The Trofile Assay identifies the HIV virus's co-receptor (tropism). But why is this important? Well, there is an HIV medication, Selzentry (maraviroc), from the class of drugs called entry inhibitors that only works on virus that has an R5 tropism. Before including Selzentry in an HIV regimen, the HIV tropism must be identified using the trofile assay. The benefit of the trofile assay is that by identifying tropism, it allows for the use of the effective entry inhibitor Selzentry. The downside of the test is the expense, over $1500 per test, and the length of time it takes for results to get to your provider—in some instances, two weeks or more. That fact and the fact that Selzentry is a twice a day medication have decreased the popularity of the medication and that has decreased the need for trofile assays as well.

Other Important Blood Tests

While not as routine as the blood tests discussed earlier in this chapter, the following blood tests are very important in assessing the health status and medical needs of people living with HIV.

Hepatitis Serologies

Like any other part of the body, the liver can acquire infections or be damaged when exposed to such things as chemicals, medications, bacteria, viruses, parasites, or alcohol. What results is an inflammation of the liver known as hepatitis. As we know from an earlier discussion, there are liver function studies that can identify inflammation and damage that has occurred to the liver. There are also blood tests that can identify specific causes of hepatitis. For instance, there are several viral types of hepatitis, each needing different approaches to treatment and cure. For this reason, it is important to identify which virus type is causing the hepatitis. In the case of hepatitis A and B, it's important to know if there is immunity from these types of hepatitis, immunity resulting from past infection or in most cases from past immunization. There are blood tests that identify immunity, past infection, chronic infection, and acute infection with the three most common types of hepatitis, hepatitis A, B, and C.

- **Hepatitis A (HAV):** This type of viral infection is primarily spread from person to person by way of contaminated food or water. It's common for these infections to originate in a restaurant whose cooks don't use good handwashing after using the bathroom and before preparing food. Two blood tests are used to identify hepatitis A, both looking for hepatitis A antibody. A positive result of either test means that the person has been exposed to hepatitis A. The two tests are:
    - *IgM hepatitis A antibody (IgM anti–HAV)*—recent or acute infection with hepatitis A
    - *Total (IgM and IgG) antibody to HAV (total anti–HAV)*—past infection or immunity from vaccination
- **Hepatitis B (HBV):** This viral infection is spread from person to person by exposure to contaminated blood by way of needle sticks, open wounds, or lacerations. There are several hepatitis B markers that can identify acute (current), chronic (ongoing), or past hepatitis B infection, some more sensitive than others. These markers seek to identify hepatitis B proteins or antibodies to hepatitis b that the body has produced after exposure to the virus. Interpretation of these results can be tricky, dependent upon medical history and the clinical setting.
    - *Hepatitis B surface antigen (HBsAg)*—acute or chronic hepatitis B infection
    - *Hepatitis B E antigen (HBeAg)*—indicates chronic or acute contagious hepatitis B infection, indicates active hepatitis B replication
    - *Hepatitis B core antibody IgM (HBcAb IgM)*—indicates acute hepatitis B infection
    - *Hepatitis B core antibody Total (HBcAb tot)*—indicates past hepatitis B infection, IgM and IgG both present.
    - *Hepatitis B surface antibody (HBsAb)*—indicates immunity after hepatitis B immunization
    - *Hepatitis B viral load (Hepatitis B DNA PCR)*—This test measures the amount of active hepatitis B virus present in a blood sample. This test is the most sensitive available for the diagnosis of hepatitis B infection.

- **Hepatitis C (HCV):** This viral infection is transmitted by exposure to contaminated blood or blood products. Exposure to HCV infected blood can occur via sexual contact, needle sticks, and sharing needles to inject drugs. HCV infection is rapidly becoming a disease of epidemic proportions. A positive HCV antibody test (HCVab) confirms the presence of antibodies to hepatitis C and therefore the diagnosis of HCV infection.
    - *Hepatitis C antibody (HCVab)*—detects antibodies to hepatitis C that are formed after being infected, used to diagnose HCV infection.
    - *Hepatitis C viral load (HCV PCR)*—The most sensitive measure of hepatitis C, this test measures the amount of active virus present in a sample of blood.

Identifying Past and Present Infections

Blood tests can be used to identify active infections or those infections that have been resolved but have left antibodies behind. When treating HIV, obviously it is important to identify current infections. However, being aware of past infections is also important for maintaining optimal health. Some infections can leave some of their genetic information behind after treatment, lying in wait in dormant white blood cells. Given the right circumstances the infection can reactivate, causing a new infection. Knowing that a person has had a type of infection in the past can give the doctor a clue that if the person is sick, reactivation of a past infection should be considered. Here are some of the most common tests used to identify past and present infections.

- **Cytomegalovirus (CMV):** At some point in their lifetime, most adults have been exposed to CMV, a member of the herpes family. In the person with a normal functioning immune system, CMV exhibits few if any symptoms. However, in a person living with HIV, their damaged immune system is not able to fight CMV, which can result in serious illness. This blood test identifies the presence of CMV antibodies, which confers past exposure and/or infection with CMV.
- **Toxoplasmosis (TOX IgG, TOX IgM):** Caused by the parasite *Toxoplasma gondii*, with which the Centers for Disease Control estimate that more than 60 million people in the U.S. have been infected. The majority of those people will have no symptoms due to the strength of their immune system. However, for those with weak immune systems (e.g., people living with HIV), symptoms of infection can occur. Toxoplasmosis is usually spread to humans by ingesting undercooked meat or coming in contact with infected cat feces while cleaning a litter box or caring for a cat with the parasite. The TOXIgM detects an acute infection while the TOXIgG detects a past infection.
- **Herpes Simplex (HSV):** There are actually two types of HSV: HSV-1, which is responsible for oral and facial herpes, and HSV-2, which is responsible for genital herpes. Differentiation between the two is very difficult but possible using antibody blood tests. HSV is transmitted by sexual contact and can cause serious illness, especially in people living with weakened immune systems, like those living with HIV. Viral cultures of existing lesions can also identify HSV. Unfortunately, once you are infected with HSV, you have the infection for life.
- **Rapid Plasma Reagin (RPR):** The RPR blood test is one of two tests for the sexually transmitted infection (STI) called syphilis. Syphilis is an infection caused by the spirochete

(spiral shape) bacterium *Treponema pallidum*. The RPR tests for syphilis by detecting what are called "Nontreponemal antibodies," antibodies the body produces to fight off syphilis. However, the RPR alone can't be used to diagnose the infection because false positive results can occur. So when an RPR detects nontreponemal antibodies (reactive result), a secondary test is done on the same blood sample, a Fluorescent Treponemal Antibody (FTA) test. The FTA tests detects treponemal antibodies, antibodies produced earlier than nontreponemal antibodies. Because the FTA is very specific for syphilis, a positive FTA confirms a syphilis infection. With every reactive RPR test there will be a ratio result as well (e.g., 1:1, 1:2, 1:4, etc.). This ratio is used to determine the amount of antibody in a sample of blood. A 1:1 ratio means that antibody is only detectable in an undiluted sample, meaning there is very little detectable antibody. The sample is then diluted from 1:1 to 1:2 to 1:4 and so on until a sample has a non-reactive result. The more antibody present in the sample the more it has to be diluted to test non-reactive. Therefore, a blood sample with a 1:1 ratio has less antibody than a sample with a 1:16 ratio. The ratio gives the doctor an idea of how much syphilis is present before treatment and is used after treatment to assess medication effectiveness. For instance, if the ratio is 1:32 before treatment and 1:1 after, the doctor knows the treatment has been effective. Keep in mind that a reactive RPR will stay reactive for a very long time after treatment, in some cases, a year or more. Syphilis is a reportable infection, meaning reactive results are automatically reported to the local health department. The health department tracks infections in order to develop safer sex education targeted to at risk populations. The health department also contacts people with reactive results to make certain they get treatment and notify their sex partner(s) that they should get tested and treated if necessary.

Blood Cultures

Anyone with a weakened immune system, including those living with HIV, are at risk for systemic infections, those infections that spread from a localized area to the entire body. Systemic infections (for instance, those infections in the bloodstream) can cause serious illness. To identify the organisms that cause these types of infections, blood is drawn and placed in special growth media. After several days, the media is examined for any organisms that have grown. The presence of organisms in the blood sample confirms the type of systemic infection. Once organisms are identified, the appropriate treatment can be initiated. The testing process used to grow and identify these infectious organisms is called a *blood culture*. Typically, blood cultures are drawn as a pair, with a blood sample taken from two different sites to guard against the results being tainted by contamination.

Urine Studies

Examining samples of urine can tell the doctor many important things about a person's health. Infections, abnormal blood sugar metabolism, problems with liver function, and the presence of sexually transmitted diseases can all be identified by taking a urine specimen. While urine tests will most likely not be done at every visit, you can usually count on your doctor wanting a sample of your urine at least a couple times each year. Let's look at four of the most common urine studies.

- *Urinalysis (U/A):* The urinalysis is a study of many components of normal, healthy urine. The urine is one way the body removes waste and unwanted substances from the body. So when the body is healthy and functioning normally, the urine will contain certain components in certain amounts. Three levels of examination are part of a urinalysis.

  - **Macroscopic:** The color and clarity of the urine are examined with the naked eye. Is the urine clear and yellow? Or is it cloudy and dark, or blood streaked? Is there any sediment? The color and clarity of the urine can identify that there is a problem somewhere in the body.

  - **Microscopic:** Examining a urine specimen under a microscope can reveal above normal levels of white blood cells, red blood cells, bacteria, or crystals. The presence of any of these among other substances can identify infections, kidney malfunction, or dietary issues.

  - **Chemical:** The chemical composition of a urine sample can test for levels of acidity, urine concentration, proteins, sugars, blood and evidence of infection.

- *Urine Culture (UC):* If the urinalysis suggests there is an infection in the urine or from the urinary tract, kidneys, or bladder, a sample of urine is cultured to see what infection causing organism is causing the problem. Once it is identified, the proper medicine can be prescribed to treat the infection. Cultures are done by taking a sample of the urine and placing it on or in a growth medium. The infectious organism is allowed to grow under controlled temperatures until the growth can be identified. Once identified the growth can be exposed to different antibiotics in the lab to see which will be most effective in treating the infection.

- *Urine Chlamydia and Gonorrhea:* Chlamydia and gonorrhea are types of sexually transmitted infections (STIs) that can be detected in a urine specimen of someone who has been infected. In parts of the U.S., gonorrhea and chlamydia are at near epidemic levels so identifying those infected and adequately treating the infections is a very important part of not only the individual's health but the public health as well. If chlamydia or gonorrhea is detected in the urine, appropriate antibiotic treatment can be prescribed and safer sex education can be provided for the patient, minimizing the spread and reoccurrence of both of these STIs. Chlamydia and gonorrhea are reportable infections, meaning that positive results are sent directly to the health department from the lab. The health department will contact the patient to make certain he or she has been treated and that their sexual partner(s) have been told they may have been exposed to an STI and should be tested and if necessary treated with antibiotics as well. Finally, the health department tracks positive results in order to develop safer sex education targeted to those populations that need it most.

STOOL STUDIES

At times people living with HIV will experience abdominal pain, diarrhea, and even blood in their feces (stool) due to a variety of causes. Most often these symptoms are caused by common issues that can be resolved with the proper treatment. Diarrhea due to viral illnesses, bad food, or medication side effects is easily addressed and is typically short-lived.

However, there are certain intestinal infections, bacterial, parasitic, and fungal, that are harder to treat and must be identified before any treatment can even begin. These infectious agents are identified by a collection of stool tests and cultures. Let's look at a few.

- *Giardia*—a parasite that lives in the intestinal tract of people and animals that causes cramping, diarrhea, and abdominal pain. The infection is diagnosed by analyzing stool specimens for the presence of giardia.
- *Clostridium difficile (C-diff)*—a bacterium that usually infects the elderly, those with weakened immune function, and especially those who have recently been on antibiotics or have been hospitalized. The infection causes severe diarrhea, abdominal pain, and weight loss. When in the intestine, *C-difficile* will produce toxins that are detected in diarrhea stool specimens.
- *Shigellosis (Shigella)*—an intestinal infection caused by a bacteria called Shigella. The main symptom is diarrhea, often bloody. The infection is diagnosed by examining a stool specimen (diarrhea) for the presence of *Shigella*.
- *Stool Culture*—there are countless infectious organisms that can cause illness in the intestinal tract. Stool specimens are sent to the lab where they are examined by trained laboratory personnel in an attempt to identify the infectious organism. Some specimens are just examined under a microscope and others are cultured on special growth plates and incubated for several days until a specific bacterium grows on the plate, thus identifying the infectious organism in the stool. One organism tested for is called Shiga-like toxin caused by the bacterium *Escherichia coli (E. coli)*, named because this type of *E. coli* bacterium produces toxins that are similar in structure to *Shigella*. *E. coli* is found in feces and is often spread as a result of poor handwashing after going to the bathroom, handling dirty diapers, or before and after preparing food. *E. coli*, depending on the type, can be harmless or can cause bloody diarrhea that in extreme circumstances can be life-threatening.

TUBERCULOSIS (TB) SKIN TEST (PPD) AND QUANTIFERON GOLD (QFTB)

There are two ways to test for active or latent tuberculosis, a skin test (PPD) and a blood test (QFTB).

- Tuberculin Skin Test (Purified Protein Derivative—PPD): While not a blood test, the TB skin test screening relies on the presence of antibodies to identify active and latent infection with tuberculosis. Just as blood tests identify the presence of antibodies from past infections, the TB skin test relies on the antibody response to identify past TB exposure and infection. The test consists of a very small amount of *mycobacterium tuberculosis* (TB), Purified Protein Derivative (PPD), being injected just under the skin. If the person has been exposed to TB in their lifetime, the TB antibodies would be present. The PPD injected under the skin is detected by existing TB antibodies, causing a localized itching, redness, and swelling that signals an antibody response to the PPD, confirming past exposure to TB. The PPD result must be read by trained medical staff so the patient must return for a second visit to the place of testing to have the test interpreted. Keep in mind that in order for an antibody response to occur, the immune system must be in working order, a requirement that makes the PPD unsuitable for those patients that are living with a weakened immune system (e.g., HIV-positive people).

- Tuberculin Blood Test (Quantiferon Gold—QFTB): The QFTB test is a blood test that exposes a sample of drawn blood to *mycobacterium tuberculosis* antigen. If the blood sample has TB antibodies present they will react with the antigen and a measureable immune response will be detected. Depending on the strength of that immune response, an active or latent TB infection will be diagnosed. The benefit of the QFTB is that it does not require a second visit from the patient to determine the result and people with weak immune systems can be tested regardless of their immune status.

Radiology Studies

In addition to the variety of blood tests utilized by the HIV specialist, there are many radiological studies ("X-rays") used to monitor and maintain your health. Typically, these X-rays are ordered in response to symptoms of illness. Some of the most common radiology tests include:

- ***Chest X-ray:*** As the name implies, a chest X-ray is a picture of the chest and the lungs using electromagnetic radiation passing through the body, being detected by a digital sensing plate, and converted into a digital image on a computer. The days of X-ray cassettes, darkrooms, and developing film are over with the advent of digital X-ray technology. This technology makes it possible to examine the lungs and other internal features without opening the body, with almost instantaneous results. With digital technology, images can be viewed at a remote location and by more than one viewer at a time. Also, patients can be given CDs with their images to take to other providers if need be. The chest X-ray is used primarily to detect fluid collections that result from a variety of lung infections, such as bacterial pneumonia or pneumocystis pneumonia (PCP). Other uses of the chest X-ray include identifying rib fractures, collapsed or poorly inflated lungs, heart size, and the presence of pulmonary disease (e.g., TB or COPD).

- ***Mammogram:*** A mammogram is a specialized X-ray that images the breast to detect masses in the breast tissue. A majority of these are done to detect breast cancer in women but men can have mammograms done as well. Many times men will feel "lumps" beneath the nipples or against the chest wall within the small amount of fatty tissue of the male breast. Men who have larger breasts, typically those men who are overweight or obese, have considerably more fatty breast tissue. In fact, some can have as much as a woman and as such can get "lumps" and cancers as women do. The female patient can actually experience some discomfort during a mammogram due to the squeezing of the breast tissue as part of the mammogram procedure. According to the American Cancer Society, women 45 to 54 years of age should get yearly mammograms and women over the age of 54 should get a mammogram every one to two years. For HIV positive women with a CD4 counter greater than 350 cells the guidelines are the same as a woman without HIV.

- *Abdominal X-ray:* As the name suggests, this is an X-ray of the abdominal cavity. While X-rays don't provide the best picture of the stomach and intestinal tract, they do identify air and fluid collections in the abdominal cavity. The presence of air or fluid is important to identify because both conditions suggest infection, abscess or perforation of the bowel. Some abdominal X-rays require patients to drink special liquids prior to taking the X-rays. These liquids don't allow X-rays to pass through them (*radio opaque*), thereby outlining the intestines and stomach, providing a more accurate exam. Most often, if an abnormality is found with an abdominal X-ray, more accurate and sensitive studies are done to confirm the results.

- *Computed Axial Tomography Scan (CT scan):* To better understand what a CT scan is, think of a fruitcake. Looking at the outside it's impossible to know the true complexity of the fruitcake. If you took a knife and cut a slice, you could see the thin outside crust as well as the goodies on the inside, different pieces of fruit, assorted nuts, and a lot of spongy cake in between. In a sense, that's exactly what a CT scan does, but instead of using a knife, the slices are done with X-rays. A CT scan creates "X-ray slices" of the body, allowing doctors to see what is happening on the inside of the body without actually cutting the body as you would a fruitcake. The resulting pictures are much more accurate, and contain much greater detail, than conventional X-rays. The increased resolution and accuracy of a CT scan allows for earlier and more accurate diagnosis. CT scans are used on almost every part of the body, but most often on the brain, the sinuses, the chest and the abdomen.

- *Magnetic Resonance Imaging (MRI):* Technically, an MRI is not a type of X-ray at all. Instead, radio waves and strong magnetic fields are used to take very detailed images of the body's internal structure. The MRI is used primarily to take high resolution images of the brain, spinal cord, abdomen and chest in order to identify infection, inflammation, fluid collections, or masses. Just as CT scans confirm the findings of general X-rays, MRIs often confirm those findings of CT scans. MRIs are able to produce much more detailed still images and moving pictures when compared to those produced by CT scans. The most advanced CT scanners can actually create 3D images of the body's internal and external structure

- *Positron Emission Tomography (PET scan):* PET scans use radioactive substances to identify abnormal tissue in the body—specifically, cancerous cells. A normal body substance, most often glucose, is "tagged" with a radioactive substance. This glucose is then injected into a vein and allowed to circulate throughout the body. After about forty-five minutes, the patient is placed in a scanner that locates areas in the body where the radioactive-tagged glucose has accumulated. Cancerous cells "take up" more of the radioactive glucose than normal tissue, causing cancerous tissue to appear brighter when compared to normal tissue. This characteristic of cancerous cells makes it possible to identify the disease by the amount of tagged glucose that has accumulated in the cancerous cells. While the PET scan is not used as often as a CT scan or an MRI, it is a very useful tool in identifying cancers such as lymphoma in HIV-infected people.

Health Maintenance Studies

There are tests and procedures that are performed on a regular basis to monitor the health of the individual and to identify early the potentially serious problems so treatment can be started as soon as possible. Performing these tests on a regular basis is an important part of an HIV-positive person's health maintenance plan. Let's take a look at three of these health maintenance studies.

- *Colonoscopy:* When people reach a certain age their risk for disease and illness increases. Since the data shows that this is true, why not work at identifying these illnesses earlier, making treatment easier and more successful. One way to identify illnesses earlier is to have a colonoscopy. This test is used to examine the lower intestine and rectum to identify polyps, masses, ulcerations, or colon cancer. To prepare for the test, laxatives are taken the night before the procedure to flush the bowel of any stool that would impede the test. After the patient is given light sedation the physician inserts a scope into the anus and advances it the entire length of the large intestine. As the scope is slowly redrawn the physician can directly examine the intestine through the scope, identifying polyps, ulcerations, masses, and areas of inflammation or bleeding. Instruments can be inserted through the scope to remove polyps or to take small samples of bowel tissue (biopsy) to examine under the microscope later. Most people do not need screening colonoscopies until the age of 50 when the risk of cancers and polyps increases significantly. People with a personal history or family history of colon diseases will need a colonoscopy more often, in some cases, every 12 months.

- *Pap Smears:* The cervix is the tip of a mother's uterus that projects into the vagina. The cervix is very susceptible to cellular changes; some of those changes can even become cancerous. In 2012 over 12,000 women were diagnosed with cancer of the cervix; in that same year more than 4,000 women lost their lives to cervical cancer. For that reason, cervical cancer screenings must be an essential part of a woman's preventative health care. Important for all women, cervical cancer screening is especially important in HIV positive women due to their increased risk of cervical cancer when compared to women without HIV. Human papillomavirus (HPV) is a sexually transmitted virus that has many different strains and types. Some HPV types are cancer causing, especially in the cervix. Because women with HIV are more at risk for human papillomavirus (HPV) their risk of cervical cancer is greater as well, necessitating regular screening for HPV and cervical cancer. The most important cervical cancer screening tool is the Pap smear or Pap test. Named for the doctor who perfected the technique, Dr. Georgios Nikolaou Papanikolaou, the Pap test is a simple but very effective test that can be performed in doctors' offices and clinics to identify abnormal cells of the cervix, cells that could progress to cancer if left unattended. To perform the test, the woman is placed on her back, legs spread slightly and bent at the knees. The doctor inserts a speculum to gently open the vagina in order to visualize the cervix. The doctor collects cells from the cervix by using a small swab or loop that removes cells from the surface of the cervix. In the lab the cells are smeared onto a microscope slide and are examined by men and women specially trained to identify cellular abnormalities that could progress to cervical cancer sometime in the future. HIV positive women should have a baseline Pap test upon entering HIV care; a follow up Pap test 6 months later; and then a test each year if the others are normal. If abnormal cells are found, the patient will need more frequent testing and may need areas of the cervix removed to rid the body of potentially cancerous cells.

• *Anal Pap Smears:* While Pap smears are an essential health maintenance tool for women with HIV, there is the male version, the anal Pap smear. As is the case in HIV-positive women, HPV poses a cancer risk in HIV-positive men as well. In women, the cancer risk is cervical cancer but in men, specifically, men who have sex with men (MSM), the risk is anal cancer. In the general population, anal cancer is a rare disease, striking about 2 people in every 100,000. That rate is considerably higher in HIV-negative MSM, about 40 cases in 100,000 people. But for HIV-positive MSM, the risk is considerable, about 80 in every 100,000 people. Anal cancer is caused by the same HPV strains that cause cervical cancer in women. So early detection is very important. One method of early detection is the anal Pap smear. Similar to a regular Pap smear, cells are collected, in this case using a Dacron swab, from the anal canal and rectum. Like the cells collected by a pap smear, the collected cells are examined under a microscope to identify cellular abnormalities that could progress to anal cancer in the future. In the event that abnormal cells are found, the patient will need high resolution testing and possible cell removal (fulguration) to reduce the chance anal cancer develops. Currently, experts feel having an anal Pap every 3 years is adequate to detect cellular changes (dysplasia) that may cause rectal cancer. It's important to keep in mind that data supporting the use of anal Paps as a standard of care is lacking so until such data supports the use of anal Paps, many practices only offer the test if one is requested by a patient.

Now that we know what tools your doctor will use to monitor your health and the health of your immune system, let's look at the medications used to treat your HIV. After all, it is the HIV medications that prevent you from getting serious opportunistic infections that can rob you of your health and eventually your life.

7

KNOW YOUR HIV MEDICATIONS

During the early years of the HIV/AIDS epidemic, people diagnosed with the disease died within a few months. Simply put, AIDS was a death sentence. In 1987 the FDA approved the first medication to treat HIV, providing new hope for everyone touched by this disease. Five years later the strongest of all HIV medications, the protease inhibitors, were developed, and death rates started to decline for the first time since the epidemic began.

It's no secret that medications have changed HIV from a death sentence to a chronic illness that people can manage and live with for a very long time. But in order for the medications to do their job, people living with HIV must understand how their medications work, how they must be taken, and the importance of adhering to prescribed regimens each and every day. This chapter discusses HIV medicines, explains the importance of adherence, provides ideas that will help you better adhere to your regimen, and discusses side effects that you may experience. But first, to understand HIV medicines, we must understand the HIV life cycle and how medications interrupt not one step in the life cycle but many. The following is a review of the HIV life cycle and how specific classes of HIV medications interrupt specific steps in that life cycle.

The HIV Life Cycle

Chapter 3 introduced the HIV life cycle in detail. Now, to better understand how each class of HIV medication works, let's review what we learned in chapter 3 with the addition of each class of HIV medication and how it interrupts the life cycle.

INTRODUCTION OF HIV INTO THE BODY

Obviously, before the HIV life cycle can begin, HIV must enter the body. As we learned earlier, exposure to infected bodily fluids during sexual contact or by sharing needles is the primary means by which HIV enters the body. While less common, HIV can also enter the body during pregnancy, childbirth or by ingesting HIV-infected breast milk. While there is no specific medication that stops the entry of HIV into the body, there is one drug that affects the ability of the virus to cause infection once it enters the body of an HIV-negative host. Truvada (emtricitabine and tenofovir) has been approved by the Food and Drug Administration (FDA) as a one pill once a day preventative medication. When used every day, it is about 90 percent effective in preventing HIV infection once the virus enters the body. But keep in mind, Truvada (emtricitabine and tenofovir) does not replace or eliminate the need for condoms.

VIRAL ATTACHMENT

Once in the body, HIV needs to attach to CD4 cells in order to replicate. At the time of this printing no medications are currently available that work on this very first step in the life cycle. There are promising medications currently in the first clinical trial stages that inhibit viral attachment. This research could lead to medications with a brand new mechanism of action, especially important for long-term survivors of HIV and those people with extensive resistance to currently available medications. It's believed that interrupting viral attachment will stop HIV replication before it even begins, thereby preserving CD4 cells and the immune system. Many feel that such a medication could be the closest researchers have come to a cure.

VIRAL FUSION

Once attached to the cell, HIV injects its own proteins into the cellular fluids (cytoplasm) of the human CD4 cell. This causes a *fusion* or joining of the human host cell membrane to the outer envelope of the HIV particle. Currently there is one class of drug that interrupts viral fusion—the *Fusion Inhibitor* also known as *Entry Inhibitors*. Fusion inhibitors prevent viral fusion and entry into the CD4 cell, thereby disrupting the HIV life cycle and preventing HIV replication.

THE UNCOATING

In order for HIV to use its genetic material (RNA) for reproduction, the protective coating surrounding the RNA strand must be dissolved. Research is starting to unwrap the mystery of uncoating and the very first steps of HIV infection. However, the process of uncoating is still in many ways a mystery, but one thing is certain—without this step, conversion of HIV RNA to DNA can't take place, and replication is halted. But until the process is understood, developing medications that target this stage are a long way off. Luckily, new technologies have made research in this area somewhat easier but still very challenging. If a way can be found, it could lead to an entirely new class of HIV medication.

REVERSE TRANSCRIPTION

Once in the cell, the single-stranded HIV RNA must be converted to double-stranded DNA. This takes place with the help of the enzyme *reverse transcriptase*. Reverse transcriptase uses proteins from the CD4 cell to help change the HIV RNA to HIV DNA. Reverse transcriptase allows genetic information to flow in the opposite direction (RNA to DNA), as opposed to the customary direction (DNA to RNA). The resulting DNA contains the viral genetic information needed for HIV replication to continue to the next step.

Two classes of HIV medications interrupt the reverse transcription stage by inhibiting reverse transcriptase.

- *Nucleoside Reverse Transcriptase Inhibitors (NRTIs)* are medications that contain faulty imitations of nucleotides found in CD4 cells. Instead of incorporating a cellular nucleotide into the growing chain of DNA, the imitation building block provided by the NRTI is inserted, preventing the double strand of DNA from becoming a fully formed and functional viral DNA.
- *Non-nucleoside Reverse Transcriptase Inhibitors (NNRTIs)* are medications that block reverse transcription by attaching to the reverse transcriptase enzyme in a way that prevents it from functioning normally.

INTEGRATION

To use the cell during replication, HIV must *integrate* or insert its newly formed DNA into the CD4 cell's nucleus. The nucleus is the brain of the cell, containing all of the RNA and DNA of that cell. Integration of viral DNA into the nucleus is accomplished with the help of a special protein called an enzyme; in this case, the enzyme is called *retroviral integrase.* Enzymes start and fuel chemical reactions. In the case of the HIV life cycle, retroviral integrase fuels the chemical reaction that inserts the viral DNA into the CD4 cell.

There is a class of drugs that inhibit retroviral integrase called *Integrase Inhibitors.* Within that class, there are three drugs that are the first to attack this part of the HIV life cycle. Because their point of attack is unique, the drugs are typically effective in patients that have resistance to other classes.

VIRAL LATENCY

Webster's Dictionary defines latency as an incubation period or a period of waiting. HIV must wait for additional proteins to be manufactured before replication can be completed. This period of waiting is known as viral latency. Latent virus, also known as provirus, can "hide" in provirus reservoirs that are difficult to reach with conventional HIV medication. The provirus waits until medication pressure eases and then awakens, beginning HIV replication outside of reservoir sites. Without eradicating all provirus as well as circulating HIV, an HIV cure can never happen. Studies are under way in an effort to better understand viral latency and how best to find and destroy latent provirus reservoirs. Some studies are investigating ways to "flush" provirus from the hard to reach reservoirs in order for current medication regimens to kill the provirus before it replicates.

FINAL ASSEMBLY

Once the viral proteins are manufactured, they must be cut into pieces and assembled into new HIV particles. This *cleavage* or cutting is accomplished with the help of another protein enzyme called *protease.* The protease enzyme cuts the proteins into smaller pieces, allowing those pieces to reassemble into new HIV particles.

There is a class of HIV medication that interrupts this stage of the HIV life cycle by inhibiting the enzyme protease. *Protease Inhibitors* bind to the protease enzyme and prevent it from separating or cleaving protein into smaller pieces. Without cleavage, HIV can't be assembled. The protease inhibitors that interfere with viral cleavage are considered the most potent of all the HIV medications.

BUDDING

Budding is the final step in the HIV life cycle. The newly formed HIV particle, complete with viral genetic material and a new outer coat made from the cell membrane of the CD4 cell, "pinches off" of the host cell and enters the body's circulation. After a period of *maturation*, a "growing up" so to speak, the newly formed HIV is ready to attach to another CD4 cell and start the process all over again. Currently, there are no FDA approved medications that disrupt HIV maturation. However, current Phase II drug trials have shown that a *Maturation Inhibitor* is closer to being a reality. A Bristol-Myers Squibb study has shown that so far maturation inhibitors seem to be potent and well tolerated. In the event their drug gains approval someday, a new drug class with a new mechanism of action will benefit all HIV-positive people, but especially those who have failed earlier regimens or have developed resistance to currently available HIV medications.

HIV Medication Drug Classes

Now that we have taken a brief look at how each drug class fits into the HIV life cycle, let's take a closer, more detailed look at each class and the drugs that comprise them.

ENTRY INHIBITORS

Entry inhibitors interfere with the fusion of HIV to the human CD4 cell it needs to replicate. There are areas on the outer surface of HIV, receptor sites (CD4, CCR5, and CXCR4), that makes it possible for HIV to fuse to the CD4 cell. The virus first attaches to the host cell (CD4 cell) using the viral CD4 attachment site. Then protein structural changes on the viral membrane allow for connection to a second site using either the CCR5 or the CXCR4 viral attachment point. *Entry Inhibitors* disrupt the attachment of HIV to the CD4 cell by interfering with viral attachment sites and structural changes necessary for attachment. Currently two entry or fusion inhibitors have been approved by the Food and Drug Administration.

- Fuzeon (enfuviritide)
- Selzentry (maraviroc)

PROTEASE INHIBITORS

During the final assembly stage of the HIV life cycle, the viral proteins must be "cut up" or cleaved into the smaller pieces that are later assembled into the new HIV particle. The enzyme protease is an essential part of this step of cleavage and reassembling. Protease inhibitors block the enzyme protease, interfering with cleavage and assembly, thereby interrupting the HIV life cycle. There are currently twelve protease inhibitors available; however, over the years the use of many of those has diminished in favor of newer medications with smaller pill burdens and fewer side effects.

- Aptivus (tipranavir)
- Crixivan (indinavir)
- Evotaz (atazanavir + cobicistat)
- Invirase (saquinavir)
- Kaletra (lopinavir + ritonavir)
- Lexiva (fosamprenavir)
- Norvir (ritonavir)
- Prezcobix (darunavir + cobicistat)
- Prezista (darunavir)
- Reyataz (atazanavir)
- Tybost (cobicistat)
- Viracept (nelfinavir)

NUCLEOSIDE REVERSE TRANSCRIPTASE INHIBITORS

A very important stage in the HIV life cycle involves the transfer of HIV genetic material into the CD4 cell. This essential step can't occur without the enzyme *reverse transcriptase*. The *Nucleoside Reverse Transcriptase Inhibitors (NRTIs)* are medications that contain faulty imitations of nucleotides (proteins) found in CD4 cells. During genetic transfer, the imitation building block provided by the NRTI is inserted into the growing DNA chain. These faulty proteins prevent the double strand of DNA from forming correctly. The resulting DNA strand is flawed, preventing effective HIV replication. Currently there are twelve NRTIs available:

- Combivir (lamivudine + zidovudine)
- Descovy (emtricitabine + tenofovir alafenamide)
- Emtriva (emtricitabine)
- Epivir (lamivudine)
- Epzicom (lamivudine + abacavir)
- Retrovir (AZT, zidovudine)
- Trizivir (lamivudine + zidovudine + abacavir)
- Truvada (emtricitabine + tenofovir disoproxil fumarate)
- Videx EC (didanosine)
- Viread (tenofovir disoproxil fumarate)
- Zerit (stavudine)
- Ziagen (abacavir)

NON-NUCLEOSIDE REVERSE TRANSCRIPTASE INHIBITORS (NNRTI)

Very similar to the NRTIs are the *Non-Nucleoside Reverse Transcriptase Inhibitors*. Like NRTIs, the NNRTIs interrupt the HIV life cycle by blocking the enzyme reverse transcriptase.

However, the mechanism by which NNRTIs block reverse transcriptase differs from NRTIs. Non-nucleoside reverse transcriptase inhibitors (NNRTIs) work by attaching to the reverse transcriptase enzyme, blocking its normal function. Without properly functioning reverse transcriptase, HIV replication is impeded. Currently there are five NNRTIs available:

- Endurant (rilpivirine)
- Intelence (etravirine)
- Rescriptor (delavirdine)
- Sustiva (efavirenz)
- Viramune (nevirapine)

INTEGRASE INHIBITORS

Integrase is an enzyme that does what the name implies; it integrates HIV genetic material into the DNA of human CD4 cells, making it possible for the infected cell to make new copies of HIV. By interfering with integrase during the HIV life cycle, the integrase inhibitors prevent HIV genetic material from integrating into the CD4 cell, thus stopping viral replication. There are currently three Integrase Inhibitors available:

- Isentress (raltegravir)
- Tivicay (dolutegravir)
- Viteka (elvitegravir)

COMBINATION MEDICATIONS

An HIV medication regimen is a cocktail of three or more medications that attack HIV at different points in the HIV life cycle. Since the advent of medications it was clear the best way to treat HIV was with a combination of many medications each interrupting a different part of the life cycle. As more medications were brought to market, these combination regimens consisted of several medications from different classes. While the concept was sound, attacking HIV at many different points in the life cycle, the regimens created very large pill burdens. Sometimes as many as 18 to 20 pills had to be taken throughout the day. Because large pill burdens make adherence very difficult, manufacturers have begun to combine several medications into a single tablet. Even medications from different manufacturers are being combined into one tablet regimens. The goal is to decrease pill burden while still offering an entire multidrug regimen in one easy to take tablet. Currently there are seven combination medications that contain an entire regimen in a single pill. They are:

- Atripla (efavirenz + emtricitabine + tenofovir disoproxil fumarate)
- Complera (rilpivirine + emtricitabine + tenofovir disoproxil fumarate)
- Genvoya (elvitegravir + cobicistat + emtricitabine + tenofovir alafenamide)
- Odefsey (emtricitabine + rilpivirine + tenofovir alafenamide)
- Stribild (elvitegravir + cobicistat + emtricitabine + tenofovir disoproxil fumarate)
- Triumeq (dolutegravir + abacavir + lamivudine)
- Trizivir (zidovudine + lamivudine + abacavir)

Decades of scientific studies have provided convincing statistics proving beyond a shadow of a doubt that HIV medications are effective. But those same studies have shown the key to an effective treatment regimen is the ability to take the medications on time each and every day. Missing even a few doses here and there can have a negative impact on the current regimen you are taking as well as future regimens. Despite advances in medications that have greatly diminished pill burden, the number of doses each day, and side effects, people still have a very difficult time adhering to the HIV medication regimens. Even those regimens that consist of one pill once a day seem to give many people a difficult time. Learning as much about your medications as possible can make medication adherence much easier. The following medication information will help the reader understand his or her medication regimen and by knowing their medications, their medication adherence will improve as well.

More About Medications: Doses/Frequency/Side Effects

Fusion Inhibitors/CCR5 Inhibitors

Fuzeon (enfuviritide)
- Form—reconstituted powder (mixed before injecting)
- Dose—90mg twice daily by subcutaneous injection
- Side Effects—most patients will experience injection site reactions after each dose (e.g., hard lumps beneath the skin)
- Special Considerations—medication must be reconstituted (mixed) before giving; each dose can be mixed separately or two doses can be mixed in the morning, with one dose injected after mixing and the second stored in a refrigerator; once reconstituted a dose must be injected within 24 hours; do not reconstitute more than one day's doses at a time; make certain to rotate injection sites.

Selzentry (maraviroc)
- Form—100mg and 300mg tablets
- Dose—300mg twice daily, with or without food; take 12 hours apart
- Side Effects—cough, fever, upper respiratory infection, rash, sore muscles, abdominal pain, dizziness, heart problems, elevated liver enzymes.
- Special Consideration—a trofile assay must be run on the patient before starting this medication; for use to treat CCR5 ("R5") trofile virus only

Integrase Inhibitors

Isentress (raltegravir)
- Form—400mg tablets
- Dose—400mg twice daily, with or without food; take 12 hours apart
- Side Effects—headache, diarrhea, rash
- Special Considerations—Call your doctor immediately if you develop a rash; severe rashes are potentially life-threatening (e.g., *Steven-Johnson Syndrome*)

Tivicay (dolutegravir)

- Form—50mg tablet
- Dose—50mg once daily, with or without food; may be prescribed twice daily if there is resistance to other integrase inhibitors
- Side Effects—diarrhea, nausea, headache, elevated liver enzymes (especially in people with liver diseases or hepatitis B or C)
- Special Consideration—do not take with antacids, iron or calcium supplements

Viteka (elvitegravir)

- Form—85mg and 150mg tablets
- Dose—85mg once daily with food (when taken with ritonavir-boosted atazanavir or Kaletra), 150mg once daily with food (when taken with ritonavir-boosted darunavir, fosamprenavir, or tipranavir)
- Side Effects—diarrhea, rash
- Special Considerations—must take 4 hours apart from antacids containing magnesium or aluminum

PROTEASE INHIBITORS

Aptivus (tipranavir)

- Form—250mg soft gel capsules
- Dose—2 capsules twice daily taken with Norvir (ritonavir) 200mg twice daily
- Side Effects—nausea, vomiting, diarrhea, rash, jaundice
- Special Considerations—should not be taken with Viagra (sildenafil) or St. John's wort

Crixivan (indinavir)

- Form—400mg capsules
- Dose—2 capsules three times daily on empty stomach; drink at least 2 liters of water each day
- Side Effects—back pain, abdominal pain, blood in urine (all signs of kidney stones)
- Special Considerations—should not be taken with Viagra (sildenafil) or St. John's wort

Evotaz (atazanavir + cobicistat)

- Form—tablet containing 300mg of Reyataz (atazanavir) and 150mg of Tybost (cobicistat)
- Dose—1 tablet once daily
- Side Effects—yellowing of the eyes and skin (scleral jaundice), itching, dark urine, nausea, abdominal pain
- Special Considerations—do not take with Norvir (ritonavir), Tybost (cobicistat), or Reyataz (atazanavir)

Invirase (saquinavir)

- Form—200mg capsules and 500mg tablets

- Dose—five 200mg capsules or two 500mg tablets twice daily with Norvir (ritonavir) 100mg twice daily; take on full stomach
- Side Effects—nausea, vomiting, diarrhea, burning in feet and/or hands
- Special Considerations—should not be taken with Viagra (sildenafil), St. John's wort, Rifabutin, or Rifampin

Kaletra (lopinavir + ritonavir)

- Form—tablets containing 200mg lopinavir and 50mg of ritonavir
- Dose—2 tablets twice daily or 4 tablets once daily with or without food
- Side Effects—fatigue, headache, nausea, vomiting, diarrhea, elevated cholesterol and triglycerides
- Special Considerations—should not be taken with Viagra (sildenafil), St. John's wort, or Norvir (ritonavir)

Lexiva (fosamprenavir)

- Form—700mg tablets
- Dose—2 tablets twice daily or 4 tablets twice daily with 200mg ritonavir twice daily; take with or without food
- Side Effects—malaise, headache, nausea, vomiting, diarrhea, loss of appetite, elevated cholesterol and triglycerides
- Special Considerations—should not be taken with Viagra (sildenafil) or St. John's wort

Norvir (ritonavir)

- Form—100mg tablets
- Dose—used in various doses as a boosting agent for other protease inhibitors; no longer used as a stand-alone medication.
- Side Effects—abdominal pain, bloating, heartburn, nausea, vomiting, diarrhea
- Special Considerations—should not be taken with Viagra (sildenafil) or St. John's wort; will affect dosing of many medications not related to HIV.

Prezcobix (darunavir + cobicistat)

- Form—tablet containing 800mg of darunavir and 150mg of cobicistat
- Dose—1 tablet once daily with food
- Side Effects—diarrhea, nausea, headache, muscle soreness, rash, and elevated cholesterol and triglycerides
- Special Considerations—should not be taken with Viagra (sildenafil), St. John's wort, birth control pills, or methadone; do not take with Prezista (darunavir) or Tybost (cobicistat)

Prezista (darunavir)

- Form—600mg and 800mg tablets
- Dose—one 800mg tablet once daily with 100mg ritonavir once daily or one 600mg tablet twice daily with 100mg ritonavir twice daily; take with food

- Side Effects—nausea, diarrhea, rash, common cold symptoms
- Special Considerations—should not take with Viagra (sildenafil), St. John's wort, birth control pills, methadone

Reyataz (atazanavir)
- Form—200mg and 300mg capsules
- Dose—one 300mg capsule with 100mg ritonavir once daily or two 200mg capsules once daily for those who can't tolerate ritonavir.
- Side Effects—yellowing of the eyes and skin (jaundice), nausea, vomiting, diarrhea, rash, abnormal heart rhythm
- Special Considerations—should not be taken with Viagra (sildenafil), St. John's wort; avoid antacids, Prilosec, Pepcid, and Nexium; if antacids are necessary separate from the Reyataz (atazanavir) by 12 hours.

Tybost (cobicistat)
- Form—150mg tablets
- Dose—one 150mg tablet once daily taken as a booster with other protease inhibitors
- Side Effects—typically the side effects of the medication it is boosting
- Special Considerations—can alter the blood levels of birth control pills, Viagra (sildenafil), and medications to manage pulmonary hypertension; do not take with St. John's wort

Viracept (nelfinavir)
- Form—250mg and 625mg tablets
- Dose—two 625mg tablets twice daily or five 250mg tablets twice daily; take with light snacks
- Side Effects—the majority of those taking this drug will have diarrhea
- Special Considerations—should not be taken with Viagra (sildenafil) and St. John's wort

NON-NUCLEOSIDE REVERSE TRANSCRIPTASE INHIBITORS (NNRTI)

Endurant (rilpivirine)
- Forms—25mg tablets
- Dose—one 25mg tablet once daily with food
- Side Effects—depression, high blood pressure, "ill feeling," rash, headache, problems sleeping; side effects typically fade after a couple weeks on the medication
- Special Considerations—do not take with Viagra (sildenafil), St. John's wort; avoid protease inhibitors, methadone, and antacids

Intelence (etravirine)
- Forms—100mg tablets and 200mg tablets
- Dose—one 200mg tablet twice daily or two 100mg tablets twice daily; take medication after a meal

- Side Effects—headache, high blood pressure, "ill feeling," nausea, and rash
- Special Considerations—Severe, potentially life-threatening skin reactions can occur (e.g., *Stevens-Johnson's Syndrome)*; call your doctor immediately if a rash develops. Avoid St. John's wort and protease inhibitors

Rescriptor (delavirdine)
- Forms—100mg tablets and 200mg tablets
- Dose—four 100mg tablets three times daily or two 200mg tablets three times daily; take with or without food
- Side Effects—nausea, vomiting, diarrhea, rash, and elevated liver enzymes
- Special Considerations—take one hour apart from antacids; some dose adjustment may be necessary with protease inhibitors

Sustiva (efavirenz)
- Forms—200mg capsules and 600mg tablet
- Dose—one 600mg tablet at bedtime or three 200mg capsules at bedtime; take on empty stomach
- Side Effects—vivid life-like dreams, rash, drowsiness, change in mood, dizziness, worsening of depression, anxiety
- Special Considerations—contact your doctor if you develop a rash; it's not uncommon to continue treatment until the rash clears; high fat meals will increase side effects; dose adjustment needed when taken with Crixivan (indinavir) and Kaletra (lopinavir + ritonavir); can't be used in pregnancy; pregnancy test should be done before starting.

Viramune (nevirapine)
- Forms—200mg tablets
- Dose—one 200mg tablet twice daily or two 200mg tablets once daily; take with or without food
- Side Effects—rash, headache, nausea, vomiting, diarrhea, fatigue, weakness; to minimize side effects start by taking 1 tablet daily for 7 days then increase to 1 tablet twice daily or 2 tablets daily.
- Special Considerations—call your doctor immediately if jaundice or right upper quadrant abdominal pain develops; will affect birth control pills so two types of birth control should be used when taking Viramune (nevirapine).

NUCLEOSIDE REVERSE TRANSCRIPTASE INHIBITORS (NRTI)

Combivir (lamivudine + zidovudine)
- Forms—tablets containing 300mg of AZT (zidovudine) and 150mg of Epivir (lamivudine)
- Dose—1 tablet twice daily with or without food
- Side Effects—headache, fatigue, anemia (low red blood cell count)
- Special Considerations—call your doctor if you develop worsening fatigue, shortness of breath, pale skin, weakness, or feeling "winded" after climbing stairs (all signs of *anemia);*

will need frequent blood counts while on this drug. Never take with the individual medications AZT (zidovudine) or Epivir (lamivudine)

Descovy (emtricitabine + tenofovir alafenamide)
- Forms—tablets containing 200mg of emtricitabine and 25mg of tenofovir alafenamide
- Dose—1 tablet daily with or without food
- Side Effects—headaches, fatigue, general "ill feeling," elevated lactic acid levels which could lead to lactic acidosis.
- Special Considerations—call your doctor immediately if you have "sick" feeling, muscle pain, fatigue, flu-like symptoms (symptoms of *lactic acidosis*); do not take with individual drugs Emtriva (emtricitabine) or Viread (tenofovir); tenofovir has been associated with kidney dysfunction so frequent blood tests to measure kidney function must be done when taking this medication

Emtriva (emtricitabine)
- Forms—200mg capsules
- Dose—1 capsule daily with or without food
- Side Effects—headache, nausea, vomiting, rash, "sick" feeling, muscle pain, weakness, fatigue
- Special Considerations—call your doctor if you develop muscle pain, weakness, fatigue, or a "sick" feeling (signs of *lactic acidosis*); never take with a regimen containing Truvada (tenofovir + emtricitabine)

Epivir (lamivudine)
- Forms—150mg and 300mg tablets; 5mg/ml liquid formulation (for renal dosing)
- Dose—one 150mg tablet twice daily or one 300mg tablet once daily; 10ml (50mg) liquid formulation once daily for renal dosing; take with or without food
- Side Effects—headache, nausea, vomiting
- Special Considerations—dose adjustment needed for patients with renal (kidney) disease or renal failure.

Epzicom (lamivudine + abacavir)
- Tablets containing 300mg Epivir (lamivudine) and 600mg of Ziagen (abacavir)
- Dose—1 tablet once daily with or without food
- Side Effects—"sick" feeling, flu-like symptoms, nausea, vomiting, rash, fatigue, headache, abdominal pain, dizziness
- Special Considerations—call your doctor immediately if you develop "sick" feeling, flu-like symptoms, or muscle pain (*hypersensitivity reaction*); must test negative for abacavir hypersensitivity blood test before starting; never take with Epivir (lamivudine) or Ziagen (abacavir)

Retrovir (zidovudine, AZT)
- Forms—100mg capsules and 300mg tablets
- Dose—three 100mg capsules or one 300mg tablet twice daily, take with or without food

- Side Effects—headache, fatigue, low blood counts (anemia), pale skin, weakness, shortness of breath, feeling "winded" after climbing stairs
- Special Considerations—call your doctor immediately if you develop shortness of breath, pale skin, fatigue, or feeling "winded" after climbing steps (all signs of *anemia*); will require frequent blood counts while taking this medication.

Trizivir (zidovudine + abacavir + lamivudine)

- Form—tablets containing 150mg of Epivir (lamivudine), 300mg of Retrovir (zidovudine), and 300mg of Ziagen (abacavir)
- Dose—1 tablet twice daily with or without food
- Side Effects—"sick" feeling, flu-like symptoms, nausea, vomiting, rash, headache, abdominal pain, dizziness, low blood count (anemia)
- Special Considerations—call your doctor immediately if you develop "sick" feeling, flu-like symptoms, or muscle pain (*hypersensitivity reaction*); call your doctor if you develop shortness of breath, fatigue, pale skin, or feeling "winded" after climbing steps (*anemia*); must test negative for abacavir hypersensitivity test before starting

Truvada (tenofovir disoproxil fumarate + emtricitabine)

- Form—tablets containing 200mg of Emtriva (emtricitabine) and 300mg of Viread (tenofovir)
- Dose—1 tablet daily with food
- Side Effects—headache, increased blood pressure, "sick" feeling, loss of appetite, rash, increased liver enzymes
- Special Considerations—call your doctor immediately if you have "sick" feeling, muscle pain, fatigue, flu-like symptoms (symptoms of *lactic acidosis*); do not take with individual drugs Emtriva (emtricitabine) or Viread (tenofovir); tenofovir has been associated with kidney dysfunction so frequent blood tests to measure kidney function must be done when taking this medication

Videx EC (didanosine)

- Form—200mg, 250mg and 400mg capsules
- Dose—one 400mg capsule once daily is typical dose but dose is sometimes adjusted based on patient weight; take on an empty stomach one hour before or two hours after a meal.
- Side Effects—abdominal pain, nausea, vomiting, burning in the hands and feet, altered taste
- Special Considerations—call your doctor if you develop abdominal pain, nausea, vomiting (signs of *pancreatitis*); call your doctor if you develop "sick" feeling, fatigue, muscle pain, flu-like symptoms, fever (signs of *lactic acidosis*)

Viread (tenofovir disoproxil fumarate)

- Form—300mg tablets
- Dose—1 tablet once daily; must take with food; take one hour before or two hours after Videx EC (didanosine)

- Side Effects—nausea, vomiting, diarrhea, elevated liver enzymes, changes in fat distribution (*lipodystrophy*); kidney dysfunction
- Special Considerations—dose adjustment and boosting of Reyataz (atazanavir) necessary if taken in the same regimen; dose adjustment of Videx EC (didanosine) when take in regimen with Viread (tenofovir); frequent blood tests to assess kidney function must be done while taking this medication.

Zerit (stavudine)

- Form—15mg, 20mg, 30mg, and 40mg capsules
- Dose—one 40mg capsule or two 20mg capsules twice daily if body weight greater than 60kg (132 lbs); one 30mg capsule or two 15mg capsules twice daily if body weight less than 60kg (132lbs)
- Side Effects—numbness, tingling, or burning in feet and hands; "sick" feeling, muscle pain, fatigue, flu-like symptoms (symptoms of *lactic acidosis*)
- Special Considerations—call your doctor if you develop "sick" feeling, flu-like symptoms, muscle pain, fatigue, fever (signs of *lactic acidosis*)

Ziagen (abacavir)

- Forms—300mg tablets
- Dose—one 300mg tablets twice daily or two 300mg tablets once daily; take with or without food
- Side Effects—"sick" feeling, flu-like symptoms, nausea, vomiting, rash, fatigue, headache, abdominal pain, dizziness
- Special Considerations—call your doctor immediately if you develop "sick" feeling, flu-like symptoms, muscle pain, fever, fatigue (signs of hypersensitivity)

COMBINATION MEDICATIONS/
ENTIRE MEDICATION REGIMENS IN ONE PILL

Atripla (efavirenz + emtricitabine + tenofovir disoproxil fumarate)

- Form—tablet comprised of 600mg of Sustiva (efavirenz), 300mg of Viread (tenofovir), and 200mg of Emtriva (emtricitabine)
- Dose—1 tablet at bedtime on an empty stomach (may be taken during the day if the medication is disrupting sleep)
- Side Effects—vivid, life-like dreams, rash, anxiety, drowsiness, dizziness, depression, fatigue, sleeping problems
- Special Considerations—a small percentage of patients will have insomnia and anxiety and should take the medication during the day instead of bedtime; frequent blood tests measuring kidney function must be done due to known kidney dysfunction with tenofovir disoproxil fumarate); can't be used if you are pregnant or thinking of becoming pregnant

Complera (rilpivirine + emtricitabine + tenofovir disoproxil fumarate)

- Form—tablet comprised of 25mg of Endurant (rilpivirine), 300mg of Viread (tenofovir), and 200mg of Emtriva (emtricitabine)
- Dose—1 tablet once daily with food
- Side Effects—depression, headache, fatigue, nausea, vomiting, anxiety, rash, dizziness, insomnia, loss of appetite
- Special Considerations—frequent blood tests measuring kidney function must be done due to known kidney dysfunction with tenofovir disoproxil fumarate; central nervous system side effects similar to those of Atripla are possible but less frequent and severe.

Genvoya (elvitegravir + cobicistat + emtricitabine + tenofovir alafenamide)

- Form—tablet comprised of 150mg of elvitegravir, 150mg of cobicistat, 200mg of emtricitabine, and 10mg of tenofovir alafenamide
- Dose—1 tablet once daily with food
- Side Effects—the most common side effect is nausea; can cause liver dysfunction in some people; may cause worsening of hepatitis B infection
- Special Considerations—call your doctor if you develop weakness, muscle pain, fatigue, nausea, or vomiting (signs of *lactic acidosis*); be alert for right upper quadrant abdominal pain, yellowing of the skin, or yellowing of the eyes (all signs of liver dysfunction)

Odefsey (rilpivirine + emtricitabine + tenofovir alafenamide)

- Form—tablet comprised of 25mg of rilpivirine, 200mg emtricitabine, and 25mg of tenofovir alafenamide.
- Dose—1 tablet once daily with a meal.
- Side Effects—nausea, headache, and a generalized "ill feeling" that fades after a few doses.
- Special Considerations—central nervous system side effects similar to those of Atripla are possible but less frequent and severe.

Stribild (elvitegravir + cobicistat + emtricitabine + tenofovir disoproxil fumarate)

- Form—tablet comprised of 150mg of Viteka (elvitegravir), 150mg of Tybost (cobicistat), 200mg of Emtriva (emtricitabine), and 300mg of Viread (tenofovir)
- Dose—1 tablet once daily with food
- Side Effects—typically tolerated very well; kidney dysfunction due to tenofovir disoproxil fumarate
- Special Considerations—blood tests to monitor kidney and liver function must be done while on this medication; must take two hours apart from antacids

Triumeq (dolutegravir + abacavir + lamivudine)

- Form—tablet comprised of 50mg of Tivicay (dolutegravir), 600mg of Ziagen (abacavir), and 300mg of Epivir (lamivudine)
- Dose—1 tablet once daily with or without food
- Side Effects—typically tolerated very well but can cause symptoms of hypersensitivity that include "sick" feeling, flu-like symptoms, fatigue, fever, muscle pain and weakness.

- Special Considerations—must have a negative abacavir hypersensitivity blood test prior to starting the medication; call your doctor if you develop "sick" feeling, flu-like symptoms, muscle pain and weakness, fatigue, or fever (signs of *abacavir hypersensitivity*)

Trizivir (zidovudine + abacavir + lamivudine)

- Form—tablets comprised of 150mg of Epivir (lamivudine), 300mg of Retrovir (zidovudine), and 300mg of Ziagen (abacavir)
- Dose—1 tablet twice daily with or without food
- Side Effects—"sick" feeling, flu-like symptoms, nausea, vomiting, rash, headache, abdominal pain, dizziness, low blood count (anemia)
- Special Considerations—call your doctor immediately if you develop "sick" feeling, flu-like symptoms, or muscle pain (hypersensitivity reaction); call your doctor if you develop shortness of breath, fatigue, pale skin, or feeling "winded" after climbing steps (anemia); must test negative for abacavir hypersensitivity before starting this medication.

The Importance of Medication Adherence

The results of countless clinical trials and years of taking medication proves beyond a shadow of a doubt that HIV medications have made an HIV infection a chronic disease much like asthma, diabetes or high blood pressure. Before the advent of medications, people were diagnosed only after symptoms of the most life-threatening opportunistic infections emerged (e.g., pneumocystis pneumonia). Without treatment options, infected people died soon after their diagnosis, within months in most cases. Fortunately, that's not the case today. HIV testing and effective medications have forever changed the futures of those diagnosed. People are diagnosed sooner in the course of the illness, often very soon after the initial infection. Treatment options have made it possible to go on living after diagnosis. In fact, the advent of HIV medications has now made the life expectancy of people living with HIV about the same as those without the disease. We have come a very long way.

But just taking HIV medications is not enough. The effectiveness of an HIV drug regimen depends a great deal on how religiously they are taken. In other words, the medications will do their job of controlling the virus only if they are taken every day exactly as prescribed. HIV experts called such commitment and diligence to an HIV regimen, *medication adherence.* Poor adherence is the number one reason medication regimens fail. But why is medication adherence such an integral part of a successful regimen? To answer that question let's look at two of the most important concepts in HIV care: *viral mutation and viral resistance.*

Viral Mutation

As discussed in an earlier chapter, HIV makes copies of itself (replicates) by using its own genetic material as well as the genetic material of its human host. In a perfect system, each HIV copy would be exactly like the last, from the coating on the outside of the virus copy to the genetic material within that copy. And because each viral copy would be exactly the same, medications would work exactly the same way on every viral copy. But in life, there is rarely a perfect system and HIV is no exception. While it's true that the majority of HIV copies are exactly like the one before, when exposed to HIV medications an occasional genetic mistake occurs. A small error is made during HIV replication, and that small error is then copied over and over, from new copy to new copy. Soon there are thousands of viral copies, each with the same small mistake. The issue is that viral mistakes often render an HIV medication or medications less effective, processes known as viral mutation and medication resistance. Let's look at a more practical example.

Imagine you have a document that needs to be copied for a big meeting. Using the office copy machine, you begin making copies of the original document. After twenty identical copies, you use one of the copies as the original. However, you place it on the machine a bit off center. Now all new copies will be a bit off center. Then you take an off center copy and use it as the original. Regardless of how straight you place it on the copier, all the new copies will be off center. The same thing happens during viral replication. One small error in genetic structure is passed on to every new copy. Soon you have thousands of viral copies, all with the same small error in genetic structure.

How Do Mutations Occur?

We know what mutations are, but how do they occur in the first place? How does a normal, functioning virus mutate by itself? The answer is that it doesn't happen by itself. In our copy machine example, the original was placed incorrectly on the copier, resulting in off-center copies. The original was acted upon by an outside force; in the case of our example it was acted upon by the person making the copies. By placing the original off-center that person was the outside force that created the error.

Many outside influences can stimulate viral mutation in HIV. The most important of those influences, ironically enough, is exposure to HIV medications. The same medications that prolong and improve the lives of HIV-infected people cause mutations that will eventually complicate HIV treatment. How can that happen? As HIV replicates in the absence of medication, small genetic errors occur naturally. Some of those small errors actually make the virus strong enough to resist medications. When the HIV medication regimen is added, it's most effective against non-mutated ("wild-type") HIV. As the amount of wild-type virus decreases due to the medication regimen, the virus that has mutated continues to replicate and grow in number. Over time as the mutated virus continues to replicate, it becomes the dominant type of virus in the body. Eventually, so much resistant virus is present that the medications become completely ineffective and a new medication regimen is necessary to treat the HIV infection effectively.

Logic tells us that if HIV medications interfere with HIV replication then the risk of viral mutation is very small. In the presence of an effective therapy, very little viral replication is occurring and therefore there is a lesser chance of mutations. By taking HIV medications every day, viral replication is so small that there is not enough mutated virus being copied to change the dominant virus in the body. For this reason, the medication regimen will continue to be effective.

However, if there are missed medication doses, the virus has a chance to replicate, increasing the number of mutated virus being produced. The more mutated virus present the less effective medications become. Eventually, mutations will render a once effective regimen ineffective. This being the case one can conclude that the key to an effective, long-lasting HIV medication regimen is taking the medications as prescribed each and every day. The key is *medication adherence.*

What Is Medication Adherence?

Steadman's Medical Dictionary defines adherence as *"the extent to which the patient continues the agreed-upon mode of treatment under limited supervision when faced with conflicting demands."* Simply put, adherence refers to the patient's willingness to take his or her medicines as prescribed each and every day, despite the daily demands of living with HIV. In an effort to place a number on adherence, experts believe that medication adherence means a person is taking greater than 95 percent of his or her scheduled doses. In other words, adherence equates to a person taking 28 to 30 daily doses each month. That sounds easy until you realize we all experience the pressures and demands of everyday life. Anyone who has ever had to take prescription medications long-term understands the fatigue and apathy that sets in at times, making it a chore just to open your medication bottle. But a person committed to medication adherence will push through the apathy and take their medications, knowing that is the only way they will be effective. If a patient is able to adhere, then the medications will do their job and the patient will live a long and healthy life.

So How Do Mutations Affect the HIV Patient?

So we know what mutations are, and we know how they occur. We also know how medication adherence affects the development of mutations. But how does all this impact the HIV-infected person? Remember, mutations are changes in the genetic structure of the HIV. HIV medications are designed with a certain HIV genetic structure in mind. Consequently, medications are effective against HIV copies that have typical genetic structures—in other words, virus that is free of significant mutations. By altering the genetic structure, medications become less effective, resulting in more mutated viral copies being made. As more and more mutated viral copies are made, the mutated virus becomes the dominant type of virus and therefore the medicines become less and less effective. Eventually the medication regimen becomes unable to slow replication at all. If this happens, a new HIV medication regimen will be needed to control the virus. Sometimes, only one medication in the regimen becomes ineffective but in some cases the mutation eliminates an entire class of HIV medications. Obviously, if that happens the patient's virus will be even harder to treat. The process of a virus mutating to make a medication or medications ineffective is a concept known as *medication resistance.*

Viral Resistance

Resistance is just that—HIV's ability to resist or be resistant to the beneficial effects of one or several HIV medications. Poor medication adherence leads to *viral resistance.* Once the virus is resistant, HIV is able to replicate freely, even in the presence of medications that at one time were effective.

Resistance to individual medications is just the tip of the iceberg. When resistance to an individual medication occurs, that resistance will often translate to an entire class of HIV medications. For instance, if resistance develops to a specific NNRTI, it's possible that resistance will translate to all of the NNRTIs, even the NNRTIs that the person has never taken. This severely limits choices for future regimens, making treatment much more difficult. Resistance to one medication can and will have far-reaching effects.

Why Do People Have Poor Adherence?

As our discussion of viral mutation and resistance has illustrated, improving medication adherence improves therapy effectiveness as well. HIV medical professionals and educators constantly reinforce the importance of adherence during clinic visits, through patient education programs, and by providing adherence tools to their patients. So why do people still have difficulty adhering to the very medications that improve and extend their lives? Even today, when a majority of patients can be treated with one pill once a day or a couple pills twice daily, adherence continues to be the number one issue among HIV positive people.

Common sense tells us that with such overwhelming evidence that adherence is important and results in effective treatment, people would gladly take their medicines exactly as prescribed. Yet reality proves otherwise. The fact is that adherence to HIV medications is not an easy proposition, despite their benefits and a person's commitment to taking medications. There are several factors that interfere with drug adherence. Let's take a look at the most common.

- *State of Mind:* It became obvious soon after the epidemic emerged that HIV affects far more than just the physical self. In fact, the emotional self is affected as much as, or in many cases, more than the physical self. Physically, people with HIV are healthier than ever. However, the same emotional difficulties that plagued HIV-positive people 20 years ago are still making life difficult today. Feelings of guilt, anger, depression, and isolation are just some of the emotional issues HIV-infected people deal with on a day to day basis. These emotional issues make medication adherence extremely difficult, more so if there are other issues the patient is trying to address (e.g., medication side effects). In fact, a few HIV medications can actually exacerbate symptoms of depression, anxiety, and insomnia. Therefore, before a person can adhere to medications, his or her emotional issues surrounding their diagnosis must be addressed and the provider needs to judge if the person is ready to commit to a daily medication regimen.
- *Medication Side Effects:* Medication side effects are not unique to HIV drugs. Most prescription medications have some type of side effect, some more severe and unpleasant than others. When HIV medications first emerged, they were notorious for their severe side effects. As the years passed, HIV drug manufacturers improved their medicines, diminishing side effects and creating new formulations of existing medications that have made them more palatable and easier to take. Today, many of the newest regimens consist of a number of medications wrapped into one pill. This has gone a long way in diminishing

side effects. Gone are the days when people report feeling worse on medications than they do off medications. The newest medications are relatively side effect free and any side effects that are present typically fade away after being on the medication for a week or so. Yet the stories of horrible side effects wreaking havoc with a person's mind and body still make their way into HIV chat rooms, support groups, and clinic waiting rooms. The reality is that severe side effects rarely occur anymore. Instead, the key to adherence these days is dispelling the myths about side effects and understanding the importance of adherence.

- *Cost of Medications:* It's no secret that HIV medications are very expensive and are getting more expensive with each new medication that hits the market. For those people without insurance or drug coverage, adhering to medication regimens is severely complicated by their cost. Even people with insurance may have difficulty paying the deductibles required by their insurer, in some cases, $100 or more each month. If a person can't afford deductibles or the price of medications, adherence is impossible. But there are resources and programs to help. The Affordable Care Act, state sponsored drug assistance programs, and manufacturer sponsored patient assistance programs are helping to defer some of the cost, helping people to better adhere to their medication regimen by deferring some of the copays.

- *Complexity of Regimens:* Thankfully, the complexity of regimens has gotten better and better with each passing year. Fifteen to twenty years ago it was not uncommon for people to take upwards of twenty-five pills each day. Some of those had to be taken with food, others without food. Different medications had to be separated from one another and others had to be taken together. Drug manufacturers have done a very good job decreasing the complexity of HIV medication regimens. In many cases, an entire medication regimen consists of one pill once a day, without or without food. The most complex regimens today are those that are taken twice a day but as new medications hit the market, a twice a day regimen is becoming less and less common. Recognizing that simple is better, providers are now changing to simplified HIV regimens in order to improve medication adherence.

- *Patient Limitations:* People living with HIV may have characteristics and traits that can make adherence difficult. Busy lifestyles, work schedules, and school schedules can complicate medication adherence. HIV positive mothers will often neglect their own health to care for their children. Social obstacles, such as the inability to read, a poor understanding of the English language, or being homeless, also contribute to poor adherence. Perhaps the best predictor of adherence is a person's desire, willingness, or commitment to take HIV medications. Without a true commitment to medications, adherence is literally impossible. It is important that the provider make the patient aware of the commitment necessary to have a successful HIV regimen. The patient must understand that the medication must be taken each and every day as prescribed to maintain adherence and as a result maintain an effective medication regimen.

- *Alcohol and Substance Use:* A 2006 study showed that about 52 percent of people who had alcohol or substance abuse issues were adherent (greater than 95 percent of doses were taken) compared to greater than 70 percent of those who did not have such issues. When people have addiction issues with alcohol or drugs, their focus is typically when and where they will get their next dose of drug or their next drink. Taking an HIV medication regimen requires commitment and focus, something that is very difficult to achieve when the person is consumed with finding their next dose or shot of liquor. The provider must identify alcohol or drug addiction issues and get them under some control before expecting medication adherence over the long term.

Tips to Improve Adherence

We have established the importance of medication adherence. But what can be done to improve the ability of HIV infected people to take their medications as prescribed? There are a number of ways to improve HIV medication adherence. Not all of them will work for everyone. The key is to find what works for you.

- *Combat the Hectic Schedule:* One common obstacle to medication adherence is a busy schedule that interferes with medication adherence. There are ways to improve adherence even for those people with hectic schedules.

  - Set up medications ahead of time using pillboxes. These important tools of adherence are usually available free of charge from your doctor's office. They can also be purchased at most retail pharmacies and on the Internet. Set up pillboxes a week ahead in advance, saving time and assuring that each day you have the proper pills in the proper doses ready to take with the least amount of effort. Pick a day and make that the day you set up your pillbox each week.

  - Pill boxes are comprised of seven individual day compartments that can be removed and carried in a pocket, lunch box, or brief case. This saves time and improves adherence by keeping your pills close at hand wherever you go.

  - Many pharmacies now offer a service called "Pill Packs." The pharmacy will take all your prescription medication, including your HIV medications, and package them together in cellophane packets, one packet for each dose of medication. The names of the medications contained in the packet along with the date and time the contents of the packet should be taken are printed on the packets. The patient takes the appropriate packet, tears it open, and takes all the pills in the packet. If the packet is gone the patient knows he or she has taken the necessary pills. Pill packs are perfect for patients that have trouble with names and doses of medication.

  - People often get busy or lose track of time, causing them to miss a dose or doses of their medication. Wearing a watch with an alarm or using the timer on your smart phone is a good way to be alerted that it's time for your medication. There are telephone applications that can assist patients with the timing of their medications, even if there are multiple medications that have to be taken several times each day. Even if your regimen is one pill once a day, it has to be taken at the right time each day so any method that reminds you to take your medication is good as long as it works for you.

- *Confidentiality:* Many fear that taking medications while at work or school will "tip off" their friends or coworkers to their HIV diagnosis. People choose to miss doses rather than risk jeopardizing their confidentiality by taking medications in a place where others may see them. To maintain confidentiality while taking all your doses, carry medications in a small pillbox. When it's time for your medication, excuse yourself to the restroom or step outside for a break. This allows you to take your medicine each and every day while maintaining your confidentiality. If you are seen taking medicines, remember you are not obligated to share your medical information with anyone; your confidentiality is protected by law.

- *We Are All Forgetful:* Being human, we all forget things—including when to take our medicine. People who are dealing with opportunistic infections may have poor short-term and long-term memory. Leave notes around your home, in places where you will be sure to see them—the refrigerator, the television or the bathroom medicine cabinet or mirror. Leave your pill bottles or pillboxes in places you will be sure to find them—the kitchen sink, next to your toothbrush, or with your car keys. If you have a friend or loved one who is aware of your diagnosis, ask them to help you remember by calling you when it is time for your pills. Finally, in many communities there are "buddy programs" that bring together people who are HIV-infected to remind each other and to offer support for one another when adherence is a problem.

- *When to Take the Forgotten Dose*: Even with your best effort, chances are you will forget a dose at times. When you forget a once a day dose, how do you know if you should take the dose late? The rule is if you remember your daily dose within 12 hours of the normal dose time, go ahead and take it late. If you remember more than 12 hours later, just wait for your next regular dose. Never double up if you forget a dose. That will only increase your chance of side effects.

- *Not Sure Where the Problem Lies:* For some people it's hard to identify problems with adherence until the medication regimen has been started. In fact, it's hard to predict exactly who will have adherence problems and who won't. There are ways, however, to identify adherence issues before starting your medicines. Take a trial run of your regimen using jelly beans, a different color for each type of medicine. Take the jelly beans as you would your medicines. Fine tune your medication schedule until you find one that results in the best adherence and fewest missed or forgotten doses. If jellybean doses are missed, make a note of the reason and remedy it before starting your medications for real. Identifying problems before starting your medications will improve your chances of adherence without the risk of mutation and resistance.

The Problem of Medication Side Effects

The biggest obstacles to medication adherence are the side effects inherent to each HIV medication. Luckily, the newest HIV medications have excellent side effect profiles, meaning most have very few and those that do often fade after just a week or two. While some HIV medications have side effects that resolve over time, others have untoward effects that last as long as the person is taking the drugs. Others cause long-term health conditions (e.g., heart disease) that we are just now discovering. Let's look at the most common side effects and what can be done to resolve the issues.

Nausea/Vomiting

Probably the most common of all side effects is nausea. Nausea is a common side effect in most any prescription medications, HIV included. While most nausea occurs when the therapy is first started, typically it will fade and resolve after a couple of weeks. Nausea can also occur when certain medications are taken on an empty stomach. That being said, there are ways to combat nausea if it does not resolve on its own.

- Change your diet, first to clear liquids, then add bland foods as you can tolerate. A BRAT diet is one that is comprised of **B**ananas, **R**ice, **A**pplesauce and **T**oast—easy to digest foods that give the stomach time to recover. Introduce each of these four foods one at a time, giving the intestinal tract and stomach time to "rest," which helps the body resolve the nausea. As the nausea decreases, add more complex foods as tolerated.

- Keep dry crackers at your bedside. Each morning before getting out of bed, eat a few crackers and lie still for a few minutes. This method is widely used by pregnant women to relieve the nausea of morning sickness.

- Drink cool, carbonated liquids such as ginger ale or clear soda pops. Pharmacies sometimes stock Coca-Cola syrup (Coke syrup without the carbonated water) that can be taken in small amounts to ease nausea. The Coke syrup is usually stocked behind the pharmacy counter, so ask your pharmacist.

- If the nausea is not relieved by the simple remedies above, your doctor can prescribe medications that will help. There are downsides to this solution, however. A prescription to combat nausea means at least one more pill to take each day. There is also a chance of unpleasant side effects from the anti-nausea medication, such as anxiety and restlessness.

- Many times, resolving nausea associated with HIV medications is just a matter of taking them correctly. If a medication is supposed to be taken on an empty stomach, do so; if it was supposed to be taken with food, eat before taking your dose. Just make note of your regimen and what medications can and can't be taken with food. If you are unsure, consult your doctor or your pharmacist.

- Often, vomiting will accompany nausea. If this occurs, use the same remedies as you would to combat nausea, but concentrate on increasing the amount of fluids you drink each day. While carbonated beverages help with nausea, once vomiting begins, plain cool water or electrolyte replacement drinks like Gatorade or Pedialyte are best to prevent the dehydration that results from serious or long-term vomiting. How do you know you are dehydrated? Be alert for the presence of these symptoms of dehydration:
  - headache
  - dizziness, especially when changing position
  - lightheadedness
  - dry skin, lips, tongue or mucous membranes
  - decreased elasticity of the skin
  - rapid heart rate (greater than 100 beats per minute)

If your nausea and vomiting is so severe that you are unable to tolerate or "keep down" oral fluids, then you should seek medical care immediately. Very often a more invasive means of fluid replacement, specifically intravenous fluids, may be needed to reverse your dehydration.

DIARRHEA

Undoubtedly the most inconvenient and uncomfortable side effect of HIV medications is diarrhea. While many HIV medications can cause diarrhea, the most notable is Norvir (ritonavir) and medications that contain Norvir. As is the case with vomiting, diarrhea can cause dehydration, therefore, those steps discussed earlier should be implemented to prevent dehydration. Fortunately, diarrhea as a result of HIV medications is either short-lived or easily treated. Plus, the newest HIV medications have excellent side effect profiles, making diarrhea the exception and not the rule. That being said, there are several ways to resolve diarrhea. They include:

- Eating foods high in *soluble fiber*—fiber that attracts water—including oatmeal, breads, and wheat products. Dietary fiber is not digestible by the human intestinal tract, but it does slow digestion, which in turn increases absorption. High soluble fiber foods help slow diarrhea by absorbing excess water normally absorbed by the large intestine.
- A method used to save millions of lives of rural children in developing countries is rice water. Prepare white rice and then let the leftover rice water cool. Once it has cooled to room temperature, drink the rice water as you would plain water. The fiber left behind by the rice will help ease the diarrhea and the water will help you rehydrate if necessary.
- Avoid foods that have *insoluble fiber*—fiber that does not dissolve in water—such as fruit and vegetable skin. Insoluble fiber holds water that will make the stool moist and loose. Obviously when diarrhea strikes, extra intestinal water is the last thing you need.
- Avoid foods that aggravate diarrhea such as greasy foods, spicy foods, and dairy products.
- As is the case with vomiting, diarrhea can cause dehydration. Fluids must be replaced as quickly as they are lost to prevent dehydration. Increasing the intake of plain water or electrolyte drinks (e.g., Pedialyte) will most likely not improve diarrhea, but it will prevent the dehydration that results from diarrhea.

DRY MOUTH

Many medications used to control HIV and prevent opportunistic infections can cause dry mouth. However, dry mouth can be combated in several ways. They include:

- Rinse your mouth with warm salt water several times per day. However, caution must be taken to avoid water that is too salty, which can actually worsen dry mouth.
- Hard candy and lozenges used throughout the day can alleviate dry mouth. For those people living with diabetes, make sure the candies are sugar free so the blood sugar is not negatively affected.
- In extreme cases of dry mouth, your doctor can prescribe medicines that will replace the mouth's natural moisture. If mouth pain occurs, or breaks in the mucous membranes of the mouth or tongue are present, notify your doctor immediately.

FATIGUE

A few HIV medications can cause feelings of fatigue or a lack of energy. Fatigue can be caused by HIV itself, similar to the fatigue one gets when you are sick with the flu or a bad cold. Sometimes, HIV can cause diminished levels of testosterone in men, resulting in fatigue. Even a vitamin D deficiency can cause some people to feel fatigue. When fatigue is caused by medications, there are ways to diminish the symptoms. They include:

- First and foremost, the body needs adequate rest and exercise. When you are fatigued you may sleep most of the day. However, this doesn't mean you are getting enough quality sleep. Eight hours of uninterrupted sleep each night is the best way to feel rested and energetic.
- When energy levels are low, as is the case with fatigue, summoning the energy to exercise is very difficult. But by increasing your level of exercise you can increase your energy level and relieve the symptoms of fatigue.
- Follow a healthy diet, one rich in vitamins, minerals and representing all the food groups. Many HIV medical practices have a nutritionist on staff or can refer you to one in order to help you put together a healthy diet that will improve your symptoms of fatigue.
- If you suffer from fatigue, never assume that it is being caused by the medications you are taking. Conditions such as obstructive sleep apnea, depression, low hormone levels, or a low blood count (anemia) can cause fatigue as well. In order to treat your fatigue, the doctor must determine the cause. If you suffer from fatigue, notify your doctor immediately.

RASH/ITCHING

Rashes with and without itching skin can have many causes, including liver disease, kidney disease, allergies to foods or medications, insect bites, and certain sexually transmitted infections. If you develop a rash with or without itching, you should notify your doctor immediately. While you are waiting to see your doctor, there are measures you can take relieve your symptoms. They include:

- Avoid hot baths or showers, which could aggravate rashes. When showering or bathing, use warm or tepid water and do not stay in the water longer than necessary. Avoid soaps that are drying or contain alcohol that can dry the skin; dry skin will make itching worse.
- Direct sunlight can cause or aggravate a rash. In fact, Bactrim, an antibiotic used to prevent and treat pneumocystis pneumonia, makes the skin much more sensitive to sunlight and can cause or worsen a rash. If you take Bactrim avoid direct sunlight by covering exposed skin and wearing a hat that shades the face.
- In the unlikely event you develop liver or kidney disease, generalized itching all over the body could be the first sign. For this reason, any time you experience widespread itching, you should notify your doctor immediately. Simple blood tests can tell your doctor if your itching is related to an undiagnosed liver or kidney problem.
- Before stopping any medications due to a rash, consult your doctor first. Some medications can't be restarted once they are stopped (e.g., Ziagen) so consult your physician

when the rash develops. Stopping a medication if it's not necessary may result in you having to change medications. The doctor will advise you when and if to stop a medication as a result of a rash.

Depression

Along with the emotional causes of depression, there are some HIV medications that can cause or exacerbate the symptoms of depression. The drug Sustiva (efavirenz) and the efavirenz containing medication Atripla have been known to cause depression in those people not previously depressed and to worsen symptoms in those people with an existing diagnosis of depression. The medication Complera can also cause symptoms of depression but less often than Atripla or Sustiva. Unlike the side effects discussed earlier, depression is one that should not be addressed by the patient alone. Instead, when symptoms of depression do arise, contact your HIV specialist, a psychiatrist or a psychologist as soon as possible. If your symptoms reach the point where you feel you want to hurt yourself or hurt others, call your local suicide prevention line or go to the nearest emergency room or psychiatric emergency room.

The one thing patients can do to combat depression is to be alert for its signs and symptoms. Know your body and recognize when you are not feeling what's normal for you. Because depression is such an important and complex issue, we will discuss how to recognize the signs and symptoms in a later chapter.

This chapter has taught us that HIV medications have been the key to longer, healthier lives since their introduction over twenty-five years ago. We have also illustrated the importance of adhering to your prescribed medication regimen, and the negative impact viral mutations and resistance can have on your health. Unfortunately, like any chronic illness, HIV will rear its ugly head now and again. What happens when HIV weakens your natural defenses? In the next chapter we will discuss opportunistic infections common to HIV, how to recognize them before they make you sick, and how to prevent and treat them.

8

OPPORTUNISTIC INFECTIONS

The purpose of every HIV medication, of all the doctors and nurses who care for HIV patients, of all things related to HIV healthcare, even the purpose of this book is to help people living with HIV stay healthy as long as possible. Obviously, if left untreated, HIV can be very detrimental to the immune system of those people infected with the virus. As the immune system becomes damaged from HIV, the body becomes at risk for certain infections and illnesses. This chapter deals with those illnesses and infections that jeopardize the health of every person living with HIV. We will look at the collection of infections that are common in HIV, learn how to recognize the signs and symptoms of those infections, and, finally, learn how to prevent them from occurring in the first place.

The Big Myth—HIV Makes You Sick

There are many myths and misconceptions surrounding HIV and AIDS, not the least of which is the belief that HIV makes a person sick. I may be exaggerating when I say this, but nothing could be farther from the truth. We all know that millions have died after becoming infected with HIV, but the truth is that HIV did not make all those people sick. Let's explain what I mean.

Earlier in this text we discussed the effects of HIV on the human body. For the sake of review, HIV uses the body's immune system to make copies of itself. Specifically, HIV uses CD4 cells to replicate, or, in other words, to make copies of itself. CD4 cells are those specialized cells that help the human body defend itself against infections and illnesses. Unfortunately, CD4 cells are damaged when HIV uses them for replication. The more CD4 cells that are damaged, the weaker our immune system becomes—eventually becoming so weak that the immune system is unable to protect the body from infection and illness. So you see, it's not HIV that makes a person sick, it's the weakened immune system that results in illness and infection. HIV does the damage to the immune system, but it's the infections and illnesses that take advantage of the weakened immune system that make the HIV-infected person sick. Is this just a matter of semantics? Possibly, but the concept is an important one. If indeed HIV does damage the immune system, then logic says that the key to keeping the HIV-infected person healthy is to limit immune system damage and prevent those infections that take advantage of the weakened immune system. Or, in other words, the key is to prevent opportunistic infections.

Opportunistic Infections

Exactly as the name implies, opportunistic infections exploit the opportunity to make a person sick when the immune system is at its weakest. Most opportunistic infections are caused by organisms that are essentially harmless in the presence of a healthy immune system. For example, most every adult has been exposed to the *cytomegalovirus* (CMV) at some time in their life. The majority of these people have a normal immune system which prevents CMV from doing any harm. But in people with a weakened immune system, such as an HIV-infected person, CMV can wreak havoc, causing serious infections in the retinas of the eyes or the gastrointestinal tract.

Opportunistic infections are caused by many organisms, including bacteria, viruses, parasites, and fungi. Let's look at these organisms and the most common infections they cause.

BACTERIAL

Mycobacterium Avium Complex (MAC)

MAC is *non-tuberculous mycobacteria,* meaning it is a mycobacterium that does not cause tuberculosis or leprosy. The bacterium is typically found in soil, water, and some wildlife. This naturally occurring bacterium usually poses no health risk to humans. However, in people with weakened immune systems, including those living with HIV, MAC can cause infection in the gastrointestinal tract, the lungs, and on the skin.

- Symptoms—Night sweats, weight loss, abdominal pain, bloody diarrhea, elevated liver enzymes (especially alkaline phosphatase).
- Risk Level—People are at greater risk when the CD4 count is 50 cells/mm^3 or less. Prophylaxis medications begin when the CD4 falls below 100 cells/mm^3.
- Prevention/Prophylaxis—The drugs Zithromax (azithromycin), Mycobutin (Rifabutin), or Biaxin (clarithromycin) are started when the CD4 count falls below 100 cells/mm^3.
- Treatment—Several antibiotics, including Zithromax (azithromycin), Mycobutin (Rifabutin), Biaxin (clarithromycin), Myambutol (ethambutol), or Cipro (ciprofloxacin), are used to treat MAC infection. To avoid resistance to antibiotics, the patient is usually treated with multiple antibiotics at the same time.

Tuberculosis (TB)

In the 1820s, TB was labeled a disease for the first time; it caused numerous deaths across the U.S. In fact, at one point, TB was the leading cause of death in the U.S. But with TB testing, effective medications, and isolation techniques (TB sanitariums) it was all but eliminated prior to the emergence of HIV and AIDS. However, after HIV came onto the scene, TB once again became a serious public health problem, the number of new cases peaking in 1994. Many people are infected with TB, but the infection remains inactive and they remain symptom free. However, TB activates when the immune system becomes too weak to protect the body from the infection any longer. More disturbing is the emergence of a resistant type of TB—a strain resistant to the antibiotics that are typically an effective treatment.

TB is highly contagious, spread from person to person by water droplets released into the air with coughing or sneezing. TB most commonly affects the lungs (pulmonary) but can infect other parts of the body (extrapulmonary) as well. TB can be active (infectious, and making a person sick) or latent (non-contagious and without symptoms of illness).

- Symptoms—Fatigue, night sweats, a cough producing blood-tinged sputum, fever, weight loss.
- Risk Level—While active TB usually strikes those people with CD4 counts less than 200cells/mm³, it can activate and become infectious at any CD4 count.
- Prevention/Prophylaxis—The drug Laniazid (isoniazid) is used to prevent latent TB from becoming active.
- Treatment—Usually a multiple drug regimen that can include Laniazid (isoniazid), Rifadin (rifampin), pyrazinamide, Myambutol (ethambutol) or streptomycin. With resistant strains of TB, susceptibility tests must be done to see which antibiotic will be effective.

TABLE 9. TYPES OF TUBERCULOSIS

Active
- Typically strikes people with weakened immune systems, including those with HIV.
- Symptoms include fatigue; night sweats; cough producing blood tinged sputum; fever; and weight loss.
- Effectively treated with multiple drug regimens.

Inactive
- TB-infected, but no signs or symptoms of illness.
- Typically will not activate unless the immune system becomes weakened for some reason.
- Medications are prescribed to prevent the TB from becoming active.

Salmonellosis ("Food Poisoning")

This bacterial infection is spread by way of contaminated food or water, thus the name "food poisoning." The risk of becoming infected with salmonella increases when raw meats or eggs are ingested. Therefore, it is important to cook those foods thoroughly before eating. Because salmonella can be found in feces, the spread of salmonella from person to person is also possible through oral to anal contact or through oral sex performed on the insertive partner.

- Symptoms—Abdominal pain, severe diarrhea, bloody stools, chills, a loss of appetite beginning one to three days after exposure.
- Risk Level—Salmonella can infect people with any CD4 count but is more common in people infected with HIV.
- Prevention/Prophylaxis—The best way to prevent salmonella is by frequent, proper hand washing, especially after using the bathroom or after handling raw meats, poultry and eggs. People with HIV should avoid foods that contain raw eggs, such as chocolate mousse, Caesar salad dressing, and raw cake and cookie batter. Poultry products, such as chicken and turkey, should be cooked thoroughly before eating. Steaks and pork should not be served rare. After preparing foods, kitchen counters and cutting boards

should be cleaned with bleach and disposable wipes. Make certain at risk foods are refrigerated prior to cooking, and that leftovers are refrigerated promptly after the meal.

- Treatment—Antibiotics, such as Cipro (ciprofloxacin), Bactrim (sulfamethoxazole and trimethoprim), Chloromycetin (chloramphenicol), and Omnipen (ampicillin), are used to treat infection.

Syphilis

Not actually an opportunistic infection, this sexually transmitted infection is caused by a worm-like bacterium called a *spirochete*. The genus and species name for this spirochete is *Treponema pallidum*. There are three stages of syphilis, each exhibiting different symptoms.

- Symptoms—*Primary infection* is characterized by a single painless lesion on the genitals called a *chancre*. This lesion will heal after a few weeks, but the bacterium that caused the lesion remains if not treated. *Secondary syphilis* is characterized by a rash, especially on the palms of the hands and soles of the feet. Other less specific symptoms can include fever, muscle pain, and hair loss. *Latent syphilis* can cause lesions on internal organs such as the brain and central nervous system. Left untreated, latent syphilis can cause mental illness, psychosis, and death.
- Risk Level—Syphilis can strike anyone regardless of their CD4 count.
- Prevention/Prophylaxis—The only way to prevent a syphilis infection is to use a latex condom during all anal, oral, or vaginal sexual encounters.
- Treatment—The treatment of choice is a series of three benzathine penicillin injections, each one week apart. For those allergic to penicillin, the antibiotics Vibramycin (doxycycline) and Rocephin (ceftriaxone) can be used.

TABLE 10. THE STAGES OF SYPHILIS

Primary Infection
- Painless lesion on the genitals.
- The lesion heals but the bacterium remains.

Secondary Syphilis
- Characterized by rash on the palms of the hands and soles of the feet; fever.

Latent Syphilis
- Can cause lesions on internal organs such as the brain and the central nervous system.
- Left untreated, latent syphilis can be fatal.

Bacillary Angiomatosis ("Cat Scratch Disease"/Bartonella Infection)

This bacterial infection is also known as "cat scratch disease," an infection caused by the bacterium *Bartonella henselae* and transmitted by cat scratches and cat bites. *Bacillary angiomatosis* is extremely rare in people who aren't infected with HIV. Often it's confused with Kaposi's sarcoma due to similarities in appearance. Bacillary angiomatosis is related to an infection called *trench fever*, common among soldiers in World War I. Left untreated, bacillary angiomatosis can be fatal.

- Symptoms—This infection is characterized by nodules or lesions on and just below the surface of the skin. As the number of nodules increases, patients may develop fever, swollen lymph nodes, chills, poor appetite, weight loss, and night sweats. The infection can also spread to the bone and bone marrow, spleen, liver, and lymph nodes. These bacteria can also cause blood vessels to grow out of control, resulting in purplish lesions that closely resemble the lesions of Kaposi's sarcoma.
- Risk Level—Bacillary angiomatosis is found almost exclusively in patients infected with HIV, most frequently in those people with CD4 counts less than 500cells/mm³. Obviously, being bitten or scratched by a cat dramatically increases the risk of acquiring this disease.
- Prevention/Prophylaxis—Avoid cat scratches and bites; if bitten or scratched, wash the wound with soap and water under pressure from a faucet for at least 5 minutes. Apply an antibacterial ointment or cream and cover with a dry, clean, dressing.
- Treatment—Granted it can be a very serious infection, but it's easily treated with several weeks of Vibramycin (doxycycline) and erythromycin if diagnosed early.

Bacterial Pneumonia

Pneumonia is a bacterial infection that causes irritation, swelling, and congestion in the lungs. This bacterial infection usually follows a cold. It is also known as *pneumonitis.*

- Symptoms—The onset of symptoms is usually sudden. They include fever, chills, difficulty breathing, a cough producing bloody or yellow sputum, fatigue, feeling tired, blue or pale lips or nail beds.
- Risk Level—Studies have shown that bacterial pneumonia can occur with any CD4 count but does occur more frequently in patients with HIV. The severity of the bacterial pneumonia is also greater in people with HIV.
- Prevention/Prophylaxis—There are vaccines available that help decrease the risk of bacterial pneumonia. Evidence suggests that Bactrim taken once each day can decrease the risk of bacterial pneumonia. Finally, people taking HIV medications have a lower incidence of bacterial pneumonia than do HIV positive patients not on HIV medications.
- Treatment—Antibiotic therapy is the treatment of choice for bacterial pneumonia. The type of antibiotic depends on the type of bacteria causing the pneumonia.

FUNGAL

Pneumocystis Carinii Pneumonia (PCP)/Pneumocystis Jirovecii Pneumonia

At one time experts thought PCP was a parasitic infection. Actually, PCP is caused by a yeast-like fungus called *Pneumocystis jirovecii.* This fungus typically infects the lungs of people with weakened immune systems. At the outset of the HIV epidemic it was PCP infection that first brought HIV-infected people to the emergency department. Even today, for many people the first symptom of their HIV infection is a diagnosis of PCP. Unfortunately, by the time PCP occurs there has already been significant damage done to the immune system. Before the use of prophylactic (preventative) antibiotics, most notably Bactrim (sulfamethoxazole and trimethoprim), PCP was common and most often fatal among HIV-infected people. It was the unusually high incidence of new PCP cases that signaled the beginning of the HIV epidemic in the early 1980s.

- Symptoms—PCP causes fever, shortness of breath, a dry cough, and difficulty breathing. Often, PCP-related breathing difficulties are only evident after mild exertion such as walking. As the infection progresses, the respiratory symptoms get worse, many times leading to hospitalization and the need for assisted breathing using a mechanical ventilator. If left untreated, PCP can be fatal.
- Risk Level—PCP rarely occurs in people with CD4 counts greater than 200cells/mm^3.
- Prevention/Prophylaxis—The risk of acquiring PCP can be diminished with the use of prophylactic antibiotics such as Bactrim (sulfamethoxazole and trimethoprim), Nebu-Pent (pentamidine), Aczone (dapsone), or Mepron (atovaquone).
- Treatment—PCP is treated with the same antibiotics used to prevent the infection. The preferred prophylactic medication and the treatment of choice is the same, Bactrim DS. However, for those with an allergy to sulfa drugs or Bactrim, other antibiotics, both oral and inhaled, are available. In severe cases higher doses and/or intravenous forms of the antibiotics are necessary. In addition, steroid therapy can be used to decrease inflammation caused by the PCP infection.

Aspergillosis

This type of fungus is most often found in soil and decaying plant life. Most often, the fungus is inhaled through the mouth and/or nose, primarily infecting the lungs or sinuses. Aspergillosis is rare, most often striking those people with significantly compromised immune systems. In addition to people living with HIV other populations at risk for Aspergillosis include cancer patients undergoing chemotherapy and transplant patients on anti-rejection medications.

- Symptoms—The symptoms of Aspergillosis are similar to those found in lung or sinus infections. If the primary site of infection is the lungs, symptoms will include cough, chest pain, shortness of breath, and fever. An Aspergillosis infection of the sinuses will cause headache, facial pain and fever. Night sweats can characterize any Aspergillosis infection.
- Risk Level—Most people who develop an Aspergillosis infection have a CD4 count of less than 100 cells/mm^3. However, infection can occur in people with CD4 counts greater than 100 cells/mm^3 under certain circumstances. People living with AIDS (having a CD4 count less than 200 cells/mm^3) often develop Aspergillosis after suffering from bacterial or pneumocystis pneumonia.
- Prevention/Prophylaxis—There is no specific prophylaxis used to prevent Aspergillosis. Instead, taking precautions when handling soil or plant life during yard work is suggested. Those at particularly high risk should wear gloves and masks when gardening or working outside. Good hand washing is also suggested.
- Treatment—Very potent antifungal medications must be used to treat Aspergillosis. Oral Sporanox (itraconazole) and intravenous Fungizone (amphotericin B) are the treatments of choice.

Candidiasis ("Thrush," "Candida," "Yeast Infection")

The most common fungal infection, candidiasis is caused by the fungus *Candida albicans*, one of many species of candida fungi. Candidiasis occurs in the moist mucous membranes of the mouth, esophagus and vagina. Candidiasis can also occur on the skin in the warm, moist skin folds of the groins, axilla ("armpits"), and abdomen.

- Symptoms—Candida infections of the mouth ("thrush") are characterized by white patches on the tongue, gums, roof of the mouth and the inside of the cheeks. These patches can cause altered taste, dry mouth, mouth soreness, and difficulty swallowing. Fungal infections of the esophagus ("candida esophagitis") cause chest pain, sore throat and, in extreme cases, difficulty swallowing and breathing. Vaginal candida infections ("yeast infection") are characterized by vaginal itching, milky vaginal discharge, and vaginal irritation and/or pain. Finally, candida skin infections (*cutaneous candidiasis*) are red, scaly patches of skin that are itchy and tender. The areas can also have a foul odor in advanced cases. These infections are more common in people who are obese or are diabetic.

- Risk Level—While anyone can have thrush regardless of CD4 count, the incidence increases when the CD4 count drops below 200 cells/mm^3.

- Prevention/Prophylaxis—Typically, prophylactic medications are not prescribed to prevent thrush. In fact, there is not much data to support thrush prophylaxis. If prophylaxis is ordered, antifungal medications such as Diflucan (fluconazole) are prescribed to be taken once per day. To prevent vaginal yeast infections, doctors suggest eating yogurt with active bacterial cultures. These bacteria help protect the vaginal area from infection. Keeping skin clean and dry, especially in the skin folds of the axilla, groins, or abdomen, can help decrease the incidence of skin candida infections.

- Treatment—Treatment for oral thrush, candida esophagitis, or vaginal yeast infections is in the form of antifungal medications. Diflucan (fluconazole) once per day, ranging from one day to two weeks or more, is common. Depending on the dose, yeast infections can be treated with as little as one dose of Diflucan (fluconazole). In some circumstances, topical antifungal medications are used to treat vaginal and cutaneous candida infections. Finally, mild cases of oral candida can be treated with antifungal lozenges that dissolve slowly in the mouth or antifungal medication suspension (liquid) that is swished in the mouth and either spat out or swallowed. However, these alternatives to oral medication must be taken several times each day to be effective. As is the case with topical creams, the reoccurrence rate of candida after using antifungal lozenges or suspensions is high.

Coccidioidomycosis ("Valley Fever")

Coccidioidomycosis is caused by the fungus *coccidioides*, a fungus found primarily in soil throughout the Southwestern United States, Mexico, Central America, and South America. As part of its life cycle, the fungus becomes airborne as microscopic spores. It's at this time that the fungus is most infectious, entering the body during inspiration and infecting the lungs. The lungs aren't the only organs that can be infected. Coccidioidomycosis infection can also involve the kidneys, lymph system, spleen and brain.

- Symptoms—Early symptoms include cough, weight loss and fatigue. If left untreated, the infection can spread to the brain and other parts of the central nervous system, causing headache, confusion, light sensitivity and fever. Without treatment, the infection can progress throughout the body. If coccidioidomycosis progresses to meningitis it can be fatal.

- Risk Level—The primary risk of coccidioidomycosis occurs once the CD4 count drops below 100 cells/mm³. Keep in mind that the lowest CD4 point since HIV diagnosis should be the value used to assess the risk for coccidioidomycosis. For instance, if the current CD4 value is 250 cells/mm³, but the CD4 count has been as low as 25 cells/mm³ since diagnosis, the risk for coccidioidomycosis should be based on the lowest value since diagnosis of HIV—in this case, 25 cells/mm³.

- Prevention/Prophylaxis—Precautions such as wearing gloves and a mask while working with soil should be employed. Currently, there is no medication that is used as a prophylaxis against coccidioidomycosis.

- Treatment—Most of the time, this infection will run its course and resolve on its own without treatment after a few months. For those who are at the highest risk, including people living with HIV, the course of treatment will typically extend for more than 6 months. Antifungal medications are used to treat this infection—oral Diflucan (fluconazole) for mild cases and intravenous Sporanox (amphotericin B) for more extensive and severe infections.

Cryptococcus

The yeast-like fungus *Cryptococcus neoformans* is found in soil all over the world, most commonly in soil contaminated with bird droppings. This fungus affects primarily the lungs and brain, but in advanced cases can affect other organs including the skin where *cryptococcus neoformans* causes lesions to form. Infection occurs when the fungus is inhaled into the lungs in the form of dehydrated spores. After lying dormant in the lungs, the fungus activates and then spreads to other tissues and organs outside the lungs, including the brain. A cryptococcal infection in the brain (*"cryptococcal meningitis"*) is often fatal if left untreated, especially in people with severely weakened immune systems (e.g., people living with HIV). In the lungs, this fungus causes cryptococcal pneumonia, a serious and potentially fatal respiratory infection.

- Symptoms—The symptoms of cryptococcus infection depend on the organs involved. Left untreated, symptoms worsen over the course of a few weeks. Cryptococcal meningitis symptoms include headache, fever, stiff neck, and sensitivity to light (*"photophobia"*). As the meningitis progresses, symptoms of brain swelling, such as nausea, vomiting, confusion, paralysis, and coma, emerge. Left untreated, a person can progress from coma to death in a short period of time. Cryptococcal pneumonia symptoms are much like those of bacterial pneumonia and pneumocystis pneumonia. These symptoms include fever, cough, shortness of breath, chest tightness and chest pain.

- Risk Level—The greatest risk of cryptococcus infection occurs once the CD4 count falls below 100 cells/mm³. It's important to note that even in HIV-positive people whose CD4 counts have risen above 100 cells/mm³, there is still a risk. To accurately assess the risk of cryptococcus infection, the lowest CD4 count since being diagnosed (*"Nadir"*) with HIV should be used, regardless of how early in the course of the disease it was.

- Prevention/Prophylaxis—Taking precautions, such as wearing gloves and a mask while working with soil or birds, is the best way to reduce the risk of infection. Wearing a mask and gloves minimizes the risk of inhaling the fungal spores that cause infection. The antifungal medication Diflucan (*fluconazole*) is sometimes used as prophylaxis when the CD4 count drops below 100 cells/mm^3. However, many practitioners are reluctant to use prophylaxis because of medication cost and the possibility that drug-resistant cryptococcal meningitis will develop. Drug resistant meningitis can be particularly serious because it does not respond to conventional anti-fungal treatment.
- Treatment—Oral medications such as the anti-fungal Diflucan (fluconazole) can be used in less severe cases. In advanced cases of cryptococcal meningitis or pneumonia, intravenous Fungizone (amphotericin B) can be used. Keep in mind that in people with severely weakened immune systems, treatment is often unsuccessful.

Histoplasmosis

An infection caused by the fungus *Histoplasma capsulatum,* a fungus found in soil contaminated by bird or bat droppings. Infection occurs when dehydrated spores are inhaled while working with contaminated soil, exploring caves or while cleaning bird cages or chicken coops.

- Symptoms—The symptoms of histoplasmosis depend on the tissues and organs infected. Most often histoplasmosis affects the lungs, resulting in fever, fatigue, difficulty breathing, shortness of breath and cough. If the infection progresses to organs other than the lungs it is said to be a *disseminated infection*—an infection throughout the body—and can cause skin lesions, weight loss, and an enlarged liver, spleen or lymph nodes. If histoplasmosis affects the bone marrow, platelet, white blood cell, and red blood cell production is compromised, resulting in low levels of these blood cell components.
- Risk Level—The risk of histoplasmosis increases when the CD4 count falls below 100 cells/mm^3. As in other types of fungal infections, the lowest known CD4 count since HIV diagnosis should be used to determine histoplasmosis infection risk.
- Prevention/Prophylaxis—The use of anti-fungals such as Diflucan (fluconazole) is not recommended in people with healthy immune systems. However, prophylaxis may be done using Diflucan (fluconazole) or the drug Sporanox (itraconazole) for those people with CD4 counts below 100 cells/mm^3. Precautions such as wearing a mask and gloves while handling contaminated soil will limit exposure to the *histoplasma,* thus decreasing the risk of infection.
- Treatment—For some people the symptoms of histoplasmosis will resolve on their own. For severe cases and for cases in immunocompromised people, treatment of histoplasmosis is a two-step process—treatment for the acute infection and maintenance therapy after the acute infection has been resolved to prevent recurrence. Mild to moderate acute infection is treated with the oral drug Sporanox (itraconazole). For more severe infections, intravenous Fungizone (amphotericin B) is required. Intravenous Fungizone (amphotericin B) requires hospitalization and unfortunately can be very toxic to the kidneys and bone marrow. Because of this, close monitoring of kidney function and blood count is necessary. After the acute infection is treated, maintenance therapy must

be initiated. In the case of those people with very weak immune systems, this maintenance therapy is often continued for life. Oral Sporanox (itraconazole) is the primary
maintenance drug, but in those people who have difficulty maintaining high enough
itraconazole blood levels to prevent reoccurrence, oral Diflucan (fluconazole) can be
added.

VIRAL

Cytomegalovirus (CMV)

CMV is a virus from the group of viruses known as *herpesviridae*. There are eight such
viruses in this group, one of which is CMV. Most people have been exposed to CMV sometime
in their life, via contact with bodily fluids or through sexual contact. Typically, CMV does
not cause symptoms of illness in people with healthy immune systems. However, in people
with weakened immune systems, such as those living with HIV, those taking anti-rejection
drugs after an organ transplant, or those receiving chemotherapy for cancer, CMV can cause
illness and infection. Initially, CMV infection causes symptoms similar to mononucleosis
including, fever, muscle aches, and fatigue. These symptoms usually resolve without intervention, and the person will feel better. CMV then lies dormant for years without causing
symptoms or illness. Later, as the immune system weakens, CMV reactivates, causing new
infections throughout the body.

- Symptoms—**CMV retinitis** (CMV that infects the retina of the eye) causes inflammation
  of the retina, resulting in visual changes, "floaters," diminished vision, blurred vision,
  and, in some cases, blindness. **CMV colitis** infects the gastrointestinal tract, resulting in
  colitis (inflammation of the bowels), *cholangitis* (inflammation of the bile duct), and
  ulcerations in the mouth, throat and/or rectum. CMV infections in the GI tract cause
  abdominal pain, fever, diarrhea, and weight loss.
- Risk Level—Most people have been exposed to CMV at some time in their lifetime but
  will experience no ill effects from the virus. However, once the CD4 count falls below
  50 cells/mm^3, the incidence of illnesses like CMV retinitis and CMV colitis increases
  dramatically.
- Prevention/Prophylaxis—Oral Cytovene (ganciclovir) or Valcyte (valganciclovir) can
  be used as prophylaxis medications to prevent the initial CMV infection in those patients
  at highest risk, specifically people with a CD4 count less than 50 cells/mm^3 or who have
  ever had a CD4 count less than 50 cells/mm^3.
- Treatment—The most effective treatment for both CMV retinitis and gastrointestinal
  CMV is the antiviral medication Cytovene (ganciclovir). Treatment is given intravenously in the acute stages of infection and then changed to the oral form as a maintenance therapy to prevent reoccurrence of the infection. In some cases of CMV retinitis,
  antiviral medication implants are inserted in the affected eye directly at the site of infection in order to treat CMV retinitis locally.

Molluscum Contagiosum ("Molluscum")

Molluscum is caused by a very common virus that is a member of the group of viruses
known as *Poxviridae*. Infection with this virus causes flesh-colored, pearl-like lesions seen

initially in the genital area and thighs in people with normal immune systems. In people with weakened immune systems, the lesions can spread over the entire body, especially the face. Molluscum can be confused with genital warts, so definitive diagnosis is made by taking a small sample of the lesion and looking at it under the microscope (a biopsy).

- Symptoms—Molluscum causes small flesh-colored "bumps" or lesions first appearing in the inner thigh and genital area, spreading to the face and the rest of the body. These lesions are typically dome shaped, dimpled, with a hard white core in the middle. These lesions are most often painless but can itch intensely. Itching leads to scratching, increasing the risk of spreading the lesions to other parts of the body.
- Risk Level—Anyone exposed to molluscum, either by coming into contact with the skin of someone infected or by sexual contact with an infected person, can get this viral infection. In other words, people with any CD4 count can become infected. However, anyone with a weakened immune system is at higher risk of having disseminated (throughout the body) infection.
- Prevention/Prophylaxis—Using condoms during anal, oral, or vaginal sex is the best way to reduce the risk of molluscum infection. If you already have the infection, refraining from scratching the lesions will diminish the risk of spreading the molluscum all over your body. Using an electric razor has been known to diminish the incidence of molluscum spread by shaving with a blade.
- Treatment—Left untreated, molluscum will resolve over the course of several weeks to months, typically without leaving scars. If treatment is preferred, lesions can be frozen with liquid nitrogen one at a time. In many cases, molluscum infection will respond to HIV combination therapy.

Oral Hairy Leukoplakia (OHL)

OHL is caused by another virus from the *herpesviridae* family known as the Epstein Barr Virus (EBV). Found in the mouth, OHL is sometimes one of the first symptoms of HIV infection. The presence of OHL is an indication that the immune system has been damaged and weakened by HIV and is susceptible to other more serious infections.

- Symptoms—Leukoplakia is characterized by white patches on the sides of the tongue appearing similar to that of corrugated cardboard. Among the many folds are hair-like protrusions from which OHL got its name. Leukoplakia can be confused with thrush upon initial observation, the difference being that patches of leukoplakia can't be dislodged, as is the case with thrush. Usually diagnosis can be made simply by visual examination, but a biopsy can be done if necessary.
- Risk Level—As stated above, OHL can be one of the first symptoms of HIV infection. While it can occur at any CD4 count, people with CD4 counts less than 200 cells/mm³ have a higher incidence than those above 200 cells/mm³.
- Prevention/Prophylaxis—Prophylaxis specifically for OHL is uncommon; however, patients taking Diflucan (fluconazole) to prevent thrush have a lower incidence of OHL. Because HIV medications can help the CD4 count rise, people on HIV medication combinations have a lesser incidence of OHL as well.
- Treatment—OHL doesn't need to be treated unless it causes pain or interrupts eating, swallowing, or speaking. If treatment is indicated, one of three herpes medications—

Zovirax (acyclovir), Valtrex (Valacyclovir) or Famvir (famciclovir)—can be prescribed in addition to an HIV medication regimen.

Human Papillomavirus (HPV)

Papillomaviruses are a group of viruses that infect the skin and mucous membranes of humans and animals. Over one hundred of those infect humans. Some of these viruses are known to cause genital warts. While HPV is often thought of as one specific virus, there are actually several viruses that are considered HPV and cause genital warts. Other types of HPV can cause cervical cancer in women, rectal/anal cancer in men, and ordinary warts of the hands and feet. People living with HIV are most concerned about the HPV that causes genital warts, cervical cancer, or rectal/anal cancer. HPV is spread from person to person during unprotected sex. In most cases this very common virus is inactive, causing no symptoms of illness. However, for people with weakened immune systems, HPV can activate, causing genital warts, cervical cancers, and rectal/anal cancers.

- Symptoms—Once HPV activates it causes warts or "bumps" on the penis, vulva, in and around the anus, or in the mouth. If HPV infection results in cervical cancer or rectal/anal cancer, symptoms of these conditions may include vaginal or rectal bleeding, vaginal or rectal discharge, and unusual appearing lesions. If symptoms of HPV infection occur, they should never be ignored and should be addressed as soon as possible. Failure to do so could result in the progression of the HPV infection to the most serious forms of cancer.

- Risk Level—HPV can affect anyone, regardless of CD4 count. In fact, by the time we reach adulthood, most of us have been exposed and infected with HPV. People who engage in unprotected sex or have unprotected sex with multiple sex partners have a higher HPV incidence. Women infected with HIV are more at risk for HPV-related complications (e.g., cervical cancer) than women not infected with HIV. Cervical lesions as a result of an HPV infection seem to occur more frequently in women with CD4 counts less than 500 cells/mm^3.

- Prevention/Prophylaxis—The primary way of preventing infection with those strains of HIV that can cause cancer is the HPV vaccine. Originally developed for use in only females, the vaccine is now given to both males and females. The vaccine is a series of three injections given over a six-month period that stimulates the body to produce antibodies to the most dangerous HPV strains, the strains that cause cancer. Ideally the vaccine is given to boys and girls before they become sexually active, about the ages of 8 to 12. However, the vaccine can be given to men and women less than 26 years old and still be beneficial. In addition to the vaccine, safer sex practices decrease the risk of spreading HPV from person to person. Regular physical exams can identify suspicious lesions early, meaning treatment of those lesions can begin earlier as well. In women, regularly scheduled Pap exams are done to identify abnormal cells. Typically, HIV-positive women, and those women with a history of previous abnormal Pap exams, should get Paps every six months. HIV-negative women should get a Pap exam yearly. There is some debate surrounding the benefits of anal Pap exams in gay men. By swabbing the anus your provider will collect a sample of cells from the rectal mucosa. These cells are then examined under a microscope and cells that are cancerous or pre-cancerous are identified. Once identified, they can be removed much like abnormal cervical cells in women are removed. The hope is that by decreasing the incidence of HPV infection, the incidence of cervical cancer in women and rectal/anal cancer in men will decline as well. But when HPV infection occurs, vaccines, safer sex, and Pap exams can help avoid the complications of HPV infection.

- Treatment—Genital warts resulting from HPV can be treated in several ways. The warts can be frozen with liquid nitrogen and removed, or can be burned off with lasers. The topical prescription drug Aldara cream (imiquimod) can be applied directly to the warts if a less invasive method of treatment is desired. Any cancers that result from HPV require traditional cancer treatments, including radiation, chemotherapy, or surgery.

Herpes Simplex Virus (HSV)

HSV is a member of the *herpesviridae* family of viruses, along with varicella zoster virus (herpes zoster, VZV) and cytomegalovirus (CMV). There are actually two types of herpes simplex virus, HSV-1 and HSV-2. HSV-1 is spread from person to person by way of oral secretions, sores on the skin, kissing, or sharing toothbrushes or eating utensils. HSV-1 causes oral HSV, more commonly known as cold sores. HSV-2 is spread from person to person during unprotected sexual encounters. HSV-2 is primarily responsible for genital herpes, and herpes outbreaks below the waist. HSV-1 and HSV-2 can be spread from person to person when herpes sores are present. But it is important to remember that both types of HSV can also be spread when sores or lesions are not present.

Another important characteristic of HSV is that once infection has occurred, HSV remains in the skin and nerve cells for life. Most often the virus is dormant and causes no symptoms. But in times of stress, when exposed to intense sunlight, or when suffering from a cold or other viral illness, HSV can activate, causing painful, fluid-filled blisters. There is some evidence that HSV-2 is a co-factor of HIV, meaning HSV-2 may facilitate HIV infection of CD4 cells. There is also evidence that the presence of genital herpes increases the transmission risk of HIV.

- Symptoms—A herpes break-out may begin as a tingling, itching, or numb sensation of the skin or mucous membranes. This sensation is a result of the virus moving via nerve tracts, making its way to the skin. At the point of eruption, very painful, fluid-filled blisters form on the surface of the skin. These blisters eventually break open and crust over. The entire cycle from the initial sensation to outbreak of the vesicles to complete healing can take up to two weeks.
- Risk Level—Herpes can strike anyone, regardless of the health of their immune system or whether or not they are HIV-infected. There is some evidence that suggests that herpes outbreaks are more frequent in people living with HIV.
- Prevention/Prophylaxis—The best way to prevent the initial infection of HSV-1 or HSV-2 is to prevent exposure to infected bodily fluids. Avoid coming in contact with saliva or mucous membranes when oral HSV lesions are present. To reduce the risk of genital herpes (HSV-2) use condoms with every oral, anal, or vaginal sexual encounter. In people who experience frequent herpes outbreaks, certain antiviral medications can be used to decrease the frequency of outbreaks. The medications Valtrex (valacyclovir)

and Zovirax (acyclovir) are two such antivirals that, if taken in low daily doses, can decrease the frequency of HSV outbreaks.

- Treatment—Oral antiviral medications such as Zovirax (acyclovir), Valtrex (valacy-clovir), and Famvir (famciclovir) are used to treat acute herpes outbreaks. Keep in mind that these medications do not "cure" infections. Rather, they can shorten the time it takes for the outbreak to heal and reduce the severity of the outbreak. In the case of severe outbreaks or outbreaks involving the face or eyes, intravenous antiviral medications and hospitalization are required. There can be cases of herpes that are resistant to traditional medications. In those cases, stronger antiviral medications, such as Foscavir (foscarnet), are needed. Unfortunately, with stronger medication comes the risk of kidney and liver toxicity.

Herpes Zoster Virus (HZV)

Another member of the *herpesviridae* family, *Varicella zoster* is also known as the "chicken pox" or "shingles." Most people are infected with this virus as children in the form of chicken pox. After the initial infection, the zoster virus lies dormant in the body, reactivating later as itching, painful, fluid-filled blisters called shingles. Because the herpes virus resides along nerve tracts, shingles outbreaks are usually along the straight line paths of nerves. Each spinal nerve that exits the spinal cord handles sensory impulse for a region of the body. These regions are called dermatomes. Dermatomes stack like poker chips from the bottom of the feet to the top of the head. Shingles outbreaks follow dermatomes, affecting the dermatome that correlates to a specific spinal nerve. Shingles outbreaks seldom cross the midline of the body. Because nerves are affected, the lesions itch and are usually very painful. In severe cases, hospitalization may be required. Varicella zoster (chicken pox) is spread from person to person when someone with the virus coughs, sneezes, laughs or even talks in proximity to another person. Tiny water droplets containing virus are inhaled, spreading the infection from one person to another. In the case of shingles, transmission from person to person occurs by direct contact with the lesions.

- Symptoms—Very painful, itchy, fluid-filled blisters appearing in linear patterns along nerve tracts of individual dermatomes that encompass the flank, back, buttocks, and occasionally the face. Over the course of several days, the blisters break and crust over. Outbreaks of HZV can be precipitated by stress, exposure to direct sunlight, or irritation to the affected areas.

- Risk Level—Anyone can get HVZ, regardless of HIV infection or CD4 count. In order for someone to have a shingles outbreak, they have to have had chicken pox some time in their lifetime.

- Prevention/Prophylaxis—As is the case with herpes simplex, people who experience frequent HZV outbreaks use antiviral medications to decrease the frequency of outbreaks. The medication Zovirax (acyclovir) or Valtrex (valacyclovir) can decrease the frequency and severity of HZV outbreaks if taken daily in low doses.

- Treatment—Oral antiviral medications such as Zovirax (acyclovir), Famvir (famciclovir), or Valtrex (valacyclovir) are used to treat outbreaks of herpes. Keep in mind that these medications do not "cure" infections. Rather, they shorten the duration of the outbreak while reducing the severity. In the case of severe outbreaks, especially those on the face and near the eyes, intravenous antiviral medications and hospitalization are required. There can be cases of herpes that are resistant to traditional medications. In those cases, stronger antiviral medications, such as Foscavir (foscarnet), are needed. But this stronger medication also has more risks, such as kidney and liver toxicity.

Progressive Multifocal Leukoencephalopathy (PML)

This viral infection of the brain is caused by the *John Cunningham virus* or the JC virus (JCV), as it is more commonly called. The virus was first identified in 1971 and was named after the initials of the patient, John Cunningham, suffering from PML at the time the virus was isolated. Most people are exposed to JC virus at some point in their life. In the presence of a healthy immune system, the virus does no harm. However, in people with weakened immune systems, such as those living with HIV, JCV causes a potentially fatal infection of the brain known as *Progressive Multifocal Leukoencephalopathy*, or *PML* for short. PML most often appears after there has been significant damage to the immune system at the hands of HIV, occurring in people whose CD4 counts are less than 100 cells/mm^3. Before the advent of HIV medications, PML was fatal within a few months of contracting the infection. The Centers for Disease Control has classified PML as an *AIDS-defining illness*, meaning that if a person is diagnosed with PML, they are said to also have AIDS.

- Symptoms—Because PML affects the brain, symptoms reflect impairment of the central nervous system—loss of memory, seizure activity, visual disturbances, speech difficulties, and numbness or weakness of the arms, face and legs. Left untreated, these symptoms can progress to coma and eventually death.
- Risk Level—HIV-infected people with a CD4 count less than 100 cells/mm^3 are at the highest risk. In people without HIV, anyone with a significantly damaged immune system, such as cancer patients receiving chemotherapy, are at risk for PML.
- Prevention/Prophylaxis—While there is no specific medication that reduces the risk of PML, HIV medication regimens increase CD4 levels, which in turn strengthen the immune system, decreasing the risk of PML. Keeping the CD4 count higher than 100 cells/mm^3 is the best way to prevent PML.
- Treatment—As stated earlier, prior to the advent of HIV medications, PML took the life of its victims in just a few short months. Today, there are HIV medications that are able to cross the blood-brain barrier and reach brain tissue, offering an effective treatment option for PML. HIV antiretroviral medications that cross the blood-brain barrier include Epivir (lamivudine), Zidovudine (retrovir, AZT), Kaletra (lopinavir + ritonavir) and Reyataz (atazanavir). If a diagnosis of PML is made, the HIV regimen prescribed should contain at least one of those medications that cross the blood-brain barrier (e.g., Epivir, Kaletra).

PARASITES

Cryptosporidiosis ("Crypto")

This intestinal parasite is caused by the parasite *Cryptosporidium parvum*. This parasite is found in food and water contaminated by animal and feces. The parasite enters its human host when that person unknowingly eats or drinks contaminated food or water or comes in contact with contaminated feces. The parasite is very resistant to chlorine and other water treatment chemicals.

- Symptoms—The symptoms are primarily gastrointestinal in nature, characterized by profuse and watery diarrhea, abdominal cramping, fever, fatigue, loss of appetite, and nausea and vomiting.
- Risk Level—While anyone can be sickened by this parasite, people with weak immune systems, including those living with HIV, are at the highest risk. The very young, the elderly, and people with weakened immune systems for other reasons are also at risk.
- Prevention—While there is no real medicinal prevention or prophylaxis, the best way to prevent infection is good hand washing before and after going to the bathroom, after touching farm animals, and before and after changing diapers or eating. When swimming in a public pool, take care not to ingest any pool water; crypto can linger in pool water for up to six months. Finally, washing raw fruits and vegetables before eating or preparing is essential.
- Treatment—In people with healthy immune systems, cryptosporidium infection usually resolves on its own after about two weeks. During that time anti-diarrheal medications can be used to ease the symptoms and fluids should be encouraged to avoid dehydration. If medication is necessary, the drug Alinia (nitazoxanide) can be used.

Giardiasis

This is the most common intestinal parasite in the United States. The infection is caused by the protozoan parasite *Giardia lamblia*. It is transmitted as a cyst that adheres to the intestinal wall. It is spread via ingesting feces contaminated water or via the fecal-oral route in day care centers and most commonly among gay men during sexual encounters.

- Symptoms—The primary symptoms are abdominal cramping and pain, and profuse diarrhea. Secondary symptoms include the symptoms of dehydration resulting from the severe diarrhea.
- Risk Level—Men who have sex with men have a higher risk of Giardia due to the nature of their sexual encounters, specifically, the oral contact with feces during intercourse or oral sex. Those living in areas without clean, sanitary water and sewage can also be at an increased risk.
- Prevention—Good hand washing before and after using the bathroom and before and after eating are essential. Also, avoiding oral-feces contact when men are having sex with other men.
- Treatment—Even though the FDA has never approved this drug for treatment of Giardiasis, Flagyl (metronidazole) is effective in treating the parasite. The medication is well-tolerated and is effective in about 80 percent to 95 percent of patients. However, it should not be used in pregnant women and those taking the drug should avoid alcohol use.

Toxoplasmosis

Toxoplasmosis is a central nervous system infection caused by the parasite *Toxoplasma gondii (T. gondii)*. *T. gondii* is found in under-cooked meat and in soil contaminated with cat feces. That being said, most patients that get Toxoplasmosis do so because an old infection is reactivated, not because they have been exposed to a new infection.

- Symptoms—The symptoms start out mild and benign, a headache and sometimes drowsiness. As the infection gets worse the drowsiness becomes an altered level of consciousness, seizures, speech problems, and confusion. If left untreated, the infection will progress to focal weaknesses, coma, and eventually death.
- Risk Level—Those HIV-positive patients with a CD4 count less than 100 cells/mm^3 are at the highest risk for toxoplasmosis. Also, those with previous exposure and infection from *T. gondii* are at additional risk as well.
- Prevention—People living with HIV should avoid handing soil that possibly could be contaminated with T. gondii. In addition, gloves and a mask should be used when changing a cat's litter box. For those with CD4 counts less than 100 cells/mm^3 should be prescribed Bactrim (sulfamethoxazole and trimethoprim) one tablet daily or one tablet every Monday, Wednesday, and Friday. If the person has a Bactrim or sulfa allergy, NebuPent (pentamidine), Aczone (dapsone), or Mepron (atovaquone) should be used instead.
- Treatment—Standard treatment consists of a combination of Daraprim (pyrimethamine), sulfadiazine, and Bactrim DS (trimethoprim-sulfamethoxazole) orally. For those people allergic to sulfa drugs (e.g., Bactrim) Cleocin (clindamycin) can be used. In addition, an effective HIV regimen should be prescribed and taken each and every day.

The AIDS-Defining Illnesses

The previous sections described opportunistic infections that can make an HIV-positive person sick when the immune system has been weakened significantly by HIV. Some of the most serious and life threatening opportunistic infections only occur after the immune system has suffered significant damage at the hands of HIV. The most serious of these illnesses are classified as *AIDS-defining*—meaning any HIV-positive person who has had one of these infections is henceforth classified as having AIDS.

At one point early in the epidemic, an AIDS diagnosis and being diagnosed with an AIDS-defining illness (e.g., Kaposi sarcoma, PCP) was a very significant milestone. There was no HIV test, so surveillance professionals used an AIDS diagnosis and AIDS-defining illnesses to monitor and track the epidemic. Tragically, an AIDS diagnosis also meant that the person was in the late stages of infection and had very little time to live. People diagnosed with AIDS or an AIDS-defining illness would usually be very sick and/or near death. Those that weren't would quit their jobs, tie up loose ends in their life and wait for death. Simply put, an AIDS diagnosis was a death sentence.

Today, HIV testing allows for earlier diagnosis and more accurate surveillance. Most people are now being diagnosed before significant immune system damaged has occurred. The advent of HIV medications has lengthened the lifespan and slowed or even stopped the progression of HIV to AIDS. In most people with an AIDS diagnosis, death is no longer imminent. In fact, people can live for years or even decades after an AIDS diagnosis, thanks to advances in HIV treatment and the treatment of opportunistic infections. In many cases, HIV medications even help the body rebuild the immune system—meaning that people at risk for AIDS-defining illnesses can actually rebound and be less at risk than they were when they were diagnosed as having HIV and AIDS.

In short, today an AIDS diagnosis is much less significant than it once was. AIDS is an outdated term that does not change treatment or prognosis. It's merely a classification that helps surveillance agencies gauge how well we are doing in our fight to end the epidemic. Nevertheless, many people living with HIV focus on AIDS as the benchmark in their own war on HIV. The media, the general public, and even some medical professionals use the terms HIV and AIDS interchangeably. But, as we have discussed, they are not the same at all.

The following is a list of those illnesses classified as being AIDS-defining. Some we have covered already; others we will cover in future chapters.

- Bacterial infections, multiple and recurrent
- Candidiasis of bronchi, trachea, or lungs
- Cervical cancer (invasive)
- Coccidioidomycosis, Cryptococcosis, Cryptosporidiosis
- Cystoisosporiasis (formally Isosporiasis)
- Cytomegalovirus disease (CMV)
- Encephalopathy (HIV-related)
- Herpes simplex (disseminated infection)
- Histoplasmosis
- Kaposi's sarcoma (KS)
- Lymphoid interstitial pneumonia, pulmonary lymphoid hyperplasia complex
- Lymphoma (Burkitt's, immunoblastic, and primary of the brain)
- Mycobacterium avium complex (MAC)
- Pneumocystis (carinii) jirovecii pneumonia (PCP)
- Pneumonia (bacterial, recurrent)
- Progressive multifocal leukoencephalopathy (PML)
- Salmonella septicemia (recurrent)
- Toxoplasmosis of the brain
- Tuberculosis (TB)
- AIDS Wasting syndrome

In the coming chapter we will discuss other illnesses not caused by HIV directly, but which are illnesses that many people living with HIV have to battle as part of their life with the virus.

9

ASSOCIATED CONDITIONS

In the last chapter we discussed illnesses and infections that arise after the body's immune system has been damaged or weakened. The opportunistic infections that were highlighted are a direct result of immune system damage at the hands of HIV. In addition to those infections and illnesses, there are other physical and mental health issues that commonly occur in people living with HIV. Some are a result of long-term use of HIV medications. Others are stress related, arising from the stress and anxiety associated with an HIV diagnosis. And finally there are illnesses that, for one reason or another, are more common in people living with HIV. Let's explore some of the illnesses and conditions that further complicate the life of people living with HIV.

Sinusitis ("Sinus Infection"/"Inflammation of the Sinuses")

On average, about 30 percent of the adult population suffers from sinusitis ("a sinus infection") at least once each year. However, some experts believe that people living with HIV have an increased incidence of sinusitis; upwards of 60 percent to 80 percent have at least one bout of sinusitis in the past 12 months. Whether those figures are accurate or not, sinusitis is still a common affliction of people living with HIV. Sinusitis, more commonly known as a "sinus infection," can be a very uncomfortable and annoying viral or bacterial infection. The sinuses are air pockets located throughout the skull. There is one on each side of the nose ("maxillary sinuses"), behind and between the eyes ("ethmoid sinuses"), in the forehead ("frontal sinuses"), and finally, one sinus farther back in the skull ("sphenoid sinus"). There are two types of sinusitis, acute and chronic. Let's look at their similarities and differences.

Acute Sinusitis—Each sinus cavity is lined with soft pink tissue called mucosa. Typically, the sinus cavities are empty except for a thin layer of mucus on the surface of the sinus mucosa. As the mucus is renewed it drains from the sinuses through small pin holes. On occasion, these pin holes get occluded and mucus accumulates in the sinus. As the mucus continues to fill the sinuses, pain, inflammation of the lining of the sinuses, and pressure develops. Because the sinuses are warm, dark, and moist the accumulating mucus becomes a perfect growth medium for bacteria, viruses, and in extreme cases, fungi. Eventually, if the sinuses do not drain, the organisms growing in the trapped mucus cause potentially severe infection. Depending whether the sinusitis is bacterial or viral the infection can last anywhere from one to two weeks or more. Bacterial sinusitis is treated with antibiotic therapy (e.g., levofloxacin) and over-the counter medications to treat any symptoms (e.g., ibuprofen for fever and pain) that are present. One the other hand, viral sinusitis is just left to run its natural course of one to two weeks, treating any symptoms with over-the-counter medications. Any acute sinusitis that has not cleared completely after 8 weeks is considered a chronic condition.

Chronic Sinusitis—It a person continues to have the symptoms of sinusitis after 8 weeks despite treatment, the condition is considered to be chronic. Chronic sinusitis is rarely caused by an infectious agent like bacteria or viruses. Chronic sinusitis can be caused by irritation and inflammation of the sinus cavity lining due to environmental allergies (e.g., pollen), cigarette smoke, and chemicals (e.g., over-the-counter nasal sprays). Chronic sinusitis can also be caused by mechanical obstructions in the nasal passages, namely nasal polyps or a deviated septum. Chronic sinusitis is typically not treated with antibiotics unless a bacterial cause is confirmed or suspected. Usually the symptoms are treated while the cause of the chronic sinusitis is identified.

The symptoms of acute and chronic sinusitis are very much alike except the symptoms in chronic sinusitis last longer. Another difference in symptoms is the lack of fever in chronic sinusitis whereas acute sinusitis often has a fever with chills. Finally, chronic sinusitis typically causes more profound fatigue than does acute sinusitis mainly because of the length of time the person has been dealing with the symptoms.

The symptoms start out very much like a typical cold or environmental allergies: nasal congestion and drainage, clogged ears and head, and a dry scratchy throat. But as the infection starts to blossom, pain develops over the cheek bones, under and behind the eyes, and in the head and both ears. The pain is worse when the doctor taps on the cheeks with his or her fingertips. The patient will also develop a fever (acute sinusitis), headache, and what initially feels like a toothache. However, the pain is actually related to the pressure of the infected sinuses on the roots of the teeth. Ear pain and pressure along with chills and night sweats will also occur as the infection gets worse. If the infection is bad enough, the sense of smell and taste can be altered and a foul odor and taste can be present.

If the sinusitis is viral in nature, there is no antibiotic to treat the problem. Viruses usually have to run their course. Over-the-counter decongestants, pain medications, and antihistamines are used to control symptoms and to make the person comfortable while the viral sinusitis runs its natural course. If the sinusitis is bacterial, a ten to fourteen-day course of antibiotics is prescribed. That, in addition to medication to ease symptoms are the treatment of choice. Treatment for chronic sinusitis is a bit different. First, remove the causative agent meaning if there is a smoker in the house, make that person smoke outdoors. If allergies are the cause, treat the allergies with antihistamines or in an extreme case monthly allergy shots. Finally, if there are nasal polyps or a deviated septum, surgery may be needed to correct those causes. Regardless of the cause, symptom management is key to getting through an episode of sinusitis. Nasal sprays or oral decongestants can relieve head and nasal congestion. Saline nasal sprays and cool mist vaporizers can ease the dry nasal passages and throat. Finally, warm compresses to the cheeks and oral over-the-counter analgesics (pain medications) can help with facial pain and headache.

While only 2 to 10 percent of acute sinusitis is bacterial in nature, it does occur and is treated differently than viral sinusitis. But the first step is to determine if it is indeed bacterial. There are a few differences in how bacterial sinusitis presents that help the provider determine whether the sinusitis is viral or bacterial. Viral sinusitis typically lasts seven to ten days and then symptoms improve on their own. In contrast, symptoms of bacterial sinusitis can be placed in one of three categories.

Persistent—The symptoms of this category of sinusitis continue more than 10 days and really never improve without intervention. Clear to yellow or green thick mucus develops along with a daytime cough.

Severe—The symptoms in this category include a high fever (e.g., 102 to 104F orally) along with thick, green mucus and nasal drainage lasting three to four days, beginning at the onset of the illness. Viral sinusitis may have a fever that resolves after a day or two and green mucus that does not occur until after the fourth day.

Worsening—These symptoms typically follow a viral upper respiratory infection. After feeling better, the person will suddenly exhibit even worse symptoms that include high fever, severe headache, and productive cough that peaks at about five days after the initial symptoms.

Once your provider decides your sinusitis is bacterial, he or she will prescribe a course of antibiotics to treat the infection. The same interventions used to relieve viral sinusitis symptoms can be used to ease bacterial sinusitis symptoms. The important part of antibiotic therapy is completing the entire course, be it seven days, ten days, or two weeks. If the antibiotics are stopped prior to completing the entire course, the infection will recur and just like HIV, resistance to future antibiotics can develop.

Sinus infections will happen but there are ways to decrease how often. Do your best to avoid colds and influenza and those things that cause irritation of the sinus cavities (e.g., cigarette smoke). Good handwashing is a must and avoiding those people who are coughing and sneezing will decrease your risk of acquiring respiratory infections that could lead to or exacerbate sinusitis. Finally, make certain you get your yearly influenza vaccine and stay updated on your pneumococcal vaccines. If after these measures you feel you have a sinus infection, contact your doctor to see if your condition requires treatment.

Lipodystrophy/Fat Redistribution

As we have discussed in previous chapters, the advent of HIV medications in the early 1990s has meant longer and healthier lives for those people living with HIV. Since those first medication regimens, HIV treatment has become easier to take with fewer doses, fewer pills, and fewer side effects. Thanks to advances in HIV treatment, there are people who have been living with HIV for decades. However, many were prescribed those earliest regimens, notorious for unpleasant side effects. Unfortunately, many of these people are now dealing with the long term effects of the earliest HIV medications. One long-term effect is *lipodystrophy*. Lipodystrophy is a condition characterized by the redistribution of subcutaneous fat of the face, arms, and legs to subcutaneous areas of the upper back ("buffalo hump"), the neck, the visceral areas of the abdomen, the surface of the liver, and even the bloodstream. Smaller fat accumulations called *lipomas* present as fatty tumors just under the skin. This process of fat redistribution gives the body a very distinctive appearance that sufferers fear will "tip-off" family and friends to their HIV diagnosis or at the very least put into question the health of the individual.

Lipodystrophy was first identified in HIV-positive people around 1996. While aspects of the condition were identified earlier in the epidemic, experts feel, true cases of lipodystrophy emerged after 1996 when three-drug HIV medication regimens became the standard of care. It was at the Interscience Conference on Antimicrobial Agents and Chemotherapy (*ICAAC*), held in Toronto in 1997, when scientists first reported on patients who had developed increased fat deposits in and around the abdomen and the back of the neck; the problem of lipodystrophy had officially arrived.

Experts noticed that the first patients with symptoms of lipodystrophy all had one thing in common: they had been treated with a drug regimen containing a protease inhibitor (see chapter 7). As more cases of lipodystrophy emerged, the link between lipodystrophy and protease inhibitors strengthened. In fact, the connection was so compelling that experts in HIV care coined the term *"protease paunch,"* referring to the increased abdominal girth characteristic of patients diagnosed with lipodystrophy. However, it wasn't long until cases of lipodystrophy surfaced in patients that weren't taking protease inhibitors. In fact, some patients had never taken protease inhibitors. Experts changed their way of looking at lipodystrophy and in doing so formulated many theories to explain the condition.

One theory places the blame on hormonal changes common to HIV-positive people. Specifically, HIV-infected men often have abnormally low levels of the hormone testosterone. While testosterone is a male hormone, both males and females produce the hormone naturally and need sufficient quantities in order to be healthy. One of the functions of testosterone is to generate and maintain lean muscle mass. With lower than normal levels of testosterone, the body produces and stores fat instead of lean muscle. As a result, subcutaneous fat is lost from the extremities, buttocks, and face. In many cases there is an increase of visceral fat, fat found around the abdomen, as well as subcutaneous fat in the upper back, the neck, and along the jaw line. Experts agree that this theory explains the body's tendency to produce and store fat instead of lean muscle, a situation seen in the lipodystrophy patient. However, scientists point out that in some cases of lipodystrophy there is no evidence of abnormal hormone levels. In those cases, what could be responsible for lipodystrophy?

A second theory suggests that HIV medications interfere with fat metabolism. This theory does not single out the protease inhibitor class. Instead, this theory suggests that all HIV mediations interfere with fat metabolism to some degree. This theory is supported by the fact that many HIV medications contribute to higher than normal cholesterol and triglyceride levels, a sign that some HIV medications do affect the way fats are metabolized in the body. But again, this theory does not explain why patients who have never been on HIV medications can develop lipodystrophy.

A third theory suggests that HIV contributes to *insulin resistance*, which in turn interferes with proper glucose metabolism. Glucose is the energy source of every cell in the human body. During glucose metabolism, sugars taken into the body are metabolized so the cells can use them as a source of energy. Insulin is a substance produced by the body that helps transport glucose into cells so it can be used for energy. Insulin resistance is a condition where the body produces proper levels of insulin but does not use that insulin effectively to move glucose from the bloodstream into the cells where it's needed for energy. As a result, glucose accumulates in the blood and is viewed by the body as a surplus energy source. In response, the body stores the excess glucose in the form of fat distributed in tissues *("adipose tissue")* throughout the body. In other words, when glucose metabolism is interrupted due to insulin resistance, serum (blood) glucose levels are abnormally high, meaning the body needs to store this excess energy and does so in the form of body fat.

One last theory contends that lipodystrophy is just another complication of HIV. Experts explain that prior to the advent of HIV treatment, people with HIV infection didn't live long enough for the signs of lipodystrophy to become evident. With the advent of HIV medications and longer life spans, the long-term effects of HIV infection begin to emerge—in this case, the signs and symptoms of lipodystrophy. In other words, lipodystrophy is just another way HIV disrupts the normal functioning of the human body.

Typically, lipodystrophy doesn't present an imminent danger to the HIV-positive person. That being said, there are some complications that occur as a result of lipodystrophy. For instance, most of us are aware that excess fat in the body can cause conditions that are detrimental to the overall health of the individual. Examples of some metabolic disorders include high blood pressure, heart disease, peripheral vascular disease, diabetes, and elevated cholesterol and triglycerides levels. In addition, physical problems can emerge as a result of lipodystrophy as well. Many people who have lipodystrophy complain of neck pain, headaches, and, in extreme cases, difficulty breathing because of fat build-up in the abdomen, under the diaphragm, and around their neck and upper back.

The obvious physical changes of lipodystrophy can have a negative effect on a person's body-image as well. In other words, lipodystrophy can have a negative impact on the emotional self, as well as the physical self. The loss of fat in the face and extremities, and the subsequent redistribution of fat to the neck and abdomen, results in an altered physical appearance that is characteristic of lipodystrophy. Much like a person who loses a leg, the patient with lipodystrophy develops an altered image of body and self. Lipodystrophy patients fear that their physical appearance makes them look "sick." Patients fear their physical appearance may spark health-related questions from friends, coworkers, or loved ones—questions that fuel the fear their HIV diagnosis will become public, arguably an HIV-positive person's greatest fear.

People living with HIV carry that burden each and every day. For many it's the first thing they think of in the morning and the last thing they think of at night. So the last thing a positive person needs is a reminder of their HIV. That's how many feel about lipodystrophy, that it's a vivid reminder of their HIV and their chronic illness. For many, living with their diagnosis means struggling to maintain a normal day-to-day life, physically and emotionally. Seeing their altered appearance in the mirror every day becomes a constant reminder of their disease. To cope with their illness, many choose not to dwell on HIV day in and day out in an attempt to lead a "normal" life. The characteristic look of lipodystrophy makes that difficult. For some, the constant reminder is too much to bear, resulting in mental health issues (e.g., depression) on top of their lipodystrophy and HIV.

Fortunately, there is hope for those people affected by lipodystrophy. While there is no definitive cure for the condition there are a number of interventions that have proven to be effective. One method of treatment is to use drug regimens that do not contain protease inhibitors. Many feel there is still a strong link between long-term protease inhibitor use and lipodystrophy. Fortunately, the development of new medications has made it easier to assemble an HIV regimen free of protease inhibitors. Limiting the use of protease inhibitors may slow or stop lipodystrophy. However, any lipodystrophy that has occurred may remain even if protease inhibitors are eliminated. By changing medication combinations and thereby eliminating protease inhibitors from HIV regimens, one possible cause of lipodystrophy is removed. For some, this method is effective, while in others it doesn't seem to help at all. In fact, some people continue to have worsening lipodystrophy even without taking protease inhibitors. While eliminating protease inhibitors can slow or stop lipodystrophy, it may return later even in the absence of protease inhibitors.

Some success has been seen in people using improved diet and regular exercise to treat lipodystrophy. By controlling the dietary intake of fats and simple sugars (e.g., soda pop) the risk of developing lipodystrophy declines. For those who can't lower their cholesterol and triglycerides by diet and exercise, cholesterol-lowering medications (e.g., Lipitor/atorvastatin) can be prescribed. There is evidence that these drugs can lessen the extent of lipodystrophy in some people. Whether a diet low in cholesterol and triglycerides along with regular exercise can help control lipodystrophy is not entirely clear. However, the overall health benefits of such a lifestyle are well documented. We will discuss this in detail in an upcoming chapter.

Some researchers believe that hormonal therapy, specifically testosterone, may be helpful in controlling the body changes of lipodystrophy. However, the value of hormonal therapy is not entirely clear. Testosterone has its share of side effects and is not always covered by prescription drug coverage, negating any small improvement in lipodystrophy that may be gained from testosterone therapy.

At one time, people living with lipodystrophy had the option of stopping their medicines to decrease the problem of fat redistribution. However, with changes in HIV treatment guidelines over the years, the experts agree that medications should be offered and recommended for all patients regardless of HIV viral load or CD4 counts. That being the case, stopping medication regimens is really not a medically sound choice in the management of lipodystrophy. What can be done is choosing HIV regimens that minimize the risk of lipodystrophy while being an effective treatment for HIV, a task that has gotten easier over the years thanks to the advent of newer medications with less effect on body fat.

While the aforementioned treatments or interventions to combat the causes of lipodystrophy can help to some degree, there are other options that address the physical changes of lipodystrophy. However, since these options do not address the underlying cause of lipodystrophy, the effects of many of these interventions are only temporary. Still, they offer choices to patients dealing with the effects of fat redistribution. Let's look at one such option, plastic surgery.

PLASTIC SURGERY

Tummy tucks, nose jobs, and breast enhancements are all the rage these days. Don't like your hips? Have them re-sculptured. Are your "love handles" getting out of hand? Just suck out a little of that extra fat. Skilled plastic surgeons can do wonders for our appearance and self-esteem. So it's not surprising that many HIV patients have turned to plastic surgeons to ease the symptoms of lipodystrophy. There are a few plastic surgery procedures that can help.

In the early 1980s, two French plastic surgeons, Dr. Yves-Gerard Illouz and Dr. Pierre-

Francois Fournier, introduced a procedure using plastic cannulas attached to high volume suction to evacuate large amounts of excess subcutaneous fat from the abdomen and thighs. The procedure, called *liposuction*, uses large amounts of fluid to break up fat deposits, and then that broken up fat is suctioned from the affected areas. In the case of lipodystrophy, liposuction has become a viable option. However, it's only effective for removing the fat that has been deposited at the back of the neck—often called a "buffalo hump." The reason is that the "buffalo hump" is subcutaneous, meaning it is deposited directly below the skin. However, the fat deposits of abdominal lipodystrophy are in the abdominal cavity (*visceral*) and are not subcutaneous. Therefore, liposuction is not an option.

So what is done with the excess fat that has been removed? In some cases, that fat can be transferred to the face to replace fat that has been lost in the face. Simply put, the surgeon does a fat *transfer* from a place of excess fat to a place where fat has been lost. However, fat transfer is not without potential problems. First, there may not be enough fat to transfer to make a visible difference. In cases where there is plenty of fat to transfer the results often appear unnatural, "lumpy" instead of smooth. Finally, there is evidence that the fat transfer procedure itself stimulates more fat redistribution, meaning that, after the transfer, redistribution reoccurs and is often worse than before the transfer procedure.

Another plastic surgery option is the use of surgical implants. Similar to breast implants, these surgical appliances can give shape and structure to the face, cheekbones, or buttocks after the body has been misshapen by lipodystrophy. For instance, the sunken appearance of the cheeks after fat has been lost can be built up with surgical implants in order to reestablish the normal structure of the face. Surgical implants rebuild the areas and give structure where there was once only an absence of fat and a sunken appearance.

Like all surgical procedures, there are risks involved. Infection, anesthesia complications, bleeding, or procedural failures are all possibilities. In addition, because most insurance companies consider these plastic surgery procedures cosmetic, they are typically not paid for by the insurance. One exception is a "buffalo hump" that causes neck pain and difficulty breathing. In this case, insurance companies will pay for liposuction but typically require a letter of necessity from your doctor in order to cover the service. That being said, surgery and the care required after a surgical procedure can be very expensive. But despite all these potential problems, people with lipodystrophy have undergone the procedures discussed here, and for many the results have been positive.

Lactic Acidosis

Early on in the era of HIV medications, the following scenario was not uncommon. Aside from the typical nausea and occasional diarrhea common with HIV medications, the person's regimen was working well. But then the HIV-positive patient began to experience symptoms that included muscle pain, weakness, and worsening nausea and vomiting. Abdominal pain became a constant companion, as did pain, numbness, and tingling in the hands and feet. Eventually, severe weakness sent the person to the emergency room, with subsequent admission to the hospital. After some blood testing, the person was diagnosed with another HIV-related illness, a condition called *lactic acidosis*.

Our bodies are made up of trillions of cells, each one needing energy to carry on cellular functions. This energy is produced by the body during glucose (sugar) metabolism. This process occurs in the "power plant" of our cells called the *mitochondria*. In normal, healthy cells, the mitochondria produce the energy each cell needs every second of every day. The process of energy production leaves behind a byproduct known as *lactic acid*. Typically, lactic acid is metabolized by the cell and eliminated as waste from the body. But in instances where the mitochondria have been damaged and the number of functioning mitochondria is diminished, lactic acid accumulates in our cells and our bloodstream, resulting in the condition known as lactic acidosis.

But how do the cell mitochondria become damaged? In the case of people living with HIV, the exact mechanism of mitochondrial damage is not fully understood. There is one predominant theory that most HIV experts feel is the reason for HIV-related lactic acidosis. Beginning a couple years ago, experts started seeing lactic acidosis in association with the class of HIV medications known as Nucleoside Reverse Transcriptase Inhibitors (NRTIs) (see Chapter 7). In order to produce energy for the cell, the mitochondria need specific enzymes produced naturally in the body. NRTIs interfere with one of these enzymes, interrupting the mitochondria's ability to produce cellular energy and carry on cellular functions. One of these cellular functions removes lactic acid from the cell. If the number of functioning mitochondria is too low the cell is unable to remove toxic lactic acid from the body. If the condition is not corrected lactic acid builds up to toxic levels within the cell resulting in lactic acidosis.

The symptoms of lactic acidosis are mild at first. In fact, they can be so mild that some people assume they are coming down with a viral illness that will resolve after a couple of days. But left untreated, these mild symptoms will soon give way to the serious, life-threatening symptoms of lactic acidosis. A mild upset stomach gives way to severe nausea, followed soon after by frequent vomiting. A typical stomach ache becomes constant, severe abdominal pain. Fatigue and feeling "winded" becomes shortness of breath and difficulty breathing. Finally, a few minor aches, muscle weakness, and muscle stiffness become severe muscle pain and profound muscle weakness. Because the symptoms of lactic acidosis can mimic or be very similar to other, less severe conditions, the most definitive way to diagnose lactic acidosis is by a blood test. The amount of lactic acid in a small sample of blood is measured in the lab. If the amount of lactic acid exceeds normal blood levels, a diagnosis of lactic acidosis is made.

Luckily, as new medications become available, the need to use the medications associated with lactic acidosis has diminished and as such the incidence of lactic acidosis has diminished. That being said, there are still people taking older medications, the ones most associated with lactic acidosis. So it's important to understand the problem so if it occurs people will know to contact their providers as soon as possible. An early diagnosis and early intervention will lead to a more favorable prognosis and outcome. Anyone taking HIV medications should know their own body and be able to identify signs and symptoms that are out of the ordinary. Learn all you can about the medicines you take, and be alert for any signs or symptoms that may signal the onset of lactic acidosis. Once the problem develops, the only way to treat lactic acidosis is to change to an HIV regimen that does not increase the risk of lactic acidosis. Some researchers are investigating enzyme replacement as a possible answer to the condition. More importantly, scientists are developing new medications and medication regimens that are less likely to cause mitochondrial damage. As new and safer HIV medications come on the market the hope is that lactic acidosis will be a problem of the past.

Peripheral Neuropathy

Some people describe peripheral neuropathy as a burning sensation in their hands and feet. Others say it's the sting of a thousand needles. It can be a searing pain or a cold, heavy numbness. Peripheral neuropathy can make each step a tenuous chore. While the experiences with peripheral neuropathy are all different, everyone who has ever suffered from the condition agrees: peripheral neuropathy is no fun.

Peripheral neuropathy (PN) is a condition of the peripheral nervous system. The peripheral nervous system is made up of the nerves outside of the spinal cord and brain. The peripheral nerves are primarily those that send impulses from the extremities, to the spinal cord, and up the spinal cord to the brain. These are the nerves that are responsible for the sensations of touch, heat, cold and pain. Peripheral neuropathy results from damage to the insulating cover of the peripheral nerves. Think of your peripheral nerves as an electric wire composed of two parts—a copper wire covered with a plastic insulating cover. The electric current travels through the copper wire from one end of the circuit to the other. If anything comes in contact with the copper wire, the flow of electric current is interrupted. For that reason, the copper wire is insulated with a plastic cover. This plastic cover keeps the electric current flowing along the intended path. Peripheral nerves are much the same. The nerve impulses travel along the inner nerve fiber, and the outer covering of the nerve insulates the nerve, keeping the nerve impulse traveling along the intended path.

Damage to the protective covering of peripheral nerves can occur for many reasons. For instance, one of the long-term effects of diabetes is damage to the insulating cover of peripheral nerves. Poor nutrition and vitamin deficiencies can also cause peripheral neuropathy. In the case of HIV, peripheral neuropathy can be a consequence of the virus itself. Another cause of peripheral neuropathy is the result of long-term HIV medications use. Less common causes of peripheral neuropathy include viruses such as cytomegalovirus (CMV) or opportunistic infections such as the serious brain infection Progressive Multifocal Leukoencephalopathy (PML).

Among the HIV population, the most common cause of peripheral neuropathy is the long-term use of HIV medications. The HIV medications most commonly associated with peripheral neuropathy are the nucleoside reverse transcriptase inhibitors (NRTIs) (e.g., Zerit/stavudine). Other medications that cause neuropathy (but not as often) include the protease inhibitors (e.g., Norvir, ritonavir). Not everyone taking these medications will suffer from peripheral neuropathy, but the possibility should be considered when putting together HIV medication regimens. Besides those HIV medications just mentioned, there are other medications commonly used in HIV care that may contribute to or cause peripheral neuropathy. They include INH (isoniazid), Myambutol (ethambutol), Flagyl (metronidazole) and Dapsone (diamino-diphenyl sulphone).

Unfortunately, there is no cure for peripheral neuropathy. Even stopping the medications suspected of causing peripheral neuropathy may not relieve the symptoms or halt its progression. In some unfortunate cases, peripheral neuropathy becomes permanent even after removing the cause. However, there are ways to ease the symptoms, both medicinal and non-medicinal. The drugs Neurontin (gabapentin) and Lyrica (pregabalin) are the most commonly prescribed drugs to relieve the symptoms of peripheral neuropathy. The antidepressants Elavil (amitryptyline) and Pamelor (nortriptyline) increase peripheral nerve impulses, easing the numbness and tingling of neuropathy. Finally, in mild cases, non-steroidal anti-inflammatory medications such as ibuprofen (Motrin, Advil) can be used to relieve the pain of peripheral neuropathy. However, in moderate to severe cases, stronger pain relievers are necessary to make the patient comfortable. The narcotic pain reliever Norco (hydrocodone + acetaminophen) can be utilized, but it must be done with extreme care and caution.

Opiate containing medications (e.g., Norco) are very effective in the treatment of acute pain but they must be used properly. Opiates are a class of medication with a very high potential for misuse, diversion, addiction, and dependence. They are very effective pain relievers but users of the medication grow accustomed to doses very quickly, meaning dose escalation becomes a very real problem soon after the medication is started. For instance, at first one tablet of Norco every six hours works well, relieving the pain of neuropathy effectively. But after a short time, a person starts to need more than one tablet every 6 hours; instead, that person needs two tablets every six hours to get the same degree of pain relief he or she used to get from one tablet. This type of dose escalation can continue unchecked if not managed closely by the physician. While this medication has a high risk of escalation, addiction, and dependence, studies have suggested that the incidence of addiction and dependence is less likely in those people who truly need something as strong as Norco for adequate pain relief. Nonetheless, physicians prescribe Norco (hydrocodone + acetaminophen) only after weighing the risks and benefits and only after other, non-narcotic options have been tried and have failed.

There are non-medicinal ways to ease the symptoms of peripheral neuropathy as well. Shoes should be loose fitting to maximize nerve impulses and blood flow to the extremities. Walking long distances or standing for long periods of time should be avoided. There have even been some documented benefits of wearing magnets in the shoes and socks of people with peripheral neuropathy. However, before investing any money on this method of symptom relief, great care should be used due to the high incidence of fraud associated with such unconventional forms of treatment.

At the earliest sign of peripheral neuropathy symptoms, patients should consult with their doctor. Typically, the sooner the peripheral neuropathy is addressed the better chance the person has to recover without lasting or life-long symptoms. The longer the cause of neuropathy is left unaddressed, the more nerve damage will be done. In other words, if left untreated the chances are good that the peripheral neuropathy will become permanent. Eliminating the cause or causes before too much damage is done to the peripheral nerve sheaths is the key to recovery.

Depression

Everyone has had days during which they feel a little "blue." We have all been "down in the dumps" or felt "blah" at one time or another. But when these feelings become your daily companion, when there are more days of feeling "blue" then there are not, you may be suffering from a condition known as depression. And you would not be alone. In fact, depression affects more than 10 million Americans each year. One in four people will have an episode of depression sometime in their lifetime. However, if the physical stresses of HIV were not enough, people living with HIV are five to ten times more likely to suffer from a mood disorder, which includes depression, than people without HIV.

By definition, depression is an alteration in mood that affects a person's ability to function from day to day. While short episodes of feeling down are considered normal variations in mood, longer-lasting feelings of despair are indicative of depression. Keep in mind the effects of depression are not only emotional. Physical manifestations, such as changes in appearance or behavior, are common. Physical illnesses such as indigestion, headaches, insomnia, and chronic pain can all be part of depression as well. Depression is a serious illness with symptoms that should not be ignored. If ignored or left untreated depression can have catastrophic consequences.

There are countless factors that can affect mood and the emotional health of an individual. Emotional stability is maintained by a delicate balance of chemicals in the brain. If those chemicals are out of balance, alterations in mood (e.g., depression) will occur. Chemical imbalances are triggered by life events such as losing a loved one, divorce, physical or emotional trauma, narcotic withdrawal, or a chronic illness (e.g., HIV). Family history and genetics can also predispose a person to the chemical imbalances that cause depression. Finally, some medications can cause alterations in mood as part of their side effect profiles. Examples include the HIV medications Sustiva (efavirenz) and those combination medications that contain Sustiva (efavirenz), namely Atripla (efavirenz + emtricitabine + tenofovir). In fact, many HIV specialists will also prescribe an antidepressant when using an HIV regimen containing Sustiva (efavirenz).

As is the case with physical illnesses, there are early signs and symptoms that signal the onset of depression. Recognizing these early symptoms is the key to a favorable outcome and in some cases recognizing these early symptoms can save a life. Diagnosing depression in its early stages means starting treatment earlier in the course of the disease. In most cases, early treatment translates to a less complicated course and a better prognosis. On the opposite end of the spectrum, untreated depression can make HIV treatment even more difficult, typically because people who are depressed have a hard time adhering to medication regimens and physician appointments. In fact, as depression worsens the person becomes less and less engaged in their health and life in general. If left untreated, depression can progress to harmful and even life-threatening behaviors, for the depressed person and people around him as well.

The Core Symptoms of Depression

There is a collection of symptoms that will occur at some point in most cases of depression. Subdued mood with a loss of energy or feelings of being "run down" are very common among those who are depressed. Often times, people with depression will lose interest in those activities they once found to be very enjoyable. People who are depressed find that concentration is difficult and that mental function slows. In addition, depressed people will feel physically ill, with significant pain and muscle soreness. And finally, depressed people report decreased appetite with significant sleep issues including problems falling asleep; episodes of waking in the middle of the night; and finally problems falling asleep after waking during the night. In fact, the sleeping issues become so bad that often times sleeping medications have to be prescribed just so people can get the sleep they need to function throughout the day. If sleeping problems are not addressed, depression can become worse due to the effects of sleep deprivation.

Physical Symptoms

In addition to those core symptoms, there are other physical manifestations of depression, including headaches, fatigue, excessive sleep, heartburn, stomach upset, indigestion, and unexplained weight loss. In addition, pain in the joints, muscles, or bones can be significant and debilitating, resulting in the inability or lack of desire to hold a job, attend school, or in the case of HIV, adhere to prescribed medications.

The Most Serious Symptoms

Depression can progress and have serious consequences if left untreated. Living day to day with such profound feelings of physical and emotional pain can become too much for a person to bear. Eventually, feelings of hopelessness give way to anxiety, guilt or helplessness. Feeling helpless and unable to shake the feelings of sadness, people search for a way to end their suffering. They try to find an escape from the pain. Many will withdraw from family, loved ones, and society in general, isolating themselves from the world around them. Some will try and run away from their problems, they will move to another city, they will run to other relationships, they will try and put their current life behind them. Others will choose drugs or alcohol in order to mask the emotional and physical pain. Unfortunately, many people choose the ultimate escape—they choose to end their life by suicide. Initially people will think about suicide as a way out but won't take the next step. However, if left untreated, the depressed person will eventually act on his feelings and attempt suicide. Unfortunately, in too many cases, suicide attempts are successful.

But there is hope for those people suffering from depression. Treatment options are available that can help people dig themselves out from under the painful weight of depression. An assortment of effective antidepressants is available; the good news is that most are covered by prescription insurance. While some antidepressants have significant side effects, many are well tolerated and very effective. But medications alone aren't the answer. Antidepressants should be prescribed in conjunction with professional mental health counseling in order to find the root cause of the depression. Think of it this way. If you break your arm you take medication to relieve the pain. However, the medication does nothing to treat the root of the pain—the broken bone. For that, a cast is needed. So it is with depression. While antidepressants can relieve the unpleasant symptoms of depression, counseling will help you identify what has caused the symptoms of depression in the first place. Discussing your depression with a professional counselor will help you identify the cause or causes of your depression and will provide you with the tools you need to deal with your feelings in a healthy manner,

It can't be stressed enough how important it is for you to recognize feelings and symptoms of depression and to make your HIV physician aware of the feelings you are having. Recognizing the following symptoms of depression can literally save your life or save the life of a loved one. If you have any of the following symptoms contact your physician immediately:

- thoughts of death, hurting one's self or hurting others;
- having suicidal thoughts or making a suicide plan;

- depressed mood that may or may not be accompanied by episodes of being tearful or frequent crying;
- decreased interest in previously enjoyable activities or events;
- being unable to concentrate;
- being unwilling to get out of bed each morning;
- excessive sleeping but feeling fatigue despite the increased number of hours you are sleeping;
- being unable to find pleasure or satisfaction in most all activities or sources of entertainment;
- feelings of anxiety, restlessness, guilt, or anger accompanied by mood swings, lack of patience, or sudden outbursts;
- and finally, problems falling asleep and staying asleep.

If you feel you have any of these symptoms or if you just don't "feel like yourself," call your doctor immediately. If you have thoughts of suicide or feel like you want to hurt yourself or others, go to the nearest emergency room or psychiatric emergency room. Finally, if you are close to someone with these symptoms and feelings, encourage them to call their doctor or go to the emergency room or psychiatric emergency room as soon as possible.

Anxiety/Anxiety Disorder

Everyone experiences anxiety now and again. Feeling anxious in certain situations is completely normal in fact. Anxiety becomes an issue when it begins to interfere with your normal lifestyle. But what is anxiety exactly? Anxiety is defined as a state of uneasiness or apprehension surrounding a future event or situation. But unlike other conditions associated with HIV, anxiety is not a medical problem. It's actually a behavioral issue, either in the way you think or the way you act with regard to a given situation. But what happens when your anxiety starts to negatively impact your lifestyle. For instance, you are anxious about a diagnostic test your doctor has ordered. Your mind becomes so consumed with the upcoming test you can't concentrate, you can't sleep, you can't perform your normal day-to-day activities. When this occurs, your anxiety has become a disorder. If your anxiety is affecting your daily life, then chances are it is affecting your medication adherence, meaning your HIV is eventually going to cause problems by weakening your immune system. For that reason, you should be able to recognize the symptoms of anxiety and how to deal with them affectively.

Regardless of whether or not your anxiety has reached the level of an anxiety disorder, the symptoms are the same. The only difference is how long they last and how much they impact your day-to-day life. Symptoms of anxiety can vary from person to person; can vary from male to female; and can vary between different age groups. The following are the most common symptoms of anxiety. The symptoms of anxiety include:

- a feeling of uneasiness;
- being worried or concerned regarding an upcoming event or situation;
- being alert and "on edge" due to a feeling of impending danger;

- over react to situations or things perceived as dangerous;
- sudden panic attacks characterized by a rapid heart rate, altered breathing, nausea, and sweating;
- tremors or nervous tics or actions (e.g., wringing the hands; biting fingernails)
- heart palpitations;
- feeling of "gloom and doom."

There are many ways to address anxiety, apprehension, and fearful behavior. The best way is to seek a professional well versed in the treatment of anxiety and anxiety disorders. Because anxiety is an issue of behavior, the key is to eliminate the root cause of the anxiety. Once you eliminate the cause of the anxiety or apprehension, the symptoms should resolve as well. Seek out therapists who are aware of the dynamics of anxiety and can provide you with tools to not only deal with the symptoms of anxiety but can help you find the root cause of your anxiety. The tendency of many people is to ask for medication, specifically, antianxiety drugs such as Valium (diazepam), to achieve a rapid fix, a quick and effortless method of relieving anxiety. While there are circumstances that could benefit from short term medication interventions, most experts agree that long-term use of drugs like Valium does more harm than good. Many of the medications used for rapid relief of anxiety have a high incidence of dose escalation, dependence, and addiction. While they do a great job of alleviating anxiety in the short-term, becoming dependent or becoming addicted to one of these antianxiety drugs will have long-term negative effects on a person's health. In fact, eventually, being dependent on these drugs could create anxiety over such things as getting to the next dose and getting to the next prescription. If at all possible, non-medicinal methods of dealing with anxiety are always preferred.

Elevated Cholesterol and Triglycerides

It's no secret: a well-balanced diet is one of the keys to a healthy life. One aspect of good nutrition is maintaining the right amount of fat in your blood. Two substances that we talk about when assessing the level of fat in your blood are *cholesterol* and *triglycerides*.

Cholesterol

Cholesterol is a naturally occurring, soft, fatty substance produced in the liver and found circulating in your bloodstream. It's a critical ingredient in the construction of cell walls and membranes throughout the body. Cholesterol also allows for the production of hormones, vitamin D, and the fat-digesting substance known as bile. Cholesterol is also found outside of the body in foods such as meats, dairy products, and eggs. While cholesterol is an important substance throughout the body, only a small amount of cholesterol is needed, and the body produces that naturally. Cholesterol from food sources is seen as extra by the body. Extra cholesterol is deposited on the walls of blood vessels around the body, especially blood vessels in the heart, the carotid artery, and the legs. Surplus cholesterol is also deposited within liver tissue.

To understand the effects of cholesterol deposited on the walls of blood vessels, think of blood vessels as drainpipes in your kitchen. When soap scum and food from your dishes builds up on the inside walls of drainpipes, the flow of water through the drain is slowed. Eventually, as more and more soap scum and food builds up on the walls of the pipes, the flow of water will stop altogether. The same is true when cholesterol clogs blood vessels. The flow of blood to a vital organ such as the heart is diminished. As more cholesterol is deposited on the vessel walls, the blood flow will eventually stop altogether, depriving the organ of blood and oxygen. This results in damage to the organ and as a result diminished function of that organ. In the case of the heart, when the flow of blood to the heart muscle is stopped, the muscle is damaged and is no longer able to pump blood effectively; the person suffers a *myocardial infarction,* commonly known as a heart attack.

When excess cholesterol deposits in the liver, the function of the liver is compromised. Liver tissue filters the blood of impurities. When the liver has fat and cholesterol deposits in the tissue, the liver's function will eventually be compromised. That being said, fatty liver is reversible by simply decreasing the amount of fats and cholesterol taken into the body and circulating in the blood. Unfortunately, the same can't be said about cholesterol deposited in the lining of blood vessels. While the amount deposited can be slowed, the cholesterol already deposited is there for good. In fact, as time passes the cholesterol on the vessel walls changes from soft and fatty, to hard plaques that can eventually block blood flow altogether, once again resulting in a heart attack.

While the body needs cholesterol, it needs only what it makes naturally. Therefore, it is important to make certain that the diet is not adding excess cholesterol to the body. By limiting fat and simple sugar intake, the amount of circulating cholesterol can be controlled and kept to only what is needed. Doing that will help avoid heart disease, liver disease, and obesity in general.

TRIGLYCERIDES

Triglycerides are the chemical form in which most fats exist, both in the foods we eat and in our body. They are often called "sugary fats" because they are composed of three fatty acids (fat molecules) and glycerol (a sugar molecule). Triglycerides in our blood are derived from fats eaten in foods or made in the body from other energy sources, namely sugars. Excessive calories that are not used for energy are converted to triglycerides and transported to fat cells to be stored. Hormones regulate the release of triglycerides from fat tissue so they meet the body's energy needs between meals. Like cholesterol, the body needs triglycerides to function normally—but only in the right amounts. Excessive triglycerides in the bloodstream increases the risk of serious health issues, particularly heart disease.

HIGH DENSITY LIPIDS (HDL)/LOW DENSITY LIPIDS (LDL)

In many respects it's often not how much fat you have in your diet but what types of fat you are eating. For instance, eating the type of fat in red meat is much less healthy than eating the type of fat in fish. Eating the type of fat in a handful of macadamia nuts is much less healthy than eating the type of fat in a handful of unsalted almonds. Experts agree that too much fat is bad for your health, but there are types of fat that are actually better for you than others. In fact, some fats have been shown to decrease your risk of heart disease. It's important to know which are the "good fats" and which are the "bad fats." There are two types of cholesterol.

- High Density Lipids (HDL)—Also known as "good cholesterol," these lipids carry harmful fatty deposits away from cells and tissues to the liver for excretion from the body. An HDL that is too low actually increases your risk of heart disease because without HDL the harmful fatty deposits aren't carried to the liver for excretion.
- Low Density Lipids (LDL)—Also known as "bad cholesterol," these lipids account for most of the cholesterol in the blood. They carry lipids to the tissues by way of the blood vessels. Bad cholesterol is deposited on vessel walls, causing the vessels to become narrowed and eventually clogged entirely. Heart and vascular disease is a result of blood vessels that have been clogged by bad cholesterol. Blood flow through narrowed and clogged vessels is diminished, making it more difficult to provide adequate oxygen and nutrients to muscles, organs, and tissues throughout the body. Tissues that do not get the needed amounts of oxygen and nutrients are damaged, the heart muscle included.

FACTORS CAUSING HIGH CHOLESTEROL

We have established that having too much cholesterol and triglycerides circulating in the blood is bad for your health. There are many factors that can affect the levels of cholesterol in your blood. Some of these factors are out of our control. These factors include:

- a family history of high cholesterol;
- a genetic tendency and sensitivity to lifestyle factors that can increase cholesterol; and
- a family history of certain diseases/conditions (e.g., diabetes) that increase cholesterol and triglycerides.

But many of the factors contributing to higher than normal cholesterol and triglycerides are under our control. They include:

- a diet high in fats and carbohydrates (sugars);
- a lifestyle with little or no exercise; and
- being obese or overweight.

Many of the factors mentioned contribute to higher than normal cholesterol and triglycerides in the HIV-positive person. In addition, certain HIV medications interfere with the fat metabolism, resulting in elevated triglycerides and cholesterol in the blood.

There is growing evidence that people taking some protease inhibitors are at an increased risk of elevated cholesterol and triglycerides and therefore an increased risk of heart disease. There is evidence that cholesterol and triglycerides are highest in people taking regimens containing a protease inhibitor boosted by Norvir (ritonavir). While most protease inhibitors can cause an elevation to some degree, it's boosted protease inhibitors that cause the most profound rise in cholesterol and triglycerides. However, drug manufacturers are developing improved protease inhibitors that do not affect triglycerides and cholesterol. One example of a protease inhibitor that does not elevate cholesterol or triglycerides is Reyataz (atazanavir). Even when boosted with Norvir (ritonavir), Reyataz (atazanavir) is less likely to elevate cholesterol and triglycerides when compared to other protease inhibitors.

There are steps you can take to keep your cholesterol and triglycerides under control. Treatment for elevated triglycerides and cholesterol usually starts with non-medicinal options—namely, diet and exercise. Typically, for people with elevated cholesterol and triglycerides, the instructions would be to reduce the amount of fats you eat. However, for people living with HIV, decreasing the amount of fats in your diet may not be so easy. Ironically, some protease inhibitors need some fat in the diet in order for the drug to be absorbed properly. Many HIV-positive people are underweight due to the effects of their disease. Limiting fat intake in these people may not be in their best interest. So in these special circumstances, changing the type of fats in the diet is a better option. The best way to do that is to learn how to read food labels. The Food and Drug Administration (FDA) requires food manufacturers to place labels on all their product packaging, itemizing what is contained in each product. The food labels list the ingredients of the product, how much fat, sugar, and protein is in the product, and how many calories are contained in each serving of the product. By reading and understanding labels, you can make sure you are eating the right types of fat in the proper amounts.

As we touched on earlier, some fats are better for you than others. For instance, animal fats, dairy fats, and foods containing palm oil contain the type of cholesterol and triglycerides that are most detrimental to your health. Limiting the unhealthiest fats in your diet will help decrease bad cholesterol and triglycerides in your body. On the other hand, certain fats, such as those contained in fish, flaxseed, and linseeds, are good for your overall health and should be eaten several times each week. Finally, replacing red meats with chicken, turkey, or tofu can cut down the amounts of bad fat that ultimately elevate your cholesterol and triglycerides.

As hard as we try, eventually it may take more than just changes in your diet to get your cholesterol and triglycerides under control. When dietary changes no longer maintain your cholesterol and triglycerides at an acceptable level, it may be necessary to consider cholesterol-lowering medications. There are several cholesterol-lowering drugs to choose from, depending on the level of cholesterol, triglycerides, HDL, and LDL. For example, there are medications that can lower your cholesterol, others lower your triglycerides, and still others lower both. There are even medications that are designed specifically to lower bad cholesterol (LDL) while elevating your good cholesterol (HDL).

Kidney Disease/Fanconi Syndrome

As people with HIV are living longer and thus taking medications longer, adverse effects of some of the HIV medications are starting to come to light. We have known for many years that many of our HIV medications have some adverse side effects: nausea and vomiting to name a couple. But as people live much longer and treatment guidelines have most everyone taking HIV medication regimens, others are starting to emerge. Arguably the most serious and potentially damaging of those adverse effects is kidney disease, specifically, *Fanconi Syndrome.*

To understand Fanconi Syndrome, we first have to have a basic understanding of how the kidneys function. The kidneys are fist-size organs that are responsible for several important bodily functions. These include:

- remove waste products from the body;
- remove drugs from the body;
- fluid balance within the body;
- regulate blood pressure;
- Vitamin D production; and
- control the production of red blood cells.

Each of your two kidneys is positioned in the low back, one on each side of the spine just below the lowest rib. Each kidney consists of millions of functioning units called *nephrons*. Each nephron consists of a *glomerulus* attached to a *tubule*. The very small blood vessels in the glomerulus allow the blood to be filtered much like coffee through a coffee filter. The fluid that remains after the filtering flows through the tubules. Water, minerals, electrolytes, and other chemicals are either added to the fluid or reabsorbed from the fluid to produce the urine that is excreted from the body. Urine is the collection of waste material left over after the filtering and reabsorption processes that take place in the glomeruli and tubules in the kidneys.

Fanconi syndrome is a defect in the functioning of the tubules. Specifically, the tubule no longer reabsorbs the electrolytes, water, and minerals, resulting in these essential substances being lost in the urine. As a result, the body becomes deficient in those essential substances, eventually causing illness and dehydration. But what causes this defect in the tubules? In many people with Fanconi Syndrome, the tubule defect is hereditary. But in people living with HIV, the first thing providers look at is the HIV medication regimen. Some HIV medications can cause tubule damage after being taken for extended periods. One medication implicated in Fanconi Syndrome in HIV positive people is Viread (tenofovir). Either taken as a single drug within a regimen, or as part of several medication combinations, Viread (tenofovir) has been implicated in Fanconi Syndrome among HIV positive people. And as such, providers are monitoring their patients' kidney function much closer when they are taking a tenofovir containing regimen.

Symptoms of Fanconi syndrome can include:

- frequent urination especially at night;
- abnormal lab findings, including glucose and protein in the urine, electrolyte imbalances in the blood, and a Vitamin D deficiency;
- bone pain; and
- muscle weakness.

The treatment for Fanconi Syndrome first centers around removing the agent that is causing the problem; in the case of HIV positive patients, removing the tenofovir or tenofovir-containing combination medication. Then, the fluid volume loss and the electrolyte imbalances must be corrected. Luckily, if the causative agent is removed, Fanconi Syndrome is reversible. However, if the offending medication is not removed, the tubule damage could be permanent.

Non-Alcoholic Fatty Liver Disease (NAFLD)

We mentioned earlier in this chapter that excess fat circulating in the body can be deposited in the liver tissue resulting in compromised liver function. With the concern over fat redistribution and lipodystrophy understanding fatty liver is important for anyone living with HIV. Let's take a closer look at fatty liver and how it can impact the lives of people living with HIV.

Non-alcoholic Fatty Liver Disease (NAFLD) is a condition of fat accumulation in the liver in the absence of excessive alcohol use. In the U.S., the incidence of NAFLD in the general population ranges from 14 to 31 percent. However, certain groups within the general population have an even higher incidence. For instance, adults who are obese have an incidence around 67 percent and those who have larger than normal waist circumferences have a high incidence of NAFLD as well. In fact, as the body mass index (BMI) increases so does the risk of NAFLD. In the HIV population, the risk of NAFLD is higher than the general population, around 40 percent. Research has shown that HIV medication regimens increase the incidence of NAFLD. In fact, studies indicate that the risk of NAFLD increases each year an HIV-positive person has been taking an NRTI-containing regimen (e.g., regimen containing Viread/tenofovir).

So how does a person know if they have NAFLD? In most cases of NAFLD there are no symptoms that can definitively diagnose the condition. If symptoms do occur, they mimic many other issues and conditions, some related to liver disease and some that are not. The non-specific symptoms you may see in NAFLD include:

- fatigue,
- weakness,
- weight loss,
- nausea,
- loss of appetite,
- abdominal pain

In extreme cases of liver dysfunction, yellowing of the skin and the whites of the eye may occur. However, this would be in the later stages of liver failure and typically is not related exclusively to NAFLD. That being said, NAFLD can cause changes to the liver tissue called *cirrhosis*. As cirrhosis progresses, jaundice (yellowing of the skin) and accumulation of fluid in the abdominal cavity (ascites) are common.

Because NAFLD lacks specific symptoms that aid diagnosis, imaging using ultrasound or CT scan is the best option when diagnosing NAFLD. Actual biopsy of liver tissue can also aid in diagnosis but is much more invasive and has more potential for complications. Biopsy is the best choice for diagnosing cirrhosis, however, and is important as indicators of liver dysfunction progress and cirrhosis becomes more likely.

The treatment for NAFLD falls into two categories, treating the development of fatty deposits in the liver and preventing the pathologic cellular changes that take place in the liver due to steatosis (fatty liver). Factors that decrease fatty liver include weight loss, medications to treat insulin resistance, and medications to treat elevated serum lipids (cholesterol and triglycerides). Bariatric surgery and weight loss medications have shown promise in decreasing the incidence of fatty liver by decreasing body fat. Medications like Glucophage (metformin) and Glucotrol (glipizide) help manage elevated blood sugar due to insulin resistance while Lipitor (atorvastatin) and Zocor (simvastatin) manage elevated serum lipids that contribute to fatty liver.

The second category of treatment is addressing the pathologic changes to the liver that occur when fatty liver is present. Simply put, this treatment category attempts to prevent the cellular changes that occur in the liver when fatty liver is an issue. Various medications address such issues as chronic inflammation and oxidative damage. For instance, the medication Urso-diol (Ursodeoxycholic acid) has been shown to have an anti-inflammatory action that helps diminish pathologic changes to liver tissue. Anti-oxidants such as vitamin E can decrease the amount of pathologic changes as a result of oxidative processes. Unfortunately, there are no currently available medications that prevent the fibrotic changes of cirrhosis, a late compli-cation of fatty liver.

Vitamin D Deficiency

Vitamin D is one of many minerals found in the body, each one necessary for the healthy functioning of the human body. In the case of Vitamin D, it's necessary for healthy and strong bone growth; for proper functioning of the immune system; for maintaining proper calcium levels in the body; and finally helping to maintain mood and emotional health. Unlike most other vitamins, Vitamin D is only found in a few food sources, namely certain fish and fortified food sources like milk and breakfast cereal. The primary method of Vitamin D production is exposure to sunlight.

So how does sunlight produce the Vitamin D we need every day? When our skin is exposed to sunlight, the ultraviolet light causes the body to release cholesterol into the blood-stream. The cholesterol travels to the liver via the bloodstream where is it converted to *25-hydroxyvitamin D (25HD)*, a precursor of active Vitamin D. The 25HD then travels via the bloodstream to the kidneys where it is converted to the active form of vitamin d, *1,25 dihydroxyvitamin D*. The newly formed Vitamin D is reabsorbed back into the bloodstream by the kidney tubules and is transported to areas of need throughout the body.

Under normal circumstances the kidneys and liver keep the blood's Vitamin D level pre-cisely at the level needed for normal body function. But situations and conditions can arise that interfere with the proper level of Vitamin D. Conditions that can result in lower than normal Vitamin D level include:

- liver or kidney disease;
- conditions that affect the proper reabsorption of Vitamin D in the gastrointestinal tract;
- Fanconi Syndrome (see previous section) that interferes with reabsorption of Vitamin D by kidney tubules;
- disrupted Vitamin D production (e.g., caused by HIV medications);
- illness and disease (e.g., HIV);
- and insufficient Vitamin D production or dietary intake.

People who have a Vitamin D deficiency in all likelihood will be asymptomatic. If there are symptoms, they mimic many other illnesses so diagnosing Vitamin D deficiency by symp-toms is not done. Instead, a blood test is done to measure the amount of circulating 25HD, the precursor to the active form of Vitamin D. Depending on the laboratory running the test, the normal range of 25HD can vary a bit. However, the typical normal level of 25HD ranges from 25ng/ml of blood to 100ng/ml, with an optimal range of 30ng/ml to 50ng/ml.

For those people whose Vitamin D levels are lower than normal, a Vitamin D supplement can be prescribed by their HIV providers. There are many ways to prescribe the Vitamin D. One such approach is to prescribe Vitamin D3 (cholecalciferol), 50,000 international units (IU) taken once each week for 8 consecutive weeks, followed by 2000IU of Vitamin D2 (ergocalciferol) once daily thereafter. You may notice that two different types of Vitamin D are being used for replacement therapy. Vitamin D3 is the type of Vitamin D found in animals while Vitamin D2 is the plant form of Vitamin D. While you can use either form, some studies suggest vitamin D3 is the form that best raises 25HD levels in your blood. Your provider will recheck the 25HD level a couple weeks after the 8-week high dose Vitamin D course is completed. Please note that at some doses, Vitamin D supplements are over-the-counter and as such are seldom paid for by medical insurance. The 50,000IU of Vitamin D3, however, is a prescription dose and is typically covered by medical insurance. Your local pharmacist can provide more details regarding doses and coverage.

While Vitamin D deficiency is very common among HIV-positive people, Vitamin D toxicity can occur. Vitamin D is one of the fat-soluble vitamins meaning you can accumulate too much Vitamin D in your blood. However, the only way to have excessive amounts of Vitamin D in your blood is by taking excessive amounts of Vitamin D supplements. Studies have estimated that an average size person would have to take 50,000IU once a day for several months before toxicity would occur. That being said, Vitamin D toxicity does occur and can cause the following:

- excessive calcium levels (hypercalcemia) in the blood;
- poor appetite;
- nausea and/or vomiting;
- muscle weakness;
- frequent urination;
- and kidney problems.

The best way to treat Vitamin D toxicity is to discontinue the vitamin supplements that have caused the toxicity. In extreme cases intravenous fluids and even small doses of steroids can be used. While Vitamin D toxicity is a very rare occurrence you are at a higher risk if you suffer from other medical conditions, most notably kidney disease. Talk to your doctor if you are concerned about your Vitamin D level, whether you think it is too low or too high. Having a normal Vitamin D level is part of a healthy body, physically as well as emotionally.

Avascular Necrosis (AVN)

The success of HIV medications, namely the longer, healthier lives resulting from Highly Active Antiretroviral Therapy (HAART) has made HIV medication regimens a constant in the homes of HIV-positive people. Since the advent of HAART, new complications associated with long-term medication use and complications associated with a long life of HIV positivity are becoming more common. One such complication is *Avascular Necrosis (AVN)*. By breaking down the two words Avascular Necrosis, it's rather obvious what the term means. "Avascular" meaning without blood vessels and "Necrosis" meaning cellular death describes a condition where cellular death occurs due to the absence of a suitable blood supply. In the case of avascular necrosis, the condition refers to cellular death of bone; most commonly death of the humeral head; the ball at the very end of the upper leg bone (femur). The humeral head is one half of the ball and socket that makes up the hip joint. There is a similar ball and socket joint that makes up the shoulder and this joint too can be affected by AVN. Over time AVN destroys bone in these joints, resulting in severe pain, fractures, and ultimately lack of function.

Since the era of HAART, the incidence of AVN is higher than the general population. The reason for the increased incidence is not entirely understood but experts have found conditions, illness, and behaviors that may contribute to the development of AVN. Those factors than can increase the risk include:

- a history of taking HAART, especially if taking long-term;
- protease inhibitors included in their HIV medication regimen;
- elevated cholesterol and triglycerides;
- steroid use;
- smoking and/or alcohol use;
- and a CD4 count less than or equal to 200 cells/mm^3.

Experts have also found that 73 percent of patients with AVN actually fall into at least two of these factor categories at the same time (e.g., smoking with an elevated cholesterol).

AVN most commonly affects the hip but can affect the shoulders, knees, feet, or hands. The onset of symptoms is very insidious meaning symptoms are slow to emerge and can be very mild at first. In fact, many people initially will have no symptoms at all. In the case of the hip joint, as the condition worsens, pain will develop but only when bearing weight. As time goes on, eventually pain will be present even when lying down and when at rest. When the hip joint is involved, pain will be gradual and typically be in the groin, buttocks, or thigh. As damage to the bone worsens and bone loss continues, the joint becomes weak and eventually will fracture, causing severe pain. Eventually, the affected bone or bones can lose so much structural integrity that they resemble honeycomb or sawdust. The damage will negatively impact mobility, especially if the person has AVN in both hips at the same time. So what happens to the blood supply and why is the bone dying in the first place?

Organs of the human body need to be well-nourished with oxygen delivered to them by the blood. The same holds true for skin, hair, muscle and even bone. When that blood flow is disrupted, the body's systems are deprived of the oxygen and nutrients that are essential to their health and well-being. Such is the case in avascular necrosis. The bone death of AVN is due to an interruption of the blood supply. Without nutrient-rich, oxygenated blood, cellular death and bone loss will eventually occur. As more cell death occurs, the structure of bones, particularly the hip bone, weakens and eventually collapses and fails, causing pain and destruction of the bone, and with it a loss of hip function. As stated, AVN typically involves the hip bone and joint but can involve most any bone, including the femur (leg), the humerus (arm), the foot, the hand, and the jaw.

There are many reasons blood flow to the hip is disrupted. For instance, vessel damage resulting from trauma to the bone and vessels themselves will disrupt blood flow. Vascular disease narrows blood vessels of the hip, diminishing blood flow, which in turn diminishes the oxygen and nutrients that reach the bone cells. Finally, there is documented evidence that long-term exposure to certain medications, including protease inhibitors and steroids, can damage the blood vessels that supply the hip, once again resulting in cellular death and destruction of the hip bone and joint.

Because symptoms appear relatively late in the condition, they are not a suitable method of diagnosing AVN. Neither are basic hip X-rays. The most definitive way to diagnose AVN is by *Magnetic Resonance Imaging (MRI)*. MRI is a specialized type of imaging that uses magnetic and radio waves instead of X-rays to examine internal structures of the body. These waves are linked to a computer which creates a very detailed image of body structures—in the case of AVN, the hip bone and joint.

Unfortunately, even after diagnosis there are few treatment options for those people found to suffer from AVN. Prescription narcotics are often needed for pain control, especially in advanced stages of the disease. There are medications that can reduce the swelling of surrounding tissues, decreasing pain and reducing the need for narcotics. Most often this intervention is only effective for the treatment of mild to moderate disease. Once the disease progresses to bones that collapse and fracture, narcotic pain relievers are necessary for comfort.

While there are a few options to treat the symptoms that result from AVN, there are very few options to actually treat the cause of the debilitating condition. And, unfortunately, once bone death occurs, that bone tissue is lost permanently. Remember, even if there was a way to grow bone to replace that which has died, the same diminished blood flow that caused the death in the first place persists. In order to halt the loss of bone due to poor blood supply, blood flow to the area must be improved or restored. The way to restore blood supply is through vascular surgery. Blood flow to the area can be improved or restored using delicate and complex vascular surgery procedures. Some people will benefit from these vascular repairs, slowing or even stopping bone cell death. However, while these procedures can be helpful in some people, they are typically a short-term solution that does not help everyone. The most effective way to manage AVN is surgical hip replacement. Bones that make up the hip joint are replaced with titanium prosthetic implants—in essence, by rebuilding the entire hip joint. While there is some rehabilitation necessary after hip replacement surgery, the procedure is the most effective and long-term way to treat AVN.

Hepatitis

The liver is the one of the most vital organs in the human body. The liver performs a variety of roles and is considered an organ and a gland. As an organ it is responsible for hundreds of chemical reactions that are essential to the health of the human body. On the other hand, it is a gland that secretes substances used by other organs in the body.

The functions of the liver are many. It produces substances that are used all over the body. Cholesterol, triglycerides, glucose, and bile are all produced in the liver. It detoxifies chemicals and medications taken in to the body. Ammonia is a toxic byproduct of the body's metabolism. The liver detoxifies this substance by converting it to the substance urea which is excreted from the body through the kidneys. The liver metabolizes ("breaks down") medications, alcohol, and insulin as well as converting glucose to glycogen, a form that can be stored in the liver for future use. Finally, the liver stores substances used as building blocks for the rest of the body. The liver stores vitamins such as Vitamin A, D, and K, as well as folic acid and iron that is used to make red blood cells. So it's obvious that the liver is an essential part of a healthy human body.

So as important as the liver is, it's easy to understand why liver disease can be catastrophic for the individual. The liver can fall victim to many types of illnesses, infections, and diseases. One such condition that is common among those people living with HIV is *hepatitis*. To understand exactly what hepatitis is, let's break down the word. The *Online Etymology Dictionary* defines the word hepatitis as follows: "*Hepatitis—from the Greek 'hepatos' meaning liver and 'itis' meaning inflammation.*"

So, as the origin of the word indicates, hepatitis is an inflammation of the liver. The reasons for the inflammation are many. For instance, exposure to chemicals or toxic substances can damage liver tissue, causing inflammation. Excessive use of alcohol, or diseases of the gall bladder or pancreas, can also cause the inflammation of hepatitis. The metabolism or breakdown of certain medications by the liver, including some HIV medications, can place stress on the liver, once again causing inflammation. Finally, one of the most common causes of hepatitis, and one that can potentially be fatal, is viral infection. In other words, viral infections cause tissue damage, inflammation, and liver dysfunction. Let's explore the types of hepatitis that most commonly affect HIV-positive people.

VIRAL HEPATITIS

There are several types of viral hepatitis, some more common than others. Some are specific to certain geographic areas, and others are found all over the world. Some have vaccines to prevent their spread, and others do not. Let's take a look at the three most common forms of viral hepatitis: Hepatitis A, B, and C.

Hepatitis A (HAV)

Hepatitis A (HAV) is a viral infection that can cause mild to severe illness almost anywhere in the world. In fact, the virus is one of the most frequent causes of foodborne illness. There can be isolated cases scattered throughout a geographical area, but usually cases of Hepatitis A appear in clusters; groups of people in the same area with certain factors in common, such as eating at the same restaurant or buying vegetables at the same farmers' market. In some parts of the world, HAV epidemics are widespread, involving large numbers of people over large geographical areas.

Hepatitis A is primarily a disease related to personal hygiene and a lack of sanitary conditions. This type of hepatitis is caused by the hepatitis A virus found in the feces of people carrying the infection. It's spread from person to person by coming in contact with hepatitis A-infected stool. Most often this occurs by ingesting contaminated food or water, a result of poor hand washing, hygiene, or sanitation. Typically, food is contaminated with HAV because an infected person did not wash their hands after using the bathroom. Their contaminated hands come in contact with food that is being served to others. Water can also carry the virus, usually a result of poor sanitation conditions and the lack of adequate water treatment.

Another, less common method of spreading HAV from person to person is by direct contact with someone infected; in many cases that contact is oral and anal sex. While it's less common among the general public, among gay men it occurs with some frequency because anal and oral sex are much more prevalent. Men who have sex with men have a greater risk of HAV because they engage in anal sex routinely. Finally, in rare cases, HAV can be transmitted by sharing needles to inject prescription medication (e.g., insulin) or recreational drugs (e.g., heroin).

Once infected, recovering from HAV can take a very long time, sometimes weeks or even months. Thankfully, HAV can be prevented and the risk of transmitting the infection to other people can be reduced by a couple different methods. First, good hand washing before and after using the bathroom, and before handling and preparing food, can reduce the spread of HAV significantly. Another means of reducing the risk of HAV infection is the HAV vaccine. The vaccine is a series of two injections administered over six to twelve months. The vaccine stimulates the immune system's antibody response, resulting in the production of protective antibodies. If enough hepatitis A antibodies are produced, immunity to hepatitis A results. This vaccine is particularly important to men who have sex with men, whether they are HIV positive or negative, because of their increased risk of hepatitis A by means of unprotected anal sex.

The symptoms of hepatitis A are similar to symptoms of many liver diseases, those of liver dysfunction and liver failure. These symptoms include:

- jaundice (yellowing of the skin and whites of the eyes);
- fatigue;
- dark urine;
- clay-colored stools;
- abdominal pain (primarily right upper quadrant);
- loss of appetite;
- diarrhea;
- nausea; and
- fever.

The treatment of these symptoms depend a great deal on their severity. Most often, treatment is aimed at easing the symptoms and providing comfort measures until the HAV infection runs its course. Depending on the severity of the illness, most people will clear the infection and be back to normal sometime between two to six months after infection. Unlike other types of viral hepatitis, HAV does not cause chronic illness.

Hepatitis B (HBV)

Unlike the limited course of HAV, the virus that causes hepatitis B (HBV) can produce life-long liver disease. Over time, being infected with chronic HBV can cause scarring ("cirrhosis") of the liver, damage to liver tissue, and if left untreated, even death. The mode of transmission differs somewhat from that of HAV. The virus is typically spread from person to person by exposure to infected bodily fluids during sexual encounters, needle sharing, needle sticks, and during childbirth by HBV infected pregnant women. While HBV can infect anyone, there are groups of people that are at a higher risk of infection. These groups include:

- people who have unprotected anal, oral, or vaginal sex;
- people who inject drugs and share needles and syringes;
- newborn children of infected mothers; and
- healthcare workers exposed to infected bodily fluids or suffering needle stick injuries.

Once infected about 30 percent of people with HBV have no symptoms at all. If symptoms do occur, they include:

- jaundice (yellowing of the skin and eyes);
- abdominal pain (primarily right upper quadrant);
- nausea and vomiting;
- dark urine; and
- fever.

As you recall, HAV is usually left to run its course untreated, lasting about two to six months. The same can't be said for HBV. There are medications available to treat HBV with the goal being to minimize HBV replication and in the process prevent damage to the liver. In fact, some of the medications used are the same medicines used to treat HIV, the only difference being the dose. For instance, Epivir (lamivudine) is prescribed at 100mg daily when used to treat HBV, but 300mg daily when treating HIV. In addition, there are medications that have been developed specifically for the treatment of HBV, namely a medication called Baraclude (entecavir).

In addition to daily prescription medications, there is a preventative vaccine much like the vaccine used to prevent HAV. The HBV vaccine is a series of three injections given over a six-month period. When given to adults, dose #1 is given at a clinic or doctor's appointment, dose #2 is given one month later, and the final dose is given six months after dose #1. The HBV vaccine is part of the standard vaccination schedule for newborn children as well: the first dose is given at birth; the second at 1 to 2 months of age; and the third dose at 6 months of age.

Typically, the three dose HBV vaccine is an effective way to stimulate the immune response that creates antibodies that protect against HBV exposures. However, because some HIV-positive people have a weakened immune response, one HBV vaccination series is not enough to produce protective antibodies. To assist the weakened immune response, providers will administer a second three dose series but at double the dose in an effort to produce an immune response, antibodies, and immunity to HBV.

Hepatitis C (HCV)

In 1975, researchers found that a large number of viral hepatitis cases were neither HAV nor HBV, the only known types of viral hepatitis at the time. So experts classified this third type of hepatitis as "non–A non–B hepatitis." By 1989, researchers were able to clone this non–A non–B hepatitis and classified it as hepatitis C (HCV). People develop HCV after exposure to the hepatitis C virus. There are two types of HCV infection, acute HCV and chronic HCV.

Acute HCV typically runs its course within 6 to 10 weeks of exposure. Approximately 80 percent of people who contract acute HCV do not exhibit any symptoms. If symptoms do occur, they are typically mild and easily mistaken for other illnesses. Vague abdominal discomfort, nausea, vomiting, weight loss and fatigue are the usual initial symptoms. These will progress to jaundice (yellowing of skin and eyes) in about 25 percent of people who are infected with HCV. Liver function studies will show varying degrees of liver enzyme abnormality but rapid, fatal liver failure is very rare with acute HCV. However, 70 to 90 percent of people infected with HCV fail to clear the infection entirely and progress to the second type of HCV, chronic HCV.

Approximately 150 million people worldwide are living with chronic HCV with 500,000 people dying from liver disease or liver cancer caused by HCV. Four million of those living with chronic HCV are from the United States. The difference between chronic and acute HCV is a matter of time: chronic infection is diagnosed if the infection is still present six months after the initial infection. Sadly, a majority of people living with chronic HCV have no idea they are infected. In fact, so many people are infected but unaware that some experts refer to HCV as the "silent epidemic." The phrase was coined to describe the asymptomatic nature of chronic HCV. The infection can persist for years without any symptoms at all. In fact, 80 percent of all people with chronic HCV are symptom free. If and when symptoms do occur they are similar to those seen in HAV and HBV, namely jaundice, abdominal pain, fever, nausea, fatigue, dark urine, and loss of appetite.

An important aspect of chronic HCV is the persistent nature of hepatitis (liver inflammation) that is characteristic of chronic HCV. This slow progressing, long-term inflammation causes cirrhosis (scarring) in 10 to 20 percent of people with chronic HCV and fatal liver failure in about 20 percent of those with cirrhosis. Chronic cirrhosis also causes hepatocellular cancer (HCC/liver cancer) in about 1 to 5 percent of people with cirrhosis. However, without cirrhosis, HCC rarely occurs. That being said, in a small number of HCV patients, liver transplantation is indicated due to total liver failure.

HCV is spread from person to person by exposure to HCV-infected blood or blood components. This typically occurs when sharing needles to inject recreational drugs; when receiving blood products prior to 1992 or clotting factors prior to 1987; by needle stick injury for those in the healthcare setting; or during childbirth involving a HCV-infected mother. While HCV infection can occur during sexual encounters the incidence of sexual transmission is low. However, if there is exposure to blood during sexual encounters, either due to mucous membrane trauma (e.g., anal sex) or during menstruation (e.g., vaginal sex during menstruation), the risk of sexual transmission increases.

The fact that most people infected with HCV experience few or no symptoms should not lead anyone to believe the infection is minor. In fact, HCV causes chronic liver disease in about 70 percent of infected people, and will be fatal in many of those cases. Furthermore, HCV liver failure is the leading indicator for liver transplant.

Unfortunately, there is no vaccine to immunize against HCV, as there is for HAV and HBV. But there are effective precautions that can be taken to prevent infection. These precautions include:

- not sharing needles or drug paraphernalia with others;
- not sharing any personal items that could be contaminated with blood (e.g., sex toys, razors and toothbrushes);
- those who choose to get a tattoo or body piercing should make certain it's done by a professional tattoo artist using accepted health practices, sterile, single use needles, and proper sanitary techniques;

- a condom should be used with each oral, anal, or vaginal sexual encounter, regardless of how slight the risk is.

Prior to 2015, HCV treatment was difficult to take and even harder to tolerate due to significant side effects. Adhering to a HCV drug regimen required a great deal of commitment and in many people, the benefit of HCV treatment was not entirely clear. When deciding if hepatitis C medications were indicated, doctors had to weigh the potential benefits of treatment versus the potential side effects. The treatment of choice prior to 2015 was a combination of two medications, PEGylated interferon and ribavirin. This combination typically suppressed the virus in 50 to 80 percent of the people for whom it was prescribed.

In October 2014, the Food and Drug Administration approved a new therapy to treat HCV, a one pill once a day combination drug that has made effective treatment easier and more effective than ever. The medication Harvoni (ledipasvir+sofosbuvir) is a combination of two antiviral medications that are effective against multiple HCV genotypes. The amazing thing about the drug is the effectiveness; some studies put that effectiveness at 90 to 99 percent after 12 weeks of treatment. That along with the ease of treatment and the low side effect profile now makes Harvoni the drug of choice for the treatment of HCV.

Prior to Harvoni, people who were coinfected with HCV and HIV typically were only treated for HIV because of the difficult, hard to tolerate nature of HCV treatment. Not to be outdone, HIV treatment had its own uncomfortable side effects, making simultaneous treatment of HIV and HCV impractical and most likely unsuccessful. But now, with the easier to take and tolerate HIV regimens and the ease of Harvoni treatment, HIV/HCV coinfected people can be successfully treated for both conditions at the same time, meaning people will be healthier and will live longer, more productive lives.

Drug-Induced Hepatitis

In addition to viral hepatitis, which we have just discussed, there are also non-viral causes of hepatitis that affect the HIV population. The most common type of non-viral hepatitis is *drug-induced hepatitis*. There are more than 900 medications, toxins, and herbs that can cause liver injury and hepatitis. The process of metabolizing these substances can place significant stress on the liver, causing irreparable damage. If enough damage is done the liver can no longer perform those essential functions needed for the body to stay healthy. Eventually, so much damage can occur that only a liver transplant will save the person's life.

Certain medications and substances are known for their increased liver toxicity. Two familiar examples include the medication acetaminophen, the main ingredient found in Tylenol, and the adult beverage alcohol (ethanol). The use of these products even in recommended amounts can put stress on the liver if taken over the long-term. Acetaminophen has been found to be so liver toxic that the Food and Drug Administration (FDA) has lowered the recommended maximum daily dose because of the high incidence of liver toxicity when using acetaminophen. When people drink alcohol in excess they develop a condition called *alcoholic hepatitis*. If excessive alcohol intake continues a more severe and life threatening condition develops, *alcoholic cirrhosis*. These two conditions cause liver dysfunction and eventually liver failure if alcohol consumption is not eliminated.

Typically, drug-induced hepatitis will resolve without permanent liver injury after the drug (e.g., acetaminophen), toxin (e.g., herbal supplements), or chemical (e.g., alcohol/

ethanol) causing the problem is discontinued. However, in some cases the damage to the liver does not resolve even after stopping or removing the causative agent. In the most severe cases of drug-induced hepatitis, liver injury can be so significant that liver failure occurs, requiring a transplant to save the person's life.

There are three reasons why drugs cause hepatitis. First, there are certain drugs that by their nature can be toxic to the liver. Taken in the prescribed and recommended dosages, the medications are non-toxic and usually will do no harm. However, if these drugs are taken in amounts that exceed recommended dosages then stress and damage to the liver can occur. Under normal circumstances, the liver metabolizes drugs into nontoxic byproducts. In the case of medications that are considered "liver toxic," damage occurs if higher-than-recommended doses are taken. Damage occurs because instead of the liver metabolizing the drug into nontoxic byproducts, the opposite occurs. When excess medication is taken the liver metabolizes the drugs into toxic byproducts that ultimately cause liver damage. Simply put, if too much medication is in the bloodstream, the liver can't metabolize all of the medication into nontoxic byproducts, meaning some of the toxic medication remains.

The second way medications are toxic to the liver is due to *hypersensitivity*. Depending on the individual, there are drugs that can trigger an unexpected hypersensitivity that results in hepatitis. This type of hepatitis is not related to dose, meaning the hypersensitivity can occur at any dose, even at recommended, FDA approved dosages. Typically, this type of hepatitis only occurs after the person has been taking the drug in question for a prolonged period of time. Just how long it takes to develop hypersensitivity to a drug depends on the specific drug and the person for whom it's prescribed. For instance, the HIV medication Ziagen (abacavir) can cause a hypersensitivity reaction in those patients with a specific genetic type (allele) known as *B*5701*. Hypersensitivity typically occurs within 6 weeks of starting therapy but can occur as early as 8 days after therapy starts.

Finally, the third way drug-induced hepatitis can occur is as a result of certain external factors. These factors include age, genetics, the presence of certain illnesses and diseases (including HIV), smoking, and the use of alcohol. Some of these factors can be controlled by the individual—smoking or drinking alcohol, for instance. Others, like genetics, age, and gender, are out of the control of the individual. The prescribing provider should be aware of factors that could increase the risk of developing drug-induced hepatitis before prescribing medications.

AIDS Wasting

AIDS wasting has been a complication of HIV infection since the epidemic emerged in the 1980s. Before the emergence of HIV medications, the thin, drawn appearance characteristic of AIDS wasting became the face of the disease during the early years of the epidemic. In addition to being a complication of HIV infection, wasting can be a complication of many of the serious opportunistic infections that occur when the immune system has been damaged by HIV. In fact, wasting is considered an AIDS-defining illness by the Centers for Disease Control (CDC), meaning that if someone is diagnosed with HIV-related wasting they are considered to have an AIDS diagnosis.

Wasting is defined as a 10 percent loss of body weight, accompanied by diarrhea, fever, and often times a CD4 count less than 100 cells/mm³ of blood. However, wasting can be seen in people with CD4 counts greater than 100 cells/mm³ as well. Wasting is the result of one of three causes.

Disturbances in Metabolism

HIV can cause hormone deficiencies that change the way food is metabolized. Changes in the way the body metabolizes food results in altered absorption of those nutrients needed to maintain body weight. In wasting syndrome, hormonal changes cause muscle to be burned for energy instead of fat. *Cytokines* are proteins that produce inflammation. People who are HIV positive have a large quantity of cytokines, which causes the body to produce more fats and sugars and fewer proteins. This lack of protein production in addition to proteins being used for energy contributes to wasting by decreasing muscle production and muscle mass. The result is the characteristic drawn, thin appearance of those with AIDS wasting.

Hormone deficiencies can also affect metabolism. The deficiency of hormones, specifically the hormone testosterone, can contribute to wasting. While testosterone is a male hormone, both males and females have testosterone in their body. One role of testosterone in both men and women is to generate and maintain lean muscle mass. Inadequate levels of testosterone, combined with changing metabolic function, result in the loss of lean muscle mass, muscle that is not easily replaced. The resulting lack of lean muscle contributes to the problem of AIDS wasting.

Poor Nutrition

Many factors contribute to a state of poor nutrition. Diminished appetite, coupled with increased caloric needs, results in weight loss. Fighting an HIV infection takes energy, energy generated by the food we take in each day. All foods have calories but in order to fight HIV, the calories needed are those from quality, healthy food sources. For instance, fast food and a piece of grilled tuna each have plenty of calories but the calories in the tuna are of a higher quality than those in the fast food. That being said, when money is tight, it is difficult to purchase high quality foods; tuna is much more expensive than fast food. So when there are limited resources, people choose the fast food because less money can go farther, and in the process nutrition suffers.

Another factor affecting nutrition is a poor appetite. When a person just doesn't feel like eating it's difficult to take in the calories needed to fight an HIV infection. In these situations, it's imperative that the food that is eaten be high quality and high in calories. For instance, if a person only eats one meal a day the food that is eaten must be high in calories even in small amounts. In other words, the food must be calorie dense food. One example is an avocado, a fruit that packs 320 calories into a 7 ounce serving size. In addition, there are 30 grams of fat needed for energy, and all of those 30 grams are heart healthy fats. Compare this to an apple of comparable size. The apple, while a healthy fruit, only has 115 calories, none of which are from fat. So by eating the same 7 ounce serving size, a person gets 200 more calories from the avocado, the benefit of calorie dense food.

Another factor contributing to poor nutrition is the body's ability to absorb essential nutrients. The nutrients provided by the foods we eat are absorbed primarily through the intestinal tract. However, there are circumstances that can interfere with absorption. Factors like chronic inflammation, colitis, and intestinal parasites or infections can all interfere with intestinal absorption of nutrients. Those nutrients not absorbed are lost in feces expelled when a person has a bowel movement.

There are other factors that affect a person's ability to consume enough calories, vitamins, and minerals to fuel the body's fight against HIV. Factors like medication side effects, difficulty swallowing or chewing, and altered taste can all make taking in calories and nutrients much more difficult, contributing to poor nutrition. Mechanical issues of the mouth such as oral candida ("thrush") and apthous ulcers ("canker sores") can cause pain, changes in taste, and difficulty in swallowing, interfering with the intake of adequate food and calories. Poor dentition including painful cavities, missing teeth, and broken teeth can negatively impact the ability to eat, making it difficult to chew food. Finally, medication side effects like nausea, diarrhea, and bloating can make eating unpleasant. All of us can relate to the effects nausea, abdominal bloating, and diarrhea can have on appetite and the desire to eat. While improvements in HIV medication regimens have decreased the number of side effects, from time to time they do rear their ugly head and when they do, it greatly affects the ability to take in the calories needed to fight the illness and maintain proper nutrition.

Reversing AIDS Wasting

While the causes of AIDS wasting are fairly evident and understood, reversing the problem isn't always easy. Treating the underlying opportunistic infections, gastrointestinal illnesses, and HIV itself will help slow and, in some cases, reverse wasting. Nutrition can be maintained with high-calorie nutritional supplements; however, those supplements can be expensive and are rarely covered by medical insurance or prescription drug coverage. Many HIV treatment programs have access to registered dieticians who can help their patients plan healthy menus, assist them with food choices, and help them obtain high-calorie nutritional supplements.

In cases of hormonal deficiency, testosterone can be replaced using hormone injections, transdermal patches, or transdermal gels. Steroids such as Megace (megestrol) have been used as well to increase and maintain lean muscle mass. Keep in mind, however, that many drug coverage programs do not cover testosterone supplements or steroids such as Megace (megestrol) without prior authorization and very strict guidelines and prerequisites.

Finally, in those patients whose poor appetite prevents them from eating a healthy diet, appetite stimulants such as Marinol (dronobinol) are sometimes prescribed in an effort to improve the appetite and by doing so increase the caloric intake. At the same time, Marinol has an antiemetic effect (anti-nausea) which could help improve appetite by easing nausea.

As this chapter has clearly illustrated, people living with HIV and AIDS deal with many illnesses and infections, in addition to their HIV. In fact, so much progress has been made in the treatment of HIV that most of the time it's associated illnesses like hepatitis and kidney disease that are the health threats for those living with HIV. As people continue to live longer, patients and their HIV specialists will face new and more challenging conditions associated with living long term with HIV. It's the myriad of associated illnesses that go along with HIV that best illustrate the need to treat the entire person—physical, mental, and emotional.

Focusing on any one of these areas does a great disservice to those living with HIV. Doing so would result in very poor outcomes and compromised health care.

Our next chapter discusses the whole body concept of treating HIV and AIDS. Since the emergence of the disease, experts have learned that the best HIV treatment programs are the ones that follow this concept: treat HIV by treating the whole person. Let's see what that entails.

10

TREATING THE WHOLE PERSON

HIV affects all aspects of a person's life—physical, psychological, social and spiritual. For that reason, HIV care should address all those areas as well. So often care is centered on the physical aspects of HIV, leaving other dimensions of the individual unattended. Since the early years of the epidemic, experts have stressed that HIV-positive people need care that encompasses all aspects of a person—physical, psychological, social, and spiritual. By focusing only on the physical manifestations of HIV, living with the disease is infinitely more difficult.

Participating in professional counseling as a member of a support group or as an individual attending one on one sessions teaches important coping skills that will help deal with the day to day stress of HIV. Less structured methods of social support—those in the form of friends and family—help cope with the various issues associated with each stage of the disease. Psychosocial support in any one of these forms decreases the incidence of mental illness including depression, and helps people cope with their new diagnosis and the adjustment period that follows. Continued support throughout the course of the illness helps the HIV-positive person flourish even with a chronic disease. With a strong support system, people living with HIV can and do persevere despite their illness. Ultimately, the person who once needed the support of others becomes the support for others

As we know, an HIV diagnosis brings with it prejudice, stigma, isolation and guilt. Psychosocial support helps the individual cope more effectively with these issues and assists those living with the disease to make informed and educated decisions regarding their HIV healthcare. Without psychosocial support, prejudice, fear and isolation will overwhelm even the strongest person, making a life with HIV one of pain, loneliness, and anger.

In addition to the obvious physical manifestations of HIV and the psychosocial issues we just discussed, HIV creates economic issues as well. Chronic illness can make it difficult to continue to work and earn a living. The resulting lost wages combined with a rising cost of living and ever-increasing healthcare costs can affect quality of life. For example, money that once went to buy groceries and pay the heating bill are now being used for doctor's visits and prescription medications. That combined with fewer hours at work and the resulting lost wages will eventually cause financial hardship.

Lack of employment or diminished hours also means medical and prescription coverage may be lost, too expensive to afford. For instance, if you are no longer able to work full time hours, it is possible you will lose your employer-sponsored insurance. At the very least, going from full time employment to part time may result in higher monthly insurance premiums and again less money for rent, utilities, and food.

Finally, without adequate income, permanent housing may be jeopardized. Having an unstable living situation will eventually impact medication adherence, nutrition, and overall health. Without stable housing there is nowhere to store prescription medication, there is nowhere to store and prepare food, and there is nowhere to get a good night's sleep in a safe, warm, and dry environment. Poor or unstable housing leaves a person exposed to unsanitary conditions that increases the risk of opportunistic infections. Without stable housing your entire life is turned upside down. Your physician can't contact you for appointments, can't call you to discuss lab results, and can't find you in the event of a medical emergency or necessary medical intervention. Lack of housing will eventually adversely affect your health: that much is for certain.

Unfortunately, poor or failing health is not the only reason employment is compromised. Even if your health is good enough to maintain full-time employment, the prejudice, fear, and ignorance of employers may interfere with employment or in extreme cases may prevent securing employment at all. Legally, a job can't be denied or taken away based on an HIV infection. That being said, once an HIV diagnosis becomes public knowledge it's not uncommon for an employer to find ways to discriminate based on an HIV diagnosis, claiming it has nothing to do with the diagnosis at all. Sadly, even after 30 years of education, still there are employers that find creative and devious ways to harass, fire, or prevent the hiring of people with HIV.

More than any other aspect of your life, your personal relationships will feel the effects of HIV. Disclosing your diagnosis to a loved one is probably the most difficult thing you will ever have to do. Unfortunately, regardless of how strong the relationship is a loving, supportive response to your HIV disclosure is not guaranteed. In fact, HIV infection can and does tear apart relationships for a myriad of reasons. For example, when a married man is diagnosed with HIV his wife is sure to ask how her husband was infected. Did the man have a sexual encounter outside of the marriage? Is there a drug problem that his wife didn't know about? What about the gay man who's done well to hide his sexual preference from family and friends? Disclosing his HIV diagnosis may jeopardize his secret or at the very least will cause questions to be asked, questions that are not easily answered. If his secret is revealed family and friends will not only have to deal with his HIV diagnosis but with the realization that their friend, brother, or son is gay. Simply put, disclosing an HIV diagnosis may necessitate revealing secrets as well, secrets that can stress or destroy a relationship.

Chronic illnesses including HIV impact relationships in countless ways. Just as newly diagnosed people experience fear, confusion, and denial, so will their loved ones as they try to accept the news of such a life-altering diagnosis. There is no question that the countless feelings and emotions associated with HIV stress even the strongest relationship. But understanding that fact will help the diagnosed and their loved ones come to terms with the diagnosis and get on with their lives. Let's look a little closer at the psychosocial aspects of HIV and how to get past the initial emotions of disclosure and go on with our lives.

Grieving After Diagnosis

Grieving is a process that most people will experience at least once in their life. When we think of grieving, most of us think about the death of a loved one or maybe a divorce from a spouse. However, grieving is an emotion that most people experience when they first learn of their HIV diagnosis. Like the death of a loved one, an HIV diagnosis is perceived as a loss—the loss of your good health, a loss of control over your future, and a loss of the life you once had. We know from previous chapters that new treatments make it possible to maintain the quality of life you had before diagnosis. However, they say perception is reality and for those first diagnosed the perception is that the life they once had is lost for good. And as such, there will be grieving. Grieving is a process we all go through to cope with a loss in our life, be it the loss of a loved one or the perception of lost health and well-being.

Dr. Elizabeth Kübler-Ross did a great deal of work in the field of grief and how people deal with loss. Her stages of grief have been applied to the grieving process since 1969 when she published her work *On Death and Dying.* The work deals with grieving and the stages we go through in times of a loss. However, there is some controversy over the application of these stages to the grief process. In fact, there has been no real proof that people experience grieving in stages at all. Another problem with the stages of grief is the implied belief that there is little a person can do to move from one stage to the other, the belief that each stage must "run its course" before moving to the next. There are several theories pertaining to the stages of grief; some involve five stages, another has seven stages. The most important things to remember about stages of grief is that first, not everyone experiences grief in stages. Second, if there are stages of grief they are not necessarily experienced in the same order. Third, the thought that each stage must just "run its course" before moving to the next is nothing more than a myth, a myth that can be damaging to a person's recovery from grief and loss. Finally, remember that the newly diagnosed man or woman is not the only person who will experience grief. Loved ones, family, and friends will experience loss and grief as well and as such may go through the following stages as well. So with these caveats in mind, let's look at Kübler-Ross's stages of grief to illustrate how they apply to a new HIV diagnosis.

SHOCK/DISBELIEF

The initial reaction to hearing bad news is typically shock and disbelief. Such is the case when first hearing a diagnosis of HIV. Initially, there may be no reaction to the bad news at all. It's not uncommon for people to sit and stare, detaching themselves from the situation at hand. Others may just nod and appear accepting of the news. Still others may act as if the news of their diagnosis is "no big deal." On the outside, a person may appear to be in total control, hearing the diagnosis and understanding and accepting his or her situation. However, internally the person is mentally blocking out the news of the diagnosis in an effort to protect themselves from something they don't wish to hear. Shock and disbelief can impede understanding and retention of any information provided at this time. Any information given most likely will need to be repeated several times before the person is actually fully aware of what is being said. Physically, this stage of grief can be accompanied by tremors, nausea, vomiting, or sweating. Have you ever heard the term "you look like you've seen a ghost"? This phrase refers to the pale appearance common to someone who has heard or seen something shocking, like the news of an HIV diagnosis. To ease the impact and duration of the shock and disbelief stage, disclosing the news of your HIV diagnosis or giving someone else their diagnosis should be done in a private setting where fears, concerns, and emotions can be expressed freely.

DENIAL

After the initial shock of learning your diagnosis the stage of denial begins. During this stage the validity of the HIV diagnosis is questioned. Simply put, the person receiving news of the HIV diagnosis refuses to believe what they're being told and carries on with their life as if nothing has happened. In fact, some people get stuck in this stage even after seeking medical care. It's not uncommon for an HIV-infected person to continue to question his or her diagnosis long after receiving the news, sometimes even after being in care for months or years. Unfortunately, this state of mind can disrupt HIV care to the point of impacting the health of the individual. We know from earlier chapters that getting into care is the key to a healthy prognosis. By denying your diagnosis you delay establishing HIV care, which will ultimately have a negative effect on prognosis. So strong is the power of denial that many times physical symptoms miraculously disappear or resolve by themselves. When loved ones deny the validity of an HIV diagnosis, it encourages and reinforces the same feelings in the person given his or her HIV test results.

ANGER

This stage is a direct result of repressing emotions that have developed during the first two stages of grief. This stage is characterized by an outpouring of emotion and grief in the form of verbal outbursts and other expressions of anger. It's during this stage that the diagnosed asks, "Why Me?" Someone learning of their loved one's diagnosis for the first time will express their anger using such terms as "How could you?" or "How did that happen?" Often they direct their anger toward the person being diagnosed. This is the stage where questions start to surface; some are uncomfortable questions about how the infection occurred and the events surrounding the infection. Loved ones may ask the newly infected "What did you do?" and may demand an explanation. As for the newly infected, their anger is usually directed toward a loved one or a person nearby, typically someone not infected with HIV themselves. Anger may also be directed toward the person providing the test results or giving them their new HIV diagnosis. It's also not uncommon for the newly diagnosed to be angry at themselves, saying things like "I get what I deserve" or "That's what I get for being so careless." If you have disclosed your status and the people you just told are angry, ask yourself the reason for the anger. Do they feel you kept something from them? Do they think you were unfaithful or were infected due to high risk behaviors? Or is their anger based on fear they may lose you due to your illness? Anger is a normal expression of grief and should be expected regardless of the reason.

BARGAINING

After the anger has subsided and the pent up emotion has been released, bargaining begins. It's at this stage in the grief cycle that the person grieving tries to make a deal with a higher power or deity. For instance, the person grieving will think something to the effect of "I'll clean up my life if you make this all go away," or "I'll eat right and exercise if you just let me be healthy." Bargaining, for the most part, is not an overt process where the grieving person stands in front of their doctor trying to make a deal. Instead, bargaining takes place in the mind, making private pacts with his or her god. It's quite common for the person to feel guilt or a sense of being punished for something they feel they've done wrong—an extramarital affair, drug use, or even their sexual preference. This sense of guilt feeds into the bargaining stage of grieving. An individual feels they are being punished for something they have done wrong. And therefore, refraining from what they feel is wrong will set things straight in their mind and in the mind of their god. In other words, the person bargains by asking his or her god for good health if they refrain from the activity they feel is wrong or immoral. Unfortunately, the guilt that emerges in this stage is often long-lasting and will eventually impede a person's progress toward accepting their disease and moving on with their life. If such guilt is not dealt with effectively it can also adversely affect the health of the individual and may even interfere with proper treatment, medication adherence, and day to day life in general.

In some cases, bargaining can take on another, less obvious face. Bargaining can also be in the form of seeking alternative therapies or experimental medications that they feel may be the cure for their disease. In other words, a person bargains for their renewed health by showing those around him or her that they will do whatever it takes to stay healthy or regain they healthy and normal lifestyle. These are the people who get their diagnosis and are overly eager to get started with their HIV care, showing few if any signs of grief or upset after hearing their diagnosis. However, it is difficult for a person to maintain this sort of commitment or drive and eventually they may revert to old habits, poor adherence, and behaviors that are more typical of the person before diagnosis. Whatever form it takes, bargaining is a request for a second chance. In actuality, it is a form of hope that the bad news, in our case the HIV diagnosis, is reversible and will just go away if we do the right things with our life.

DEPRESSION

While bargaining is a product of denial, depression signals that the grieving person is moving toward acceptance. The inevitability of their new diagnosis "sinks in," and reluctantly the person accepts what has happened and what is going to happen. While anger and bargaining are very animated and outgoing, depression is isolated and lonesome. They turn away from support, treatment, or any outside help being offered to them. In this stage, people become very pessimistic, seeing very little hope for their future, seeing only illness, suffering, and despair before them. This stage can be a dangerous one. The depression in this stage can be so profound that people seek an escape from their diagnosis and their suffering. Some choose substances such as alcohol or drugs. Some run away, turning to isolation and escape from reality. Sadly, others will seek the ultimate escape—suicide. People in this stage are vulnerable to such extreme actions because they feel hopeless, isolated, and withdrawn. Because these feelings are so prevalent, it's important for loved ones to continue offering support even when those grieving refuse any help that is offered to them. Without a place to turn for support, feelings of hopelessness and isolation worsen, opening the door to worsening depression and an uncertain prognosis and future. If you or a loved one are depressed, you should seek professional counseling or psychiatric care immediately. Speak with your HIV physician at the first sign of feeling depressed.

Testing

It's during this stage that the grieving person begins to realize that he or she can't stay depressed forever. There comes a realization that surviving their new diagnosis or supporting their loved one who has disclosed their diagnosis will only be possible if there is some degree of acceptance. The person searches for actions that can be taken in an effort to cope with their new diagnosis. The grieving person takes small steps in an effort to test the waters, to find a way out of their grieving. For instance, during this stage the newly diagnosed reluctantly begins their HIV care as a first step in dealing with their diagnosis. The person who has just learned of a loved one's diagnosis tries to open a dialogue to discuss how the newly diagnosed is coping or feeling about the new diagnosis. In most cases this stage can progress only with the support of loved ones and professionals. As the grieving person takes steps that prove beneficial and successful, he or she realizes that the steps being taken are better than the depression and grieving that they had been experiencing. Each successful step toward acceptance breeds another step.

Acceptance

This final stage of grieving is one of stability. The grieving person has advanced to a point where he or she is ready to move on with life. In the case of the newly diagnosed, they will continue their HIV care and strive to incorporate their illness into their lives. As their grief process stabilizes, they will be ready to offer support to others. In some instances, the newly diagnosed become the support for the people to whom they've disclosed their illness. On the other hand, now having passed through all the stages of grieving, the loved one can offer support to the newly diagnosed.

Keep in mind that people who are grieving can move in and out of stages more than once. Many times people will experience the stages of grief out of order or will experience more than one stage at a time. People can get stuck in one stage or skip a stage altogether. There is really no right or wrong way to grieve. While there are stages we all go through, the manner in which we pass though those stages is unique to each of us. The most important thing to keep in mind is that grief after learning of an HIV diagnosis, be it yours or a loved one's, is perfectly normal. Working through that grief will take time but rest assured it will pass. For those newly diagnosed, living a healthy, productive life with HIV should not be a possibility—it should be the expectation.

Fear and Anxiety

Fear and anxiety are two common emotions experienced by the HIV-positive person. Especially in those early days immediately following diagnosis, fear and anxiety can be overwhelming for many people. The root of fear and anxiety in the HIV-positive person stems from the unknown. How will HIV change my life? How long will I live? Will I be sick all the time? All these questions are common for the newly diagnosed person. Not knowing the answer to these questions causes anxiety. Assuming the worst creates fear. Not knowing what to expect after an HIV diagnosis, and fearing what others may think of you after having been diagnosed, only adds to the fear and anxiety.

While fear and anxiety are emotional conditions, they also cause physical symptoms. An elevated heart rate; rapid, shallow breathing; nausea; and interrupted sleep patterns can all occur in the midst of fear and anxiety. Additionally, a person suffering from fear and anxiety can experience profuse sweating, agitation, nervousness, shortness of breath, and dizziness. There are ways, however, to control or limit feelings of fear and anxiety. They include:

- Learn as much about HIV and AIDS as possible. Understanding the disease will ease the fear and anxiety by shedding some light on the unknown. Understanding the biology of HIV and its typical course will give some hint as to what the future with HIV holds for the diagnosed. Fear is a product of the unknown. Decreasing the unknown will also decrease your fear.

- You will have questions about your disease. Make sure you get them answered to your satisfaction by your HIV specialist at your next visit. When questions arise, write them down. Take the list of questions to your next doctor's appointment. The adage "knowledge is power" is absolutely right. By better understanding your illness you are better able to control your fear and anxiety.

- Seek out emotional support in the form of friends, family, or loved ones. Find HIV-related support groups in your community. It's always helpful to speak with people experiencing feelings and emotions similar to your own. Learn from their experiences, and they can learn from yours.

- Once you have learned to manage your fear and anxiety, reach out to others and offer to help. Volunteer at an HIV agency or in a community advisory group. Helping others and being active in the HIV community empowers you, which in turn helps further manage your fear and anxiety and allows you to advocate you and others living with HIV.

- If fear and anxiety persist after trying the above interventions, it may be time to seek professional mental health counseling. Doing so is not a sign of weakness or illness. Mental health counseling is just another avenue available to you and others living with the disease. There are medicinal options but they can cause more problems than they solve. Anti-anxiety medications (e.g., benzodiazepines) such as Xanax (alprazolam), Ativan (lorazepam) or Valium (diazepam) can help temporarily, but they have many side effects and the potential for dependence and addiction is very high. Because of potential problems, drugs like Xanax, Ativan and Valium are the last resort and are prescribed for short-term use only. Your HIV specialist should consider these risks before prescribing benzodiazepines for your anxiety. Taking medications such as benzodiazepines is like putting a bandage on a laceration. It will cover the open wound but will do nothing to close the laceration. On the other hand, mental health counseling can identify your fears and anxieties and help you find ways to cope with them. If necessary, there are medications that, when used in conjunction with mental health counseling, treat your anxiety and fear rather than just masking their symptoms.

Stress

We all experience stress in our everyday lives: the stress of a traffic jam; the stress of debts that need to be paid on time; the stress of raising three teenage daughters. Stress can be uncomfortable and unpleasant, but in many ways stress pushes us to succeed and helps us get things done. Stress can be an incentive to push forward, but only if we are able to control the way we react to the daily stressors in our life.

The causes of stress are in many ways unique to each one of us. We need to recognize what causes our stress and learn to cope before it gets the best of us. As you learn to recognize your stressors you will develop coping mechanisms that help manage stress. Learning what causes stress in your life allows you to take measures to minimize those causes and, in turn, decrease your stress. Here are just a few ideas how you can manage your daily stressors.

- Physical activities, such as exercise, walking, or swimming, can help relieve the anxiety, nervousness, and anger characteristic of stress. Physical activity can help relieve tension created by stress, and it's an excellent way to improve your health at the same time.

- Take care of your body. Eat healthy; exercise at least three times each week; and do your best to get eight hours of sleep each night. Many HIV programs have access to dieticians that can help you choose healthy foods and a healthier diet. Never exceed your physical limitations when exercising. Exercise only to your ability. If stress is interrupting your sleep patterns, talk to your doctor. He or she can suggest ways to improve your sleep and, if needed, can prescribe medications that will help you get the sleep you need.

- Develop a support system of people you trust and who care about you. Talk to them about your stress. Talking about your stress with others is therapeutic, and the people in your support system may suggest ways to deal with stress that you have not tried or considered.

- A good cry can be very helpful. It's a means of releasing the tension that builds during periods of stress. Relieving tension is the key to relieving stress. Tension prevents the body and mind from relaxing. Relaxation allows us to recharge our batteries, so to speak, and in doing so it allows us to more effectively cope with our stress. Crying excessively or at the first sign of a problem can be a sign of depression but a "good cry" now and again can go a long way to relieve the stress of the day.

Coping with the Emotions

After learning of your HIV diagnosis, the typical response would be one of shock, disbelief, fear, and sadness. Fortunately, these feelings do resolve in time. An emotional reaction to a new HIV diagnosis is expected and is completely normal. That being said, there are methods the HIV-positive person can use to better cope with the emotional aspects of an HIV diagnosis. These methods include:

- Share your feelings with trusted family members, loved ones, your doctor, or a professional counselor. Keep in mind that in order to share your feelings, you will most likely have to disclose your HIV diagnosis. As we learned earlier, disclosing your status is a very emotional and fearful time. Disclosure is difficult, but can be done. Review Chapter 4 to learn how to disclose your diagnosis with the least amount of stress possible.

- Find an effective means to relieve your stress, such as exercise, swimming, or finding a hobby. Join a support group for those living with HIV. Such a support group brings together people going through the same thing; in this case, living with HIV. Joining such a group allows you to share feelings and emotions with people experiencing those feelings and emotions themselves. Support groups make it possible for you to learn ways to deal with your emotions from people who have already learned to cope. As the saying goes, "There's strength in numbers." Support groups help you take advantage of that strength and illustrate that you are not alone in your fight against HIV.

- Get plenty of sleep each night, allowing your body and mind to rest and recharge. Adequate rest is essential to a physical and emotional recovery. Learn and employ relaxation techniques, such as meditation and deep breathing exercises, to assist with sleep issues. Because caffeine and nicotine are stimulants, limit the amount you ingest, especially before going to bed.

Dealing with the emotional aspects of HIV is very difficult. Even the most emotionally stable person will eventually need some sort of emotional support, if only for a short period of time. The easiest way to find the support you need is through support groups. Support groups are comprised of people from all walks of life who share a common illness or issue. This commonality works in favor of the group's members, each learning from the experiences of others within the group. These groups can be found in medical practices, community agencies, churches, schools or anywhere there are HIV-infected people coming together to help one another. Let's look a little closer at support groups and what to look for when trying to find a group that is right for you.

Support Groups

In many ways, HIV is like any other chronic disease. The emotional impact of chronic illnesses can be devastating—many times as devastating as the physical effects of the illness. Feelings of fear, anger, and isolation are commonly felt by people with chronic disease. However, for all the similarities, in many ways HIV is unlike any other disease. As an example of how HIV differs, let's look at another serious chronic illness—diabetes. When a person learns they have diabetes, there will be feelings of fear, anger, and isolation. But in the case of diabetes, the person living with diabetes seldom has to face these feelings alone. When a person is diagnosed with diabetes, people gather around to offer love and support in any way they can. The person with diabetes doesn't have to worry about being labeled or stereotyped because they have diabetes. Prejudice is seldom predicated on the basis of a person's blood sugar. However, when a person is diagnosed with HIV, people tend to move away, unable or unwilling to offer support. Many times the newly diagnosed are unable to turn to anyone for support, not even their family and loved ones. Many people attach morality to an HIV diagnosis or end relationships because of an HIV diagnosis. So you can imagine anyone newly diagnosed would be very reluctant to reach out for help for fear of prejudice and rejection. You would be hard pressed to find another chronic illness that creates that type of fear.

Support groups provide HIV-positive people with the emotional support they so desperately need. Support groups can also be a benefit to loved ones, caregivers, and family members of the HIV-positive person as well. These groups provide a safe, non-judgmental atmosphere in which HIV-positive people and their family and friends can discuss feelings, concerns, and fears surrounding an HIV diagnosis. Support groups are generally relaxed and informal, an atmosphere that encourages participation of the members. For people dealing with the emotional aspects of HIV, supports groups provide an atmosphere of acceptance so members realize they are not alone in their struggle to cope with their diagnosis. Support groups bring together people who are experiencing the same difficult situations to encourage sharing and mutual support of one another. HIV support groups can be open to a variety of people or just to specific groups. For instance, there are groups that allow anyone HIV-infected to join: women, men, gay, or straight. There are also groups that are only open to specific people: HIV-positive women, teens, or gay men. Still other groups are for HIV-affected people: those people who are HIV-negative but are impacted by the disease. Members of this type of group include loved ones, caregivers, and medical professionals. Support groups provide a place where people can interact with their peers to discuss the impact HIV has on their life.

Support groups can be especially beneficial for the HIV-infected person. As illustrated earlier in this chapter, people are often alone in those first days after learning of their HIV diagnosis. Support groups offer a place of acceptance amid a world of rejection and prejudice. So many emotions confront the newly diagnosed and those around them. Changing medical, social, and financial situations cause fear and worry; rejection and prejudice cause depression, anger, and isolation. Support groups can help cope with all those feelings.

Countless studies have demonstrated the benefits of a support group for people infected with and affected by HIV. One study showed that 86 percent of people who attended an HIV support group showed dramatic improvement in how they handled the stress of the disease. It's also been shown that people attending HIV support groups showed more improvement in their depression symptoms when compared to standard psychotherapy sessions. Finally, evidence suggests that members of HIV support groups make better choices with regards to safer sex practices than those who don't attend peer-type support groups. Brett Grodeck, author of the book *The First Year—HIV: An Essential Guide for the Newly Diagnosed*, summed up the benefits of support groups in one sentence: "Talking with other people in similar situations can help you come to terms with your own situation."

SUPPORT GROUP TYPES

Support groups fall into one of four types according to the rules that govern them and how they are formatted and facilitated. In other words, does the support group have specific rules, guidelines, structure, and a leader? Keep in mind that some groups take on traits of more than one type. Let's look at the four types.

- *Structured Format*—These groups feature a very structured, almost ritualistic format, following written guidelines and rotating facilitators (facilitators being the person who leads the group). Each group session follows the same schedule led by a different member each session.
- *Free Form*—These groups can have rotating facilitators or no facilitator at all. If there is a format, it's very loose, allowing the meeting to progress in a free-flowing manner without having to adhere to a structured format. The flow of the meeting is governed by the discussions within the membership.
- *Trained Volunteers*—These groups are led by people who donate their time and are trained in the proper way to facilitate support groups. These groups usually have written

agreements and ground rules on how group sessions will be conducted. Members agree in writing as to what can be discussed, how members treat one another, and how the meetings run each session.

- *Professional Facilitators*—The guidelines and format of this type of group vary according to the style of the professional who is facilitating the group. These facilitators are typically trained, professional counselors, social workers, or health care professionals. The involvement of the facilitator often changes as the group becomes more established. The goal of some facilitators is to eventually have the group be facilitated by its membership, with the professional just there to oversee the group or to answer questions or concerns that arise.

The Role of the Facilitator

Most support groups do have a facilitator that guides the activity of the group. Some facilitators are members of the group, while others are paid or volunteer to be an outside observer and leader. The facilitator performs many roles for the group, including:

- working to make sure the group operates effectively and according to written guidelines and formats,
- assuring that discussions adhere to written rules and approved topics,
- setting meeting boundaries and determining topics to be discussed.

Many times there will be co-facilitators in a group. This could be a male and female, a nurse and social worker, or HIV-positive and HIV-negative facilitators. Studies have found that co-facilitated groups are very effective because they provide two perspectives and two areas of expertise.

Finding a Support Group

One look at the Internet will tell you there are literally hundreds of support groups from which to choose. But like a kid in a candy store, having such a large number of choices can make it more difficult to find a group that provides what you need. Luckily, there are proven ways to find the group just right for you.

- Speak with your HIV specialist, nurse, or social worker to see if one of them can recommend an HIV support group in your area. Better yet, do any of your HIV care team facilitate a support group?
- If you're seeing a psychiatrist, counselor, or psychologist, ask if they can recommend a support group and suggest characteristics your group should possess.
- Using the Internet, search for support groups in your area. Remember to make certain you are using reputable websites when looking for information.
- Speak with the community-based organizations in your area. It's possible that one of the local HIV agencies will offer a support group as part of their services. If not, they should be able to direct you to an agency that does.

Characteristics of a Good Support Group

Different people are looking for different things from a support group. Are the group meetings nearby? Can family members attend group sessions with me? Is there child care available while the group meets? What makes a support group beneficial to an individual varies from person to person. But there are characteristics that all support groups should have. These include:

- The group should have regularly scheduled meetings in a safe, easily accessible location (e.g., the location should be on a bus route).
- The support group should have access to mental health and medical professionals that are willing to participate in the support group from time to time. The best way to find these types of support groups is through hospitals or mental health practices in your community.
- The group should have a clearly defined confidentiality policy to protect the privacy of each member. Each member must understand that discussions within the group never leave the group.

Things to Keep in Mind

So now you know the traits common to a quality support group. But what other factors should you keep in mind when choosing an HIV support group?

- Understand what you want out of a support group before choosing one for you. Do you want medical information? Are you looking for peer interactions? Are you looking for emotional support?
- Have an idea how you want the group to be run. Do you want a group run by professionals or by its members? Are there strict guidelines and rules or is the group free flowing?
- Have an idea how far you are willing to travel for your support group. How far from your home is the support group located? How much time are you willing to devote to travel?
- If you have children finding a source of child care should be considered when choosing a group. Is there child care available during meeting times? If provided, is there a fee for the child care?
- If you have family members or a loved one who wants to participate, you need to consider that when choosing a group. Who is allowed to attend support group meetings with you? Can different people come with you each week? Are there restrictions limiting who can attend or how many can attend with you in any one session?

Relationship Issues

Life is meant to be shared with someone you love. But the first step in love is dating, looking to find that special someone with whom to share your life. One of the most common myths surrounding HIV is that, once diagnosed, you must give up any chance of meeting your special someone and give up on the dream of having a family. In fact, every day I hear from newly diagnosed people telling me that because they are now HIV-positive they intend to give up dating for good. That doesn't need to happen. With the right precautions and a lot of honesty, people living with HIV can date, have sexual relationships, and find that special someone to share their life. Let's look at dating and the potential issues that arise when living with HIV.

DATING WITH HIV

In Chapter 4 we discussed HIV disclosure. To review, most states have laws that require that any potential sexual partner be made aware of your HIV status before any sexual contact occurs. Is there a perfect time to disclose your HIV status? Probably not. Disclosing your HIV status is frightening whenever you choose to do so. In fact, it may be the hardest thing you'll ever have to do. But what if your relationship hasn't reached that sexual stage? What if sex has yet to enter the picture? Some fear disclosing too early in a relationship will end the relationship and at the same time jeopardize confidentiality for no reason. Others fear that disclosing late in the relationship will be perceived as dishonest. There are two schools of thought regarding when HIV disclosure should take place.

- ***Kiss and Tell***—The people who choose to "kiss and tell" will go on a few dates before disclosing their HIV status. This does have its advantages. It allows you to wait and see if the relationship is going to get serious before disclosing. If the relationship stalls, your status was not disclosed needlessly. In other words, people who "kiss and tell" feel this option limits the number of people who become aware of their diagnosis, preserving confidentiality.

- ***Tell and Kiss***—The people who choose to "tell and kiss" will disclose very early in the relationship, in some cases on the first date. Early disclosure occurs at a time of very little emotional attachment between the two people. It's a fact of life that some people will not be ready or willing to date an HIV-positive person. For many, it's less painful to be rejected early in the relationship before any emotional attachment has occurred. An added benefit of early disclosure is the honesty it implies. Delaying disclosure may be viewed by some as dishonest, as if you are trying to hide something that could have a very significant impact on the relationship. A final consideration regarding early disclosure is what it says about the relationship in general. If you disclose early and the relationship succeeds, you know that success has a foundation in honesty. You can take comfort in knowing that your new partner, girlfriend, or boyfriend accepts you and your diagnosis.

Regardless of when you choose to disclose, it can't be emphasized enough that disclosure must take place prior to any sexual contact—oral, anal, or vaginal.

DATING TIPS FOR HIV-POSITIVE PEOPLE

It goes without saying that the first time you date after being diagnosed with HIV is going to be a very stressful and frightening experience. There are a few things to keep in mind that will make the situation much easier for you and your prospective partner.

- *Serosorting*—some people employ a dating concept commonly referred to as *serosorting*. The practice of serosorting involves dating and having physical relationships with only those people who are the same serostatus as you; HIV positive dates positive and HIV negative dates negative. The idea is that if you date only those people who share your serostatus you are practicing safer sex and therefore condoms are not necessary. This line of thinking has major flaws. The biggest issue with serosorting is accurate information. A person's serostatus can't be determined by age, gender, race, or outward appearance. Some people may mistakenly believe they are HIV-negative. Unless the two parties are presenting some type of proof of their serostatus the information is just not reliable. In addition, even if serostatus has been determined correctly this concept offers no protection from other sexually transmitted infections like chlamydia, gonorrhea, or syphilis. If serosorting is your choice, make certain you share test results with your prospective partner and they share them with you.

- *Online Dating*—There are HIV-positive dating services on the Internet that can be helpful when it comes to looking for a date who is positive. But you need not limit yourself to only HIV-positive people. With the right precautions and honest discloser, you will find that special someone. Keep in mind that many social networking sites are primarily used for anonymous sexual "hook-ups." These types of encounters carry considerable risk of exposure to sexually transmitted diseases, including HIV. Some people consider taking personal ads in publications targeted at HIV-positive people, or at groups with a high incidence of HIV, such as the gay population. It's important to note that whether you date HIV-positive or negative people safer sex is still necessary. The risk of sexually transmitted diseases such as chlamydia, syphilis, and gonorrhea as well as the risk of HIV re-infection (see chapter 2) means safer sex and condoms are a must with each and every sexual encounter even between two HIV positive people.

- *Talk to Those Who Have Been There*—Talk to other HIV positive people who have resumed dating. Ask how they disclosed their diagnosis; what the experience was like; and if they have any advice for someone entering the dating world for the first time since being diagnosed with HIV.

- *Reactions to Your Diagnosis Will Vary*—Be prepared for a reaction after you disclose. It is hard to predict what that reaction will be, as it can range from supportive and understanding to rejection and abandonment. Rest assured there will be a reaction, so be prepared and keep in mind the reaction may not be what you expected or were hoping for at that time.

- *What Will You Gain*—Before disclosing your status, assess the relationship you have with the person with whom you are about to disclose. What will you gain from disclosing? Is the relationship the two of you have worth risking your confidentiality? Again, keep in mind, in most states disclosure is required if a sexual encounter is likely to occur, regardless of what you think of the relationship.

- *Be Prepared for Anything*—Be prepared for rejection, being let down, or feeling discouraged. With that being said, don't be afraid to get your feet wet. Nothing ventured, nothing gained.

- *Never Let HIV Define You*—HIV does not define who you are or what type of person you are. HIV does not rob you of your desires, your goals, or your personality. Healthy, rewarding relationships are possible for people living with HIV. Don't compromise your standards or settle for anyone less than you desire for fear of that person being your only choice. HIV does not mean you are desperate. Don't let the disease rob you of your self-esteem.

- *Be Cautious*—If you choose to use online services to find a date, take precautions to stay safe. Your first meeting should be in a public place. Do not divulge too much personal information too soon. Do not let your guard down until you are sure the person you have met online can be trusted and are who they claim to be.

So your first date leads to a second date, then a third. Before you know it, the two of you are a couple in a full-fledged relationship. Sounds like the perfect scenario, doesn't it? It can be, but there are situations that can stress any relationship. One type of relationship that has its share of unique challenges is one comprised of one HIV-positive partner and one HIV-negative partner. This type of relationship is described as *serodiscordant*.

THE CAUSE OF STRESS IN SERODISCORDANT RELATIONSHIPS

In an age when HIV-positive people are becoming more readily accepted by those around them, relationships that include one HIV-negative and one HIV-positive partner are becoming more common. One would be safe in saying that serodiscordant relationships can be riddled with anxiety, fear, confrontation, and a great deal of stress. One would think that in a relationship where a partner is HIV-positive, the cause of stress would be obvious. However, there are stressors that are not as obvious as one would think.

Transmission vs. Care Giving

In couples with two HIV-negative partners, the goal of both partners is the same: to stay HIV negative. However, in couples with one HIV-negative partner and one HIV-positive partner the goal or focus of each partner is different. The positive partner is concerned about transmitting the virus to the negative partner. In other words, the goal is to keep the negative partner HIV-free. The negative partner, on the other hand, typically devotes his or her attention to the health of their positive partner. In other words, they become the caregiver in the relationship, with the goal being to keep the positive partner healthy. This small difference in perspective, goal, and focus can cause emotional conflict within the relationship, ultimately increasing the level of stress and anxiety between the two partners.

How Did This Happen?

If one partner in a relationship becomes HIV positive, the first question the other partner will ask is, *"How did this happen?"* If the new infection is the result of unprotected sex outside the relationship, or a consequence of sharing needles while injecting drugs, it's possible the negative partner had no idea either behavior was occurring. The stress caused by the new HIV diagnosis is compounded by feelings of anger, betrayal, and sadness as the reality of their partner's infidelity and drug becomes evident.

Overly Cautious

In any serodiscordant relationship, there is concern and fear at the prospect of spreading HIV to the negative partner. Because of fear, the couple may become overly cautious in their sexual relationship, putting an end to any sexual or intimate contact for fear of spreading the infection. While it's not the most important part, sexual intimacy is an essential aspect of any loving relationship. Without intimacy, feelings of frustration, longing, and resentment will surface, and, as a result, the relationship will suffer. If a couple decides to be less intimate in an effort to protect the negative partner, at some point frustration and resentment may become an issue that will cause stress in the relationship.

Survivor's Guilt

Guilt can be a powerful but destructive emotion. Typically, survivor's guilt is a product of a traumatic event, such as a car accident, in which one person survives while many others die. The sole survivor feels guilty for having lived while so many others died. In a serodiscordant relationship the negative partner feels guilty for being healthy while his or her partner is living with HIV. The guilt becomes more intense if the positive partner has medical issues or becomes sick as a result of their HIV infection. In extreme cases, the guilt becomes so great that the negative partner wishes to be HIV-infected, feeling that being infected would relieve the guilt and, with it, the stressors related to that guilt.

The Desire to Have Children

Most couples in a loving, committed relationship will consider having a family at one time or another. The decision to start a family is a stressful one for any couple. But the concerns of a serodiscordant couple are unique. Obviously, outside of artificial means, unsafe sex is the primary way couples try to get pregnant. And as we all know, unsafe sex carries a considerable HIV risk for the negative partner. This, along with concerns over the risk of HIV transmission to the unborn child, creates a very stressful atmosphere at a time when couples should be enjoying the prospect of becoming parents. For serodiscordant couples, the decision to have children is much more complicated than for those couples without the risk of HIV transmission.

Keep in mind that ninety percent of the issues that strain a serodiscordant relationship are no different than those in any other relationship. However, it's the other 10 percent that can be the most challenging. What are those issues unique to the serodiscordant couple?

ISSUES FACING SERODISCORDANT COUPLES

Money/Employment

Money problems affect most any relationship at one time or another. But when it comes to serodiscordant relationships, the cause of money problems can be unique. The cost of HIV care and HIV medications is astronomical. Staying healthy requires regular trips to your doctor, sometimes as often as once each month. These visits can be very time consuming and can limit the number of hours that can be worked. As we all know, time is money, and while you can't put a price tag on your good health, the fact of the matter is that when you are at the doctor you're not working, and if you're not working your income will decrease accordingly. In addition, holding down a regular, full-time job can be extremely difficult, depending on the health of the individual. As money becomes scarce, unpaid bills, credit card balances, and late mortgage payments can accumulate, adding even more stress and anxiety to the relationship.

All the stress and anxiety related to financial difficulties can lead to resentment from the healthy partner. He or she can begin to question their partner's contributions to the household finances. Questions like "Why am I doing all the work?" can surface at some point. On the other hand, it's not uncommon for the positive partner to harbor a tremendous amount of guilt when he or she is unable to pull their share of the financial weight. Along with the guilt, the positive partner can harbor anger and resentment, realizing that it's his or her HIV infection that is causing the couple's financial difficulties.

To Disclose or Not to Disclose

Disclosure is stressful. That much we know. But it becomes a source of relationship stress when each partner has a different idea of who should be told about the HIV infection and who shouldn't. In this situation, one rule applies to every couple: except in circumstances of medical emergency or medical necessity, who is to be told about the HIV infection and when they are told is at the sole discretion of the positive partner. If the positive partner says no to disclosure, then the negative partner must abide by his or her wishes without question. The negative partner should never make independent decisions regarding disclosure.

Sharing Medical Information

Some positive people want their partner with them at every doctor's visit. Other positive people prefer to keep the medical part of their life private. At times, some negative partners have a hard time understanding this. It's natural for people in a committed relationship to want to be included in all aspects of their loved one's life, including medical issues. Leaving a loved one out of medical decisions spawns fear and doubt, two emotions that will undermine any relationship. Some people see that reluctance to share medical information as dishonest and an attempt to harbor secrets. Eventually these feelings can fester into major relationship issues.

Differences of Sexual Comfort and Desire

In a serodiscordant relationship there will be differing opinions regarding sex and intimacy. How much exposure risk is each partner willing to take? What type of safer sex practices will be used? In what sexual activities is each partner willing to participate? A good rule of thumb is that if either partner does not want to engage in an activity or take a risk with unsafe sex, then then the activity or risk in question should be avoided until a discussion and joint decision is made. Regardless, differences in sexual drive and risk-taking can become divisive in a serodiscordant relationship.

Fear of the Future

As is the case with any person living with a chronic illness, there is a significant amount of fear and uncertainty surrounding the future. The positive partner is uneasy, fearing the prospect of deteriorating health and an uncertain future. The negative partner dwells on questions such as *"How long will my loved one be healthy?"* or *"How long will he or she be alive?"* Fortunately, advances in HIV care has resulted in promising futures and life spans that match or exceed the life spans of HIV-negative people. As people continue to live longer and healthier, couples become more optimistic about what their future holds, and the prospect of losing a partner to HIV becomes less of a concern. However, in many circles, HIV is still considered a very real risk to the future of an individual and his or her relationship. In that case, these types of concerns will definitely impact the health of a relationship.

Dealing with Struggles—Making It Work

For as many barriers and issues that exist in serodiscordant relationships, they can be fulfilling and successful. The fact of the matter is that, like any relationship, it takes hard work and commitment from both partners to succeed. Psychologist Robert Remien of the HIV Center for Clinical and Behavioral Studies in New York City has done extensive research on the issues facing serodiscordant couples. He reminds us all that there are ways to work through the rough spots and enjoy the good ones. Here are a few ideas.

- Never stop talking to one another about the relationship issues that may arise. Share your feelings, regardless of how sensitive or painful it may be. While the pain is short term, the benefits from openly discussing issues will have lasting, positive effects for the relationship.
- Consider seeking professional counseling whenever issues arise that can't be worked out alone. Whether it's individual counseling, couples counseling, or both, it can be beneficial to have an impartial, trained ear to help you through the tough times.
- Keep issues in perspective. Obviously, the difference in your HIV status is significant. After all, one of you is positive and one is negative. But that difference should not define your relationship. It's only one of many characteristics that define you as a couple and as individuals. Celebrate the things you have in common and only those differences that add to the relationship.
- Take care of one another. All relationships need partners who are willing to care for one another, treat one another with respect, and show the loving emotions that brought you together in the first place. Many times it is the small gestures that make or break a relationship. Bring your partner a cup of coffee; buy them their favorite treat; and if they desire, accompany them to medical appointments to lend support.
- Remember that you love one another. There is a reason you are together in the first place. Never be afraid to remind one another now and again. Small reminders of the feelings you have can do wonders to get you through a stressful time in the relationship. Leave a little note with their lunch; send an "I love you" text during the day. Again, sometimes the little gestures can make the biggest difference.
- Be realistic about your situation. Don't fool yourself into thinking the difference in your HIV status will not affect the relationship in some way. There will be times that one partner or the other will feel like they can't take the stress any longer. Don't fake it; if you are unhappy, say so.
- Stay sexually safe and create sexual guidelines that you can both live with. Plan to discover new ways of eroticizing your lovemaking. Make it fun, laugh more, and don't be so serious. Share any fears, concerns, or feelings you may have related to sexual activities. Remember, if either partner is not comfortable with a certain sexual act, don't force the issue; find sexual techniques both of you are comfortable with and enjoy. The key to a successful relationship is to be open and honest.

We have talked about the physical and emotional aspects of HIV and AIDS. Clearly, HIV does indeed impact the entire person, and therefore, should be treated with that in mind. So, naturally, if HIV affects the whole person, the best way to stay healthy and live with HIV is to make healthy lifestyle choices that affect the entire person.

The following chapters look at lifestyle choices, both healthy and not so healthy. Let's start with an unhealthy choice—substance use and abuse.

11

Substance Use and Abuse

As you have just learned, this text devotes an entire chapter to the psychosocial aspects of HIV. That illustrates the significant impact HIV has on the emotional health of HIV-positive people. Since early on in the epidemic, experts have recognized the effect HIV has on the entire person—emotional as well as physical. In fact, many feel the psychosocial effects of HIV can be as detrimental as the physical aspects of the disease. Especially today as treatments are much improved and people are feeling much better physically, the psychosocial aspects of HIV have, for the most part, remained an issue and continue to interfere with the day-to-day lives of those infected. Different people handle the emotional aspects of HIV in different ways. Some turn to support groups in an effort to deal with the psychosocial stresses of HIV. Others engage in individual counseling to help adjust to their new diagnosis. And others turn to family and loved ones to receive the emotional help they need. But, sadly, there are many people who seek solace in a liquor flask, a pill bottle, or a needle and syringe. It's for these people that this chapter was written.

Ironically, substance use is a means by which HIV-positive people try to cope with their diagnosis, while contributing significantly to the number of people living with the disease. In fact, since the epidemic began, intravenous drug use (IVDU) has directly or indirectly been responsible for about one-third of all HIV/AIDS cases in the United States. Of those cases related to IVDU, one in every four persons is a member of a minority group, such as African-Americans or Hispanics. It's obvious that substance use plays a very significant role in the spread of HIV—so much so that the Health Resources and Services Administration's HIV/AIDS Bureau (HRSA/HAB) has devoted considerable funds from the Ryan White HIV/AIDS Program to the treatment of substance abuse and recreational drug use. HRSA/HAB recognized early on in the epidemic that because substance use contributes significantly to the growing number of HIV-infected people, drug treatment would be necessary to keep people healthy and to slow the HIV epidemic. The funds provided by the Ryan White HIV/AIDS Program not only support substance abuse treatment but also make it possible for people with substance abuse issues to access HIV care.

Needle Sharing and HIV

We've established the fact that intravenous drug use is a contributing factor to the HIV epidemic. Sterile needles and syringes are seldom available to IVDU (here meaning intravenous drug users). In fact, most states require a prescription to purchase needles and syringes. Because most IVDU have no medical need for their needles and syringes, they are unable to get a prescription to purchase the needle and syringe they need. Unable to get them legally, IVDU will obtain needles and syringes any way they can—either from illegal and unreliable sources, or by sharing the needles and syringes of other drug users. Because sterile needles and syringes are so difficult to come by, it's common practice for IVDU to share their needles and syringes with one another. In fact, in drug user circles, not sharing your needles and syringes is viewed as selfish, anti-social behavior. An IVDU who won't share is looked upon in a negative light, often resulting in theft or violence.

Sharing injection tools or "works," as they are called, exposes all IVDU to blood borne illnesses, including HIV. To inject recreational drugs into a vein, the user inserts the needle through the skin and into a vein. To make certain the needle is in the vein, users will pull back on the syringe plunger. If blood is pulled into the syringe the user knows he or she is in the vein and can inject the drug. After injecting the drug, some of the blood remains in the needle and syringe. When that needle and syringe are loaned to another user the remaining droplets of blood are incidentally injected along with the recreational drug into the person who borrowed the needle and syringe. This incidental injection of blood exposes the borrower to blood borne illnesses of the person from whom they borrowed the needle and syringe. It's this type of repeated sharing and reuse that drives the HIV epidemic among IVDU.

One obvious solution to the problem of needle sharing is abstinence from injecting drugs. However, kicking a drug addiction is very difficult, even when there is the desire to quit. Sadly, any desire to quit that may exist is usually outmatched by the power of cravings and withdrawal symptoms. In the event that the desire to quit does overpower the addiction, the process involves a long detoxification process, followed by a long period of group and individual counseling. In other words, it requires a long-term commitment.

In a perfect world, drug users would kick the habit and stop sharing needles. Consider this: if people stop using drugs there would be no need to share needles. If there is no needle sharing, then HIV risk would be reduced dramatically. To an HIV prevention specialist such a scenario is the perfect solution to the HIV problem among injection drug users. Unfortunately, a scenario of universal drug use abstinence is neither probable nor realistic. Just as sexual abstinence is an unrealistic way to prevent sexual transmission of HIV, so is abstinence from injecting illegal drugs and sharing needles. The concept of risk reduction applies to those who inject illegal drugs as well as those who engage in risky sexual behavior. Needle exchange programs incorporate risk reduction education in addition to swapping out used needles and syringes. While studies have shown needle exchange does decrease HIV transmission, the concept is clouded in controversy.

To those opposing needle exchange, it's believed to be nothing more than a means for addicts to get what they need to inject more illegal drugs. Most politicians view needle exchange as the hot button issue that could spell political suicide for anyone publicly supporting the practice. As a result, political support and financial resources for needle exchange programs are scarce. The situation begs the question: if needle exchange is as effective as studies have shown, why is there so little support from the people who hold the purse strings?

Needle Exchange Programs

The simple fact remains that sterile needles and syringes are not easy to get your hands on if you're an IV drug user. And because they're so hard to come by, IVDU resort to sharing dirty needles in order to satisfy their need for opiates. Even in those rare circumstances when clean needles and syringes are available by prescription, most IVDU do not have the financial means or medical need to get them legally. The criminalization of drugs and drug paraphernalia makes IV drug users reluctant to seek out sterile needles and syringes through exchange programs. So one of the few options available is using dirty needles and syringes borrowed from fellow injection drug users. Because needles and syringes are desperately needed to satisfy the powerful urges and cravings characteristic of an opiate addiction, refusing to share those items is considered bad etiquette among drug users. In fact, refusing to share sometimes places the user at considerable risk of retaliation from other users desperate to get their next opiate fix. Think of it as an extreme case of peer pressure. Unfortunately, on many occasions, the fear of physical violence pressures the user to share his or her needles and syringes even if they would rather not do so.

To combat the health risks of needle sharing and to offer drug users a less risky alternative, needle exchange programs have been developed. These programs are based on the concept of risk reduction—if the risk can't be eliminated entirely, then the next best thing is to reduce the risk. Because kicking the opiate habit is unrealistic for many people, the next best thing is to reduce the risk of intravenous drugs by using only sterile needles to inject drugs.

Needle exchange programs reduce the HIV infection risk by providing sterile needles and syringes in exchange for used ones. Drug users bring their dirty needles and syringes to a needle exchange site and are given a new sterile needle and syringe in return. Not only does this decrease the HIV risk of the person exchanging the needle, but it actually decreases a number of people's HIV risk. By taking one needle and syringe out of circulation, the HIV risk for several people is decreased. Depending on where the injection was done and how many people are in the social environment, one used needle and syringe potentially could cause many HIV infections. In addition, taking the used needle and syringe out of circulation decreases hepatitis C infections transmitted by needle sharing.

Needle exchange programs are most often part of community-based HIV agencies offering such services as HIV testing and prevention and medical case management. To maximize accessibility, these programs are sometimes mobile—housed in motor homes, buses, or trucks, making it possible for the agency to take the needle exchange program into the community where it's needed most. For instance, in large urban areas you may find a needle exchange van parked near food banks, homeless shelters or halfway houses, any place IV drug users are known to frequent. Often, drug users are reluctant, unwilling, or unable to go to the HIV agency where the needle exchange program is housed. Therefore, in order for needle exchange to be successful it has to be taken to those hard-to-reach people, which means going into the community where they live, hang out, and inject their drugs.

Typically, a needle exchange program is much more than a place where dirty needles and syringes are exchanged for new. The agencies that operate these programs take advantage of the time they have with the IV drug user by incorporating other important services into the needle exchange program. It's a concept borrowed from the retail industry. Retail stores will have big sales in order to get buyers into the store. Once in the store, buyers will purchase other items along with the sale item. In the case of needle exchange, the offer of free sterile needles and syringes brings the IV drug user to the needle exchange professionals. Once with the program staff, the IV drug user is offered other services in addition to the needle exchange. For instance, a drug user can meet with an HIV test counselor, case manager, or addiction counselor. Some programs require an assessment by these other professionals in order to get the sterile needle and syringe. In many cases, medical examinations are also offered in an attempt to get HIV-positive drug users into HIV care if they are not in care already. In essence, the needle exchange program serves a two-fold need: it's a means to decrease needle sharing, and it's a way to reach an otherwise hard to reach population, bringing to them the other services they so desperately need.

However, HIV professionals walk a very fine line between offering additional services and scaring people away from the program altogether. For instance, those people reluctant or afraid to be HIV tested will shy away from any needle exchange program that requires HIV testing as part of the exchange. The services must be presented as a recommended option, not a requirement that will scare people away. But for those IV drug users who are willing, HIV testing, counseling, and medical care are additional benefits of the needle exchange programs.

Decades of HIV surveillance data has provided scientific evidence that needle exchange is an effective means of decreasing the spread of HIV. So one would assume that government entities would be eager to fund such programs. After all, it's a simple way to cut infection rates and slow HIV transmission. But despite recommendations from the Centers for Disease Control (CDC), the World Health Organization (WHO), and the U.S. Surgeon General, support for needle exchange programs is sometimes difficult to find in the political arena. In the United States, politicians and government leaders are very reluctant to support and promote funding for such programs. In fact, since 1980, it has been against the law for the U.S. government to provide funding for needle exchange programs. Why, you ask? The answer is simple. It's politics. The politics of needle exchange is a major barrier to this effective HIV risk reduction method.

The Politics of Needle Exchange

The truth is that needle exchange has been proven to be an effective HIV risk reducing method. If that's the case, then why are the politicians and government officials who hold the purse strings so reluctant to take a stand and provide the funding necessary to make needle exchange programs a reality? One would think people would jump at the chance to slow the HIV rate. After all, common sense tells us that programs proven to be effective in slowing the HIV epidemic, like needle exchange, for instance, should be funded and put in place across the country. Unfortunately, it doesn't seem to be that easy.

The fact of the matter is that needle exchange is a politically charged issue that very few politicians are willing to have their name attached to. In fact, up until recently, federal law made it illegal to use government monies to fund needle exchange programs. Only about half of all states even permit needle exchange in their state. In 2009, Congress lifted the ban just to have it reinstituted by the House of Representatives in 2012. Finally, in 2016, the ban was lifted somewhat. While it is still illegal to use government monies for needles and syringes, government funds can now pay for program staff, administration costs, and facility rental. Still not perfect, but it is a step in the right direction. Money saved on what government funds can cover will be available for more needles and syringes. So until the laws change, needle exchange programs rely primarily on private funding sources and the few state and local funding opportunities that exist. Unfortunately, because these sources are closely tied to changes in the economy, they can be very tenuous and short-lived, and ideally shouldn't be relied upon to keep programs afloat for long periods of time.

THE ARGUMENT SUPPORTING NEEDLE EXCHANGE FUNDING

Proponents cite several reasons why needle exchange laws preventing government funding should be repealed:

- Data shows that nine out of every ten cases of heterosexually transmitted HIV are related to IV drug use and sharing needles.
- HIV surveillance data shows that around the world, HIV transmission increases in areas where needle sharing and injection drug use is common.
- Numerous studies have demonstrated that needle exchange programs contribute to decreased rates of HIV transmission rates among IV drug users.
- Studies have concluded that needle exchange does not increase the probability that a person will start using injection drugs.
- Finally, studies have shown that the number of people entering drug treatment programs increases in the presence of needle exchange programs.

THE ARGUMENT AGAINST NEEDLE EXCHANGE FUNDING

Opponents of needle exchange are quick to point out dozens of reasons why they feel funding needle exchange is a mistake. Opponents have expressed many concerns. According to opponents:

- Funding needle exchange sends the "wrong message" to children. Opponents are concerned that the concept of needle exchange conveys to children and young people that IV drug use is an acceptable behavior with few consequences.
- Needle exchange enables IV drug use, especially among those populations already ravaged by drug addiction. Opponents believe that removing a barrier to IV drug use will result in more people injecting drugs. In turn, if more people inject drugs, it follows that more people will become HIV-infected. However, if more people are injecting drugs and sterile needles and syringes aren't available, then needle sharing is the only alternative. The fact of the matter is users will inject drugs whether the needle is used or not. A sterile needle will not cause someone to inject drugs if they weren't already injecting drugs. In other words, the reasoning is flawed and contradicts itself.
- The practice of needle exchange is in stark contrast to the U.S. government's fight against drugs. The government's commitment to reducing drug use includes decreasing the number of needles and syringes on the streets. Any federal funding of needle exchange will increase their numbers on the street—a practice that would contradict the govern-

ment's stance on drug use. However, needle exchange is a one-to-one proposition: one old needle gets one sterile needle. If that's the case, theoretically the number of needles in circulation does not change. Again, the reasoning is flawed.

- If needle exchange programs are funded by the government, it means your tax dollars would be funding an illegal activity—in this instance, injection drug use. Few officials are willing to have their name associated with such a practice.

- Distributing drug paraphernalia in the form of needles and syringes is in stark contrast to the accepted morals of our society. These morals say that drug use is bad, and no one, including the federal government, shall do anything to make it easier for people to engage in the activity. Actually exchanging dirty needles does not make it easier to inject drugs. Dirty or clean, the drugs will be injected. Needle exchange makes it safer to inject, not easier.

- According to opponents, needle exchange promotes risky behavior and undermines efforts to stem the problems of substance abuse and HIV infection among IV drug users. Again, the reasoning is flawed. Exchanging a dirty needle for a clean one actually decreases risky behavior, in this case sharing dirty needles. In fact, a number of studies have proven that needle exchange programs do not increase drug use. In fact, a 5-year study in San Francisco showed that not only did the number of daily injections among users go down from 1.9 to 0.7 but the number of drug users taking their first injection went down as well, from 3 percent of users to 1 percent.

Where Do We Stand

In 2015, the small town of Austin, Indiana, had 200 new HIV infections due primarily to an epidemic of needle sharing to inject heroin. In the same year, the Drug Enforcement Agency (DEA) placed a new emphasis on combatting the abuse of prescription opiates, including hydrocodone (Norco/Vicodin) and OxyContin. The resulting changes to the practice of prescribing pain medications had an unanticipated side effect. While decreasing the number of opiate prescriptions is a good thing it caused an explosion in heroin use among people addicted to opiates but unable to get their prescriptions. To quench the powerful cravings of opiate addiction, people began turning to cheaper, more widely available heroin for their "fix." The resulting increase in heroin use and the infections in Austin prompted Congress to lift the ban prohibiting the use of federal funds to support needle exchange programs, to an extent. Starting in 2016, federal funds can be used to fund needle exchange program staff, facilities, office supplies, etc. It's still against the law to use federal monies to purchase needles and syringes but allowing federal money to be used for administrative costs is a start. The federal government has also permitted states to make their own decisions regarding needle exchange funding, and as a result, some states are now funding needle exchange.

In 2014, there were about 200 needle exchange programs in 33 states. By softening rules prohibiting the use of federal funds for needle exchange, the hope is that the number of programs will rise dramatically. Federal funds can now be used for purchasing vans to take programs on the road or for renting space for needle exchange clinics. However, even with the dramatic increase in heroin use in states like Kentucky, Virginia, Indiana, and Ohio, new programs are slow to emerge, especially in cash-strapped rural areas. However, in the larger cities exchange is occurring. The *Columbus Dispatch* reported in March 2016 that in five of the largest cities in Ohio, 54,000 needles are being exchanged each month. While each needle costs those programs about 97 cents, it is a far cry from the almost $400,000 it takes to care for an HIV positive patient for his or her lifetime or the $100,000 to care for a person living with hepatitis C. As you can see, 97 cents for a sterile needle is money well spent.

Understanding Substance Use and Addiction

Substance abuse continues to be a major public health issue in the U.S. and around the world. When people talk of addiction and abuse, typically they're referring to illegal drugs such as cocaine, heroin, or methamphetamine. But the fact of the matter is that prescription drug abuse and addiction is as much a problem as is addiction to illegal drugs. In a 2005 survey, more than 6 million Americans reported using prescription drugs in the previous month for non-medicinal purposes. That number exceeds the number of people who abuse heroin, crack, hallucinogens, and inhalants combined. But the scales may be tilting in the other direction. As we mentioned previously in this chapter, efforts to quell the prescription drug abuse and diversion problem in the U.S. have caused a dramatic increase in heroin use. Many are turning to cheaper, easier to obtain heroin now that physicians have slowed the use of prescription narcotics and opiates by writing fewer prescriptions. Unfortunately, doing a good thing like decreasing prescription drug abuse has caused a growing problem in another area of drug use and abuse. Once a person becomes addicted and dependent on opiates, that person will go to any and all lengths to get that next dose and avoid withdrawal, even using heroin if that's what it takes.

Addiction and abuse do not necessarily refer to illegal substances. Alcohol, for instance, is a legal substance available at any carry-out or grocery store. Yet people around the world abuse alcohol and fight one of the hardest addictions to beat. The World Health Organization (WHO) estimates that more than 170 million people worldwide suffer from alcohol addiction. Unlike cocaine, heroin, and crystal meth, alcohol is legal and readily available to anyone who wants it, making addiction more likely and kicking the habit much more difficult. Don't let the legality of alcohol fool you into believing its addiction and abuse are less dangerous than illegal drugs. Alcohol addiction is as devastating to the individual and his or her loved ones as any illegal substance. And the sad fact is that of the 170 million people struggling with alcohol addiction, an estimated 78 percent go untreated.

Substance abuse and addiction are not limited to alcohol and drugs alone. In fact, there are addictive substances all around us. For instance, according to a recent survey, nearly 42 million people say they smoke cigarettes every day. Smokers become addicted to the nicotine they take in with each puff. Or consider this fact. Research being done at Johns Hopkins reports that caffeine, the substance found in coffee, soft drinks, energy drinks, and tea, is the most abused drug in the world. Amazingly, in North America alone, 80 to 90 percent of all adults and children consume caffeine on a daily basis. And finally, people even have addiction issues with food. *Compulsive eating* (overeating), *anorexia nervosa* (starving oneself), and *bulimia nervosa* (binging and purging) are all types and degrees of food addiction. It's obvious from these examples that addiction is a very powerful disease that can touch even the most basic aspects of our life. Let's look at addiction and why it occurs.

The Science of Addiction

The concept of addiction can be a very confusing one. Terms like addiction and dependence are used interchangeably, and, in fact, are often used incorrectly. The misuse of these terms can cloud our understanding of addiction and dependence. In order to fully understand substance abuse, we have to understand the difference between drug dependence and drug addiction.

PHYSICAL DEPENDENCE

Physical dependence is defined as the adaptation by the body to a substance to such an extent that when that substance is absent, the body experiences physical withdrawal symptoms. Physical symptoms such as tremors, anxiety, and acute pain result when the body is deprived of the dependent substance. While these symptoms can be very unpleasant at times, they do not confer addiction to a substance. The key point to remember is that you can be physically dependent on a substance and experience withdrawal symptoms when deprived of that substance and yet not be addicted to that substance.

PSYCHOLOGICAL DEPENDENCE

Psychological dependence is defined as the compulsion to use a substance for its pleasurable effects. This can last far longer than physical dependence—weeks, months, years or, in some cases, a lifetime. It's related more to the person's habits and lifestyle than it is to the substance itself. It's rooted in memories of pleasure associated with the substance. People long for those memories, and their drug is merely the means by which their longing is fulfilled. Think of it in another way. Psychological dependence is a "craving" that is psychologically based, as opposed to the physical feelings of withdrawal that accompany physical dependence. That being said, physical withdrawal symptoms can also occur with psychological dependence as well as physical dependence.

TABLE 11

Physical Dependence
- Defined as the adaptation by the body to a substance to such an extent that when that substance is absent, the body experiences physical withdrawal symptoms.
- Physical symptoms such as tremors, anxiety, and acute pain result when the body is deprived of the dependent substance.
- Physical dependence does not confer addiction.
- You can be physically dependent and not be addicted.

Psychological Dependence
- Defined as the compulsion to use a substance for its pleasurable effects.
- Lasts far longer than physical dependence—weeks, months, years or, in some cases, a lifetime.
- Rooted in memories of pleasure associated with the substance.
- A craving that is psychologically based, as opposed the physical feelings of withdrawal that accompany physical dependence.

ADDICTION

Addiction is defined as a behavioral syndrome that's characterized by repeated, compulsive use of a substance or substances, despite adverse physical, psychological, and social consequences. Addiction and the probability of a person becoming addicted are dependent upon genetic, psychological, environmental, and social factors. This serious condition is typically characterized by diminishing effectiveness of the drug. In other words, addiction produces the need for increasing amounts of a substance to achieve the same affect. For instance, if you once achieved the desired "high" from two tablets of Norco (hydrocodone + acetaminophen), as your addiction progresses it will take three or four tablets to achieve that same "high." Eventually, the euphoria that was once a product of the medication will be gone and the sole effect of the medication is withdrawal symptom relief.

Understanding the difference between addiction and dependence can be very difficult. Try to think of it this way. Addiction is a behavioral syndrome in which drug use and procurement dominates a person's normal motivation. The user devotes all their energy to finding that next dose of medication. In fact, the addicted person ignores negative social consequences associated with their drug use in order to get more medication. Many will resort to criminal actions, such as stealing or writing fraudulent prescriptions, in order to get more drug. But despite the overwhelming power of drug addiction, the user may or may not experience the physical symptoms of withdrawal commonly experienced in physical dependence. So why do drugs have such a profound effect on certain people? What do drugs do to the brain that causes responsible, law-abiding people to risk everything for their next dose of Norco, Oxy-Contin, or heroin?

How Do Drugs Work in the Brain?

Think of the brain as the body's communication hub where messages are sent, received, and processed millions of times every second. The brain has to process all these messages and tell the body what it should or shouldn't do in response to the message. The brain does all this work using specialized chemicals (neurotransmitters) naturally manufactured in the body. Different nerve endings send different messages to the brain. If you put your hand in cold water, a message is sent telling you the water is cold. If that water is hot, the same type of message tells the brain the water is warm. The brain interprets these messages and issues a response appropriate for the message. If the water is too cold the brain tells your body to remove your hand from the cold water. If the water is too hot, the brain also tells your body to remove your hand from the water. It's a perfect system of message received and acted upon, working perfectly every time. However, abusive drugs can alter that intricate system of communication, and if addiction occurs the damage can be permanent.

Abusive drugs like heroin tap into the brain's communication system and mimic the action of the naturally occurring neurotransmitters. Certain drugs have molecular structures very similar to naturally occurring neurotransmitters. Because of their similarity they can access neurotransmitter receptors and activate nerve cells. In doing so they can send messages that normally would not have been sent. However, they don't stimulate nerve endings in the same way as natural neurotransmitters, so the messages sent through the neural network are typically intensified and abnormal. For instance, some drugs will cause very large amounts of natural neurotransmitter to be released, resulting in amplified messages being sent across the neural network. Others will cause abnormal messages to be sent across the network that affect the normal processing and recycling of neurotransmitters, prolonging and intensifying the effects of the neurotransmitter.

At first glance one may think that intensifying the effect neurotransmitters have would be a good thing, or at the very least would not be harmful. After all, if a little is good more would be better, right? Unfortunately, that is not the case. Prolonged unnatural stimulation of nerve endings by abusive drugs can eventually disrupt the proper functioning of the nerve cells and break down communication channels altogether. So obviously, if this is true then addiction can cause serious changes in brain chemistry and function. Since the brain is responsible for who we are and how we function, addiction can and does change the person we are and as such should be prevented at all costs. Unfortunately, there are a variety of factors that increase the risk of addiction and substance abuse; some we can change and some we can't.

Factors That Increase Risk of Addiction

We know drug addiction is a result of unnatural stimulation of our brain's communication system. So why are some people more prone to addiction than others? Why do some people suffer from addiction while others seem to have no addictive potential at all? There are many factors that increase the probability a person will have problems with addiction. They generally fall into one of three categories.

- *Biological*—the risk or probability of becoming addicted can be affected by such biological factors as gender, ethnicity, genetics, and mental status. For instance, if a person is suffering from depression or anxiety, their tendency to take abusive drugs and become addicted to them increases. The presence of certain genetic markers can predict an increased risk of addiction when compared to people who do not have those markers. Finally, certain stages of brain development are more prone to addictive behaviors than others.
- *Environmental*—there are factors in a person's environment that can increase the risk of addiction and substance abuse. For instance, a family history of addiction or substance abuse is a predictor of those same behaviors in the children of addictive parents. This is particularly true for alcohol use and abuse. Young adults with poor academic performance or poor social skills also have an increased risk of addiction. Finally, drug use and abuse by peers increase the risk of addiction and abuse by young adults trying to "fit in or belong" to their group of peers.
- *Other Factors*—there are a number of miscellaneous factors that can also increase the risk of abuse and addiction. Using drugs or alcohol at an early age increases the risk of continued addiction. Early disruption of the brain's reward system can lead to addictive tendencies as one ages. Exposure to physical or sexual abuse or belonging to a dysfunctional family situation can increase the risk of substance use and addiction. Finally, the mode of drug administration will increase addiction probability as well. Because smoking or injecting drugs has an intense and rapid onset of euphoria, the effects also dissipate

quickly. This means the user must take their next dose sooner to recapture the desired euphoria. Rapid dosing can lead to dose escalation, addiction and abuse.

Our Reward System

The human brain is an amazing organ, controlling millions of physiological processes every second. Over the course of evolution, our brains have developed specialized systems that ensure the survival of the human species. One such system involves "rewards" for those behaviors the body believes are essential and must be perpetuated for survival. Activation of this reward system produces changes in mood, affect, and motivation in such a way that the body repeats the behavior in hopes of getting the reward again. These changes can range from a slight mood elevation to intense pleasure and euphoria. In response to these "rewards," the body will direct behavior in hopes of being rewarded once again. As a result, this system assures that behaviors essential for survival are repeated over and over.

The essence of the body's reward system rests in specialized cells deep within the brain. When these cells are stimulated they trigger the release of a specialized substance known as *dopamine*. Dopamine is a naturally occurring neurotransmitter that sends nerve impulses from cell to cell within the brain. There are specialized receptors in the brain waiting to be "filled" by dopamine. When dopamine fills these receptors, mood is elevated and feelings of euphoria flood the brain. The euphoria experienced with the release of dopamine is the brain's reward for the body's essential behaviors. Like giving your dog a treat when he sits on command, your brain treats your body when you engage in a behavior the brain recognizes as important and necessary for survival.

To simplify the concept of a reward system, think of the dopamine receptor as a lock, and dopamine as the key. The only way to unlock the lock is to have the key. Once the key is in the lock, the lock can be opened. The same is true for the brain's reward system. Once dopamine has attached to its receptor in the brain, the reward system can be unlocked, elevating mood and causing euphoria. And like a dog repeating a behavior that wins him a treat, the body will repeat the behavior that elicits mood elevation and euphoria.

Experts believe the body's reward system may be at the root of drug addiction. A drug's ability to cause the release of dopamine that stimulates our reward system makes that drug potentially abusive and addictive. As we have already discussed, the purpose of our reward system is to reinforce certain behaviors and assure that they are repeated. So it's logical to assume that any drug stimulating our reward system—a reward system that produces euphoria and mood elevation—has the potential for addiction. Each time a drug stimulates the body's reward system in response to a specific behavior, that behavior is reinforced. In the case of addiction, taking your drug of choice and the euphoria that goes along with it is the behavior being reinforced, and one that your brain wants repeated over and over.

So if the reward system causes addiction to drugs like cocaine, why doesn't addiction occur with other things that stimulate our reward system—sex, for instance. When we engage in sexual activities, dopamine is released and our reward system is stimulated and we feel good. The problem is that drugs like cocaine cause the release of dopamine in amounts two to ten times greater than the naturally occurring release during activities such as sex. In other words, the euphoria produced by sex is small compared to the euphoria caused by cocaine because of the much larger amount of dopamine being released into our reward system after using cocaine. The euphoria is so much greater the body wants to take cocaine over and over to regain the unnaturally enhanced feeling of pleasure and euphoria.

The Long-Term Effects of Drugs on the Brain

Drugs like hydrocodone (e.g., Lortabs, Norco), cocaine, heroin, and other opiates have an unnatural effect on the dopamine receptors in the brain. Prolonged used of opiates can actually change the chemical make-up and physiology of the brain. These drugs affect the amount of dopamine released and the way in which receptors use that dopamine.

Different drugs affect our reward system in different ways. Under normal circumstances, cells of the dopamine system are always active, constantly releasing small amounts of dopamine into the brain. The steady release of dopamine is believed to play a role in mood stability. The introduction of certain drugs into the body affects the cells that stimulate the release of dopamine. For instance, heroin increases the amount and the rate at which dopamine is released into the brain, meaning the levels of dopamine in the brain also increase. The increased levels of dopamine cause the mood elevation and euphoria characteristic of heroin use. However, the body will eventually eliminate the heroin from the brain, meaning dopamine levels return to normal and the euphoria and mood elevation subside. But the body "remembers" the pleasant effects of heroin and is very motivated to use heroin again and again. However, in between "hits" of heroin, the user finds that the normal levels of dopamine aren't enough and feels depressed, hopeless, and without pleasure in anything they do. Their priority becomes getting their next dose of heroin so the feeling of euphoria returns. Unfortunately, the levels of dopamine that once caused euphoria are now necessary just to maintain a stable mood; the feelings of euphoria the user craves are gone so they use more heroin in hopes of achieving that feeling again. This "dose escalation" is necessary to achieve the "high" they so badly crave.

Cocaine has a somewhat different effect on the dopamine receptors of the brain. Instead of stimulating more dopamine to be released, cocaine slows the elimination of dopamine from the brain. As the body continues to produce dopamine at a normal rate, the cocaine slows its elimination, meaning the amount of dopamine increases. Think of it as a glass being filled with water. If water runs into it at a steady rate but does not empty out, the glass fills with water. Dopamine is produced at a steady rate, but because cocaine has slowed its elimination from the brain, the amount of dopamine rises. Dopamine builds up in the brain, and mood elevation and euphoria result. Once again, the brain "remembers" the effects of cocaine and is very motivated to use the drug again.

After being taken for extended periods of time, drugs such as opiates can change the way the dopamine system works. Repeated or prolonged use of substances that affect the dopamine system actually deplete the amount of dopamine in the body. In addition, prolonged drug use can cause the breakdown of dopamine receptors in the brain. With less dopamine and fewer receptors, the reward system breaks down and the euphoria and pleasure once derived from enjoyable activities is lost. With less available dopamine and dopamine receptors, stimuli that normally caused an elevation in mood and motivation no longer do so. In essence, there is no longer enough dopamine for the reward system to function properly.

More About Why People Become Addicted

We now understand how the body becomes addicted to certain substances. We understand the difference between addiction, physical dependence, and psychological dependence. Now let's take a closer look at the big question: why do people become addicted to substances like cocaine and heroin?

Factors Contributing to Addiction

Genetics

One factor that contributes to the risk of addiction is genetics. Experts have found that certain genes in the human genome can increase the probability a person will have addiction issues. In fact, studies have found that approximately 50 percent of drug addiction is related to genetics. In 2003, scientists concluded the *Human Genome Project*—a project to map the 3 billion gene pairs that make up the human genome. As part of that project, scientists mapped about 400 different genes that influence the probability of addiction.

There are plenty of genetic studies that confirm the role of genetics in addiction. Over all about 50 percent of addiction can be attributed to genetics. One study looked at 861 pairs of identical twins. The study found that if one twin was struggling with addiction, the other twin had a much higher chance of addiction as well. Another study found that children of addicted parents had an 8 times greater risk of addiction than children without addicted parents.

If that's the case, why do we have addiction genes when the results of addiction can be so catastrophic? Ironically, addiction is hard wired into our survival as a species. There is an evolutionary advantage to addiction. For example, if an animal eats a food it likes, genes of addiction urge the animal to eat that food again in order to survive. Think of it this way. How many times have you eaten too much of your favorite food despite knowing it will make you gain weight? It's our addiction genes prompting us to eat that food again and again, in an evolutionary sense, so we survive.

Environment

Studies have shown that genetics alone do not determine a person's probability of addiction. In other words, just because a person has the genetic markers for addiction doesn't mean that person is doomed to a life of drug abuse. Environmental factors, combined with genetic predisposition, determine the probability of addiction. Studies have shown that environment accounts for about 50 percent of a person's chance of becoming addicted, the other 50 percent being primarily determined by genetics. The environmental share of addiction generally falls into three domains.

The Community Domain—The community in which a person is raised or lives plays a significant role in addiction or substance abuse. For instance, in those communities where crime, violence, alcohol and drugs are prevalent, the risk of addiction is higher. If the incidence of drug addiction and the availability of recreational drugs in the community is high the risk individuals will fall prey to drugs and addiction is also high. In addition, the views a community has toward drug use and drug rehabilitation play a big role in the addiction potential of a community member. For instance, if the community has a structured network of addiction prevention and treatment services, the risk of addiction by a community member is less than if the community has no such network. Finally, in communities that have fewer financial resources or lack activities connecting individuals to the community, there is a higher risk of addiction and substance use. In fact, it is these types of communities have shown the highest prevalence of drug use and addiction.

The Peer Domain—One of the most significant factors to consider when assessing addiction risk, especially among adolescents, is peer pressure. Often times, recreational drugs are tried in order to feel part of the peer group. Members of the group use drugs and encourage others to try them. Experimenting with a certain drug is thought to be harmless: "Just once won't hurt." Unfortunately, ten percent of people who try recreational drugs will become addicted after the first experimentation. For example, the drug crystal methamphetamine ("crystal meth") is a drug used at parties in order to stay awake, increase sexual stamina, and to experience the euphoria of drug use. For these and other reasons, many people try it for the first time in a party situation and sadly, become addicted after a single use.

The risk of addiction can also be increased by having friends or associates who are addicted to drugs themselves. Having friends who encourage others to use drugs also increases a person's risk of addiction. Adolescents are especially influenced by peer pressure. Adolescents place a very high value on belonging to a group of friends and being socially accepted. Many young adults would risk the negative effects of drug use and possible addiction in order to feel they are popular, that they belong, and that they are one of the gang. Having peers that have favorable opinions about drug use will increase the risk of addiction and misuse by their friends.

In addition to peer influence, the age at which one is exposed to drugs or alcohol plays a major role in that person's risk of addiction. The earlier a person starts using drugs or alcohol the higher the risk of addiction. The developing brain of an adolescent or a child is especially vulnerable to drug addiction. The neurotransmitter dopamine is not only involved with pleasure but with memory and learning as well. Coincidentally, learning and memory along with our pleasure system are responsible for addiction. So as the brain of an adolescent develops, learns, and produces memories, it is very vulnerable to developing addiction. For instance, there is research data that offers proof that kids drinking alcohol regularly by the age of 14 years were more likely to be alcoholic by age 21.

The Family Domain—The family environment, specifically a lack of stability in the family, plays a large role in the risk of addiction. For instance, family conflict or addiction within the family can increase the risk of addiction for each family member. In families with supporting and nurturing parents and siblings, the risk of their children becoming addicted is less than those families where children lacked the support and involvement of at least one of their parents. While males in the family have a higher incidence of addiction, females seem to progress to addiction related disorders much faster than do males. When parents struggle with addiction, the children in that family will have an increased risk of addiction. The same is true of siblings. An addicted sibling increases the risk of an addicted brother or sister. The reason for this is twofold. First, children learn by example, typically by the example of those closest to them, siblings and parents. So observing a parent or sibling struggling with drugs increases the chance that the child will also have issues with addiction later in life. The other factor is genetic. Researchers know that there are many human genes that have an impact on addiction. Children are a product of genes from their mother and father. Those addiction genes mentioned earlier in this chapter are passed down from parents to children, meaning the risk of addiction is passed down as well. Finally, individuals who live impoverished or are subject to physical or emotional abuse have an increased risk of addiction, turning to illegal drugs in an attempt to mask the physical and emotional pain in their lives. Fewer financial resources means living in neighborhoods where violence and drug use are common. The stress of limited financial resources combined with exposure to a violent, drug-filled environment is a perfect recipe for drug addiction.

Mental Illness

It's not uncommon for a person to have a dual diagnosis of mental illness and drug addiction. Mental illness and addiction are related in a complex way. Of those people with addiction, 50 percent will develop mental illness. Of those with mental illness, 20 percent will develop addiction. Simply put, addiction can cause mental illness and vice versa. There are certain mental illnesses that are frequently associated with addiction.

- *Depression*—while more common in females than males, both sexes turn to illegal drugs or alcohol to deal with symptoms of depression. The drugs or alcohol mask the unpleasant and uncomfortable symptoms of depression, a short-term solution that eventually becomes a long-term problem.
- *Bipolar Disorder*—those suffering with bipolar disorder will experience emotions ranging from severe depression to a severely elevated mood ("manic"). Drugs and alcohol are sometimes used to temper the severe mood swings that people living with bipolar disorder have to endure. The illegal drugs "smooth out" the ups and downs of bipolar disorder.
- *Anxiety*—as is the case in depression and bipolar disorder, alcohol and drugs are often used to mask the symptoms of anxiety. In many instances, drugs and alcohol are used to help the individual sleep, something that can be very difficult when one suffers from anxiety.
- *Schizophrenia*—the auditory and visual hallucinations common in schizophrenia can be very disturbing and difficult to tolerate. Sufferers will often use drugs and alcohol to block those symptoms, masking them in hopes of shutting off the "voices" in their head. The "voices" are so real they can cause people to go as far as harming others or even harming themselves.

Another factor to consider is the uninhibited nature of people living with mental illness. Those who are uninhibited are more likely to engage in high risk behavior such as buying illegal drugs or frequenting drug houses and areas where drug use is rampant. These people also tend to use more alcohol and drugs due to impaired judgment and the lack of willpower. These types of behavior are the perfect precursors to drug and alcohol use and abuse. In addition, because of impaired judgment and lack of inhibitions, substance abuse treatment is more difficult because the person is unable to make rational decisions about their health.

Experts explain that addiction and mental illness are related to changes in the same region of the brain. The area known as the *amygdala* is involved with the generation of emotions, including fear, anxiety, and happiness. Because mental illnesses such as anxiety, bipolar depression, and schizophrenia are related to the amygdala as well, addiction and these mental illnesses are common bedfellows. In situations of high stress, tension, loneliness, anxiety, or depression, people often turn to drugs for a short reprieve. Unfortunately, what starts out as a short-term solution for the trials and tribulations of everyday life becomes a long-term problem with life-long consequences.

There is also a similarity in brain chemistry with addiction and certain mental illnesses. For instance, the decreased levels of the neurotransmitter *serotonin* in the brain of those addicted to alcohol as well as those with anxiety disorders may be the reason why alcoholism and anxiety disorders are commonly found together. A second example is the evidence that mental illness and addiction are associated with the dysfunction of brain chemicals known as *monoamine oxidases*. Monoamine oxidase is an enzyme that metabolizes monoamines, such as serotonin, norepinephrine, and dopamine, chemicals that play a big role in mental illness and addiction.

Experts feel it is crucial, when a person suffers from mental illness and addiction, to sort out which symptoms are related to which condition. It can be difficult to identify the type of mental illness present because many of the mental illness symptoms are being masked by the alcohol or drug use. However, it is imperative that the mental illness is identified so it can be treated at the same time as the addiction. If the mental health illness is not treated the treatment for addiction will fail. The two disorders must be treated simultaneously for either treatment to be successful.

Addiction Treatment

Despite what many believe, drug addiction is an illness—specifically, an illness seated in the brain and its function. Drug addiction does not imply weakness, immorality, or a lack of self-respect. It's an illness, and being an illness it can be treated. And while treatment is typically long-term and emotionally difficult, it can be successful. But there are some key principles common to all successful treatment programs. These principles include:

- There is not a standard treatment plan applicable to every person. Not all treatment programs will be effective for all individuals. For addiction treatment to be effective, it must be individualized to the person, his or her circumstances, and specifics of their addiction. What's the drug of choice; what are the triggers for drug use; how much does the person use; and how long has that person used drugs are all factors that determine which course of treatment is best for them.

- Treatment needs to be readily available for all who want it, addressing all needs of the individual, not just the addiction issues. In other words, the treatment plan must take a holistic approach, addressing the entire person, not just their drug use.

- An individual's treatment plan must frequently be re-assessed and updated. Drug treatment is not something you can start and forget. The effectiveness of the treatment plan must be constantly assessed and reassessed, then changes are made to address issues that arise once treatment begins. Successful addiction treatment is a dynamic, ever-changing process. Most importantly, when it comes to substance abuse treatment, *"one size does not fit all."*

- Counseling and behavioral therapy are essential parts of any successful treatment program. Remaining in treatment for an adequate amount of time is necessary for the treatment plan to be successful. Long-term abstinence from drug use depends on long-term treatment, complete with emotional as well as physical interventions, interventions taken to combat or prevent the unpleasant effects of alcohol or drug withdrawal.

- While the treatment of withdrawal symptoms is important for successful addiction treatment, it alone will do little to resolve the addiction problem. Feeling free of withdrawal symptoms allows a person to concentrate on the root cause of his or her addiction problems. Eliminating withdrawal symptoms alone does not mean the addiction issue has been resolved. However, it does allow for the person to concentrate on identifying and eliminating the root cause of the addiction. Withdrawal symptoms can be so severe and unpleasant that the person is totally consumed with eliminating the withdrawal symptoms however he or she can. If that means using drugs or alcohol, then that's what is done and in the process the whole effort to end the addiction fails. Rid the person of withdrawal symptoms or prevent them altogether and the chance of success is much greater.

- Treatment of co-existing conditions, especially mental illness, must be part of any effective addiction treatment program. As was mentioned earlier, mental illness often diminishes a person's inhibitions and willpower. As such, people with untreated mental illness often engage in risky behaviors, increasing the risk of drug or alcohol use. Without a holistic approach that addresses mental illness, successful addiction treatment is rare.

- Addiction treatment does not have to be entered into voluntarily for it to be successful. Whether a person is ordered into treatment, or feels treatment is the only way to save a relationship, job, or family, treatment can be successful without being entered into voluntarily. However, once in treatment the person has to be committed to kicking their habit in order for the treatment to be successful. A half-hearted effort at addiction treatment has little chance for success.

Effective Treatment Approaches

As stated earlier, the best approach to addiction treatment is a holistic approach, one that addresses more than just taking illegal drugs. To that end, treatment of addiction is generally a three-part procedure: detoxification, addiction treatment, and relapse prevention. The therapeutic process is a combination of medical treatment, mental health treatment, and behavioral therapy. While these approaches can be used alone, experts agree that a holistic approach using all three modalities is the most successful.

DETOXIFICATION

Before any behavioral therapy can begin, the body must be free of the abused drug. The detoxification process can be a very difficult and uncomfortable one. As the amount of drug decreases in the bloodstream and the effects of the drug fade, withdrawal symptoms will emerge, a result of empty dopamine receptors in the brain. Anxiety, nausea, insomnia, and profuse sweating are just some of the withdrawal symptoms one may experience during the detoxification process. And as you can imagine, those symptoms can be quite severe at times. It's withdrawal symptoms that most often interfere with the treatment process. As was the case before the person sought treatment, drug-seeking behavior dominates a person's thought processes. In some cases, fear of withdrawal symptoms will push the addicted person to do whatever it takes to obtain their next dose of drug. People who normally would not dream of doing anything illegal will cross that line if that's what it takes to get their drug of choice. Simply put, as long as there are withdrawal symptoms, addiction treatment failure is a possibility. While a person struggles through withdrawal symptoms there is little time or motivation to be involved in an addiction treatment program. If anything, the urge to misuse their drug of choice will be the only thing on their mind until they get that next dose.

In an effort to minimize the effects withdrawal has on addiction treatment, medications have been developed that help relieve the symptoms of withdrawal while allowing a person to complete the detoxification process. Without withdrawal symptoms, the person is free to focus on treatment and behavioral therapy. These medications have made it possible for drug-addicted people to get the treatment they need while being relatively free of the withdrawal symptoms or drug cravings that make overcoming an addiction so difficult.

Suboxone (Buprenorphine + Naloxone)

In August 2010, the Food and Drug Administration approved a combination drug that made it possible for opiate addicted people to detox from their opiate of choice without the cravings or withdrawal symptoms that typically sabotage even the best attempts of breaking an addiction. Suboxone (buprenorphine + naloxone) is used in the physician's office and as an outpatient option for those wanting to break their addiction to opiates such as hydrocodone, OxyContin, and heroin. The 2010 approval of this drug was an important step forward in the treatment of addiction because it offers an option for those opiate-addicted people who are unwilling or unable (e.g., no insurance/finances) to get involved with in-patient detoxification and treatment programs. This important treatment option is actually two drugs in one pill, each drug playing a very important role in the treatment process.

Buprenorphine—This is the active ingredient in Suboxone (buprenorphine + naloxone). Buprenorphine is a *partial opioid agonist*, meaning that depending on the clinical situation it can both activate and block the opiate receptors. Buprenorphine can produce the effects and side effects of other opiates, but because it is a partial agonist, its maximum effects are less than those of full agonists. At low doses, buprenorphine produces enough opiate effect that people who are addicted can abstain from opiates without withdrawal symptoms or cravings. Being free of the unpleasantness of withdrawal and cravings gives the opiate-addicted person the opportunity to detox.

Like all opiates, increasing doses of buprenorphine will produce increased effect—but only to a certain point. Unlike other more addictive opiates, buprenorphine has a "dose ceiling," meaning that the effect of buprenorphine increases as the dose increases, but only to a certain point. When the dose ceiling is reached, additional dosing will not elicit more effect. This characteristic means buprenorphine has a lower risk of overdose, addiction, and side effects when compared to full opiate agonists such as hydrocodone or OxyContin that do not have dose ceilings.

Finally, buprenorphine has a prolonged effect on the brain. The drug binds strongly to the brain's dopamine receptors, meaning the drug is long-acting and does not leave the dopamine receptors easily. For this reason, there is no need for re-dosing, as is the case with other opiates. People who use cocaine or heroin must re-dose frequently to maintain the drug's euphoric effect. Frequent re-dosing will lead to dose escalation, accidental overdose, and in some cases coma and death. But because of buprenorphine's long-acting properties, dose escalation or accidental overdose is unlikely.

Naloxone—This drug is an opiate antagonist, meaning it blocks the effects of opiates. When taken as prescribed, Suboxone is dissolved slowly under the tongue. When Suboxone (buprenorphine + naloxone) is taken properly, naloxone is not absorbed in sufficient amounts to have any clinical effect. In other words, the naloxone is "inert," meaning it doesn't have a therapeutic effect. It does not block the effects of the buprenorphine. Since buprenorphine is an opiate agonist (triggers dopamine receptors) it can produce euphoria. As such, there will be people who try to abuse the drug to achieve that euphoria they crave so much. Specifically, the abuser will crush tablets containing the opiates, melt them down, and inject the resulting liquid. However, the addition of naloxone to the buprenorphine blocks its opiate effect when the tablets are taken improperly (crushed and injected or swallowed whole). In fact, if the tablets are swallowed whole or crushed and injected instead of dissolved under the tongue, the naloxone is absorbed, blocking the opiate effect of the buprenorphine. The naloxone that is absorbed blocks the effect of the buprenorphine, just the opposite of what the abuser is seeking. Simply put, the addition of naloxone to the buprenorphine prevents the misuse of Suboxone while quenching the opiate withdrawal symptoms and cravings during addiction treatment.

How Suboxone Helps Beat Addiction

So as we just learned, Suboxone (buprenorphine + naloxone) is much like an opiate. It can produce euphoric effects similar to those of methadone or hydrocodone. Granted, the effects are less intense and limited, but at the very least, Suboxone (buprenorphine + naloxone) can quell withdrawal symptoms and the powerful hunger for drugs one will experience when trying to detox from opiates. So if Suboxone (buprenorphine + naloxone) can cause euphoria, then why give the drug to someone addicted to opiates? Isn't doing so just feeding their addiction? At first glance, that's how it appears. But actually, the addition of Suboxone (buprenorphine + naloxone) to addiction treatment plans has in many cases made it possible for addicts to get substance abuse treatment free of craving and withdrawal symptoms. Here's how that is accomplished.

- When opiates are taken into the body, they attach to receptors in the brain, causing dopamine release and feelings of euphoria.
- Eventually, those opiates vacate the receptors, the euphoria fades and the symptoms of withdrawal begin.
- As more receptors empty, the withdrawal symptoms worsen. When the withdrawal symptoms are at their peak, Suboxone (buprenorphine + naloxone) therapy can begin. In fact, if the initial dose of Suboxone (buprenorphine + naloxone) is taken before withdrawal begins, the small amount of naloxone that is absorbed will block the opiate receptors resulting in a sudden cascade of severe and unpleasant withdrawal symptoms.

- As the dose of Suboxone (buprenorphine + naloxone) dissolves under the tongue, buprenorphine enters the bloodstream and makes its way to the dopamine receptors previously occupied by opiates. As buprenorphine fills the receptors, the withdrawal symptoms begin to fade.

- Buprenorphine attaches firmly to the receptors, blocking other opioids from occupying those receptors. Most opiates have a relatively short duration of action, requiring frequent doses and escalating doses to achieve the same euphoric effects. Buprenorphine has a much longer duration of action, meaning its effects do not wear off quickly. Longer action means frequent and escalating doses is not necessary to remain withdrawal symptom free. Because the buprenorphine bonds are so strong and last so long, the craving for opiates and withdrawal symptoms from lack of opiates is eliminated, making detox from the abused opiates much easier.

Suboxone (buprenorphine + naloxone) has proven to be a very effective adjunct to addiction treatment. One particular study examined opiate abstinence in people taking Suboxone (buprenorphine + naloxone), compared to those given a placebo (a pill with no medicinal effect). In a 4-week study, almost 21 percent of those patients taking Suboxone (buprenorphine + naloxone) had an opiate-free urine specimen at the end of 4 weeks. Only about 6 percent of the placebo group had a negative urine screen in the same time frame. In addition, investigators measured opiate cravings using a self-reporting survey. Participants taking the Suboxone (buprenorphine + naloxone) reported about 50 percent fewer cravings by the end of 4 weeks, while those taking the placebo reported no change in their level of craving. Finally, participants were more likely to finish 4 weeks of behavioral therapy when taking Suboxone (buprenorphine + naloxone), compared to those people not taking the medication. It's obvious from this study that Suboxone (buprenorphine + naloxone) can be a very effective addiction treatment tool that improves both treatment compliance and opiate abstinence. But it's not as easy as just taking a pill; there is a proper way to begin Suboxone (buprenorphine + naloxone) therapy.

The Suboxone Treatment Plan

While Suboxone (buprenorphine + naloxone) has been proven to be an effective part of drug rehabilitation and detoxification, it's not as simple as taking a pill a couple of times a day. Suboxone (buprenorphine + naloxone) alone is not a cure for drug addiction. Experts agree that stopping opiate use is only the first step in kicking an addiction. Treatment specialists have developed treatment programs that use Suboxone (buprenorphine + naloxone) and behavioral therapy to end drug addiction. Experts agree that behavioral therapy is absolutely essential if the treatment plan is to be successful. With that in mind, the typical Suboxone (buprenorphine + naloxone) treatment plan is comprised of five steps.

Intake—It's during this initial phase of the plan that your addiction doctor gets to know you and the extent of your drug use. The doctor will conduct a medical and psychological exam to identify any medical issues or past mental illnesses that may affect your recovery. For instance, because it's not uncommon for recovering addicts to experience symptoms of depression, it's important for the doctor to know if you have been diagnosed with depression in the past.

Depending on the program, you may have an addiction nurse and mental health specialist assigned to your case. They, too, will do assessments in order to better understand your addiction. The nurse will be responsible for administering and monitoring your Suboxone therapy, while the mental health counselor will support you from a psychological perspective.

Your doctor must be certain you are physically healthy. Blood will be drawn to assess the functioning of all your major organs including the kidneys, liver, pancreas, and gall bladder. Years of drug use places a great deal of stress on the body. For instance, prolonged alcohol abuse will eventually damage the liver, eventually to the point of complete failure. Prolonged use of recreational drugs like cocaine will eventually result in damage to the heart muscle, potentially leading to hearts attacks or heart failure even in people as young as their early twenties. Even the normal metabolism of drugs taken into the body can put stress on the liver and kidneys. Most drugs, including alcohol, must pass through the liver where chemical changes occur, breaking down the drug into smaller compounds that are used by the body. The compounds that are not used are excreted by the kidneys. While this is a very natural process, having to metabolize dose after dose of recreational drugs will eventually destroy the liver and kidneys. Assessing for this kind of damage to the body is essential when planning addiction treatment.

Why is it important for the addiction treatment program to assess the physical health of their patient? Remember, Suboxone has become an important adjunct the addiction treatment. Another adjunct therapy to addiction treatment is methadone, a medication that in a sense fills the void left by the absence of recreational opiates. In the event the liver or kidneys have been damaged by extensive drug use, alcohol use or some underlying disease (e.g., hepatitis C, renal disease), Suboxone or methadone will not be broken down and excreted properly. Over time, the drugs will accumulate, eventually reaching toxic levels. Excessive blood levels of any drug, Suboxone and methadone included, can cause serious health issues and further damage to the body.

In addition to blood tests, a urine drug screen will also be a part of your initial work-up. It's not uncommon for people with addiction issues to withhold information or provide false information regarding their drug use. Drug addiction is a powerful illness, causing people to lie, cheat or steal to get their next "fix" or dose. Addiction professionals realize that a person's drug use is not always as it is portrayed by the patient. It's very important that the addiction team has an accurate picture of the patient's drug use. Unidentified or underestimated drug use by the person in recovery can undermine the entire addiction treatment process. A urine drug screen will help identify drug use not revealed voluntarily by the patient. The screen will identify any drugs or alcohol ingested, and will give the treatment team a rough idea of when it was ingested. As the treatment plan progresses, a urine drug screen can identify those patients who are not adhering to the treatment plan.

Finally, the doctor will ask you questions about your opiate use in order to assess the type, amount, and frequency of your drug use. It's absolutely essential that you be completely honest regarding the drug you use, how much you use, and how often you use. Many drug users try to deceive their treatment team, but addiction professionals have heard just about every lie, excuse, and attempt at deception. "Pulling the wool over their eyes," so to speak, would be difficult, and in the long run will only undermine your efforts to get healthy and drug free.

Induction—This phase of treatment is to transition the addict from his drug of choice to Suboxone. This is not as simple as it sounds. It's more complex than just taking a dose of

Suboxone and beginning therapy. It is important to be in mild-to-moderate withdrawal when you take your first dose of Suboxone. If you have high levels of another opioid in your system, Suboxone will compete with the other opioid molecules, knocking them off the receptors. Suboxone replaces those opioid molecules on the receptors, but because Suboxone has less opioid effect than the person's drug of choice, you will experience sudden, rapid onset withdrawal and develop severe, intolerable withdrawal symptoms. Suboxone is used is to minimize the symptoms of withdrawal. But given too early, Suboxone will cause sudden withdrawal, defeating its purpose altogether.

The first dose of Suboxone will be given under direct observation of the treatment team. The Suboxone tablet is placed under the tongue and allowed to dissolve, slowly over five to ten minutes. Usually, the withdrawal symptoms begin to ease after about one hour after the dose; however, some people experience relief of their mild withdrawal symptoms within a few minutes. Depending on how well the first dose suppresses or does not suppress withdrawal symptoms, a second dose may be given.

The key point to remember is that Suboxone must be allowed to dissolve under the tongue to be effective. If it's chewed, crushed or swallowed whole, naloxone becomes bioavailable, knocking opiates and buprenorphine from the opiate receptors, causing sudden withdrawal. When dissolved under the tongue, naloxone is not bioavailable, and much more buprenorphine is absorbed, meaning the Suboxone effectively eases the symptoms of withdrawal.

The induction phase of treatment can last as little as one day or as long as a week. During this time, daily visits to your doctor are not uncommon. Direct-observed dosing, meaning the treatment team observes each dose being taken, is used by many programs during this phase. In these programs the treatment team holds onto the Suboxone, giving the patient just enough doses to get them through the night. Urine drug screens are usually included in these daily visits as well.

Stabilization—During the next phase of treatment the Suboxone dose is adjusted to find the lowest possible dose that totally suppresses withdrawal symptoms and drug cravings. Depending on the individual, this phase can take a week or more. This phase is also the time when patient and doctor discuss treatment options—specifically, the advantages of short-term and long-term Suboxone treatment plans. Most addiction programs have a system of counseling and treatment in place with minimum requirements that each participant has to meet in order to remain in the program.

For instance, each participant must attend a minimum number of group therapy sessions to remain in the treatment program. The participant must prove to the addiction treatment staff that they are committed to the process of addiction treatment. Because commitment is necessary for success, a participant must prove they are committed to the process. A less than 100 percent investment in the program is nothing more than a waste of time and precious resources. The number of sessions required is based on the needs of the individual. In essence, when the patient presents him or herself for outpatient addiction treatment, they are contracting with the program and are bound to the rules of the plan. Addiction programs adhere to their treatment plan, with very few exceptions. If individuals miss required meetings or have difficulty adhering to the plan, the program will take issue and act accordingly. In some cases, the addict will be asked to leave the program or change to an inpatient program where personal freedom is very limited and the rules are even more strict.

An important decision during this phase is how long to use Suboxone in the treatment plan. Some people use the drug only during the detoxification period, slowly withdrawing and discontinuing it soon after the body is clear of opiates. Others use Suboxone throughout the entire treatment period to diminish the risk of relapse. Maintenance dosing, as it is called, can continue for weeks, months, or even longer in order to reduce cravings and the risk of relapse. Keep in mind there is more than one right approach when planning Suboxone maintenance therapy. Some people need to stay on a low dose of Suboxone as a maintenance medication. Others do well discontinuing the drug soon after detoxification has been completed. The key to success, however, is not discontinuing Suboxone too soon. If the Suboxone is discontinued before the patient has the tools to resist the powerful drug cravings of opiate addiction, the chance of sustained abstinence from recreational drugs is slim.

Maintenance—Suboxone can be used throughout treatment and recovery; however, the importance of substance abuse counseling can't be emphasized enough. In fact, studies have proven without a doubt that Suboxone alone is not an effective way to beat a drug habit. The chance for treatment success is greatly improved by attending professional substance abuse counseling after you have stopped taking opiates. For those who choose, Suboxone can be used throughout the recovery process in conjunction with substance abuse counseling. The counseling is typically a combination of group and individual sessions. Suboxone will be prescribed at the lowest dose that suppresses withdrawal symptoms and opiate cravings. If necessary, this phase can last months or even a year or more.

People may not realize but, because it's a partial opiate agonist, Suboxone can cause physical dependence after long-term use. However, withdrawing Suboxone treatment is considered to be less difficult than most other opiates including hydrocodone, OxyContin, and even methadone. Regardless, the potential for dependence remains and should be considered by the patient and physician when deciding upon maintenance dosing (long-term Suboxone) versus medically supervised withdrawal (short-term Suboxone).

Medically Supervised Withdrawal—For those who decide Suboxone maintenance dosing is not for them, the drug must be tapered down slowly in order to avoid uncomfortable withdrawal symptoms. If the drug is stopped abruptly, withdrawal symptoms and cravings similar to those experienced at the time of Suboxone induction will occur. During this phase your doctor will slowly decrease your dose, being careful to do so in a manner that produces the fewest withdrawal symptoms or opiate cravings. The eventual goal of this phase is to stop Suboxone treatment altogether.

This can be a dangerous time for the recovering patient. The patient realizes that all he or she needs to do to relieve withdrawal symptoms is to take a dose of opiate. Without the therapeutic effects of Suboxone, patients will be at the mercy of their opiate cravings and withdrawal symptoms. Hopefully, the patient will have the tools necessary to resist the temptation and remain abstinent. Giving in to the cravings will land the person in relapse, and their attempt at stopping their drug use will fail. For this reason, treatment teams must be aware of their patient's commitment to abstinence and their ability to resist. The Suboxone should not be stopped faster than the patient's ability to resist.

The Role of Counseling

While Suboxone treats the physical issues of recovery, professional counseling is an essential adjunct that treats the emotional aspects of addiction, the root cause of the addiction.

Experts agree that addiction counseling is essential during and after your Suboxone treatment. Think of it this way. Every morning you wake up with a headache. You take an aspirin to relieve the pain and soon the headache is gone and you feel much better. However, you wake the next morning and the headache is back. The aspirin treated the pain but did nothing to find the root cause of the headaches and therefore, the headache returns again and again. The same is true for addiction. Suboxone can remove the physical manifestations of addiction—namely, drug cravings and symptoms of withdrawal. However, Suboxone does nothing to treat the psychological root cause of the addiction. Just like with our headache example, if you don't find the cause of the addiction, relapse will occur. Believing Suboxone alone is the "cure" for addiction is a big mistake that will most certainly lead to relapse down the road. Counseling and group sessions explore the root causes of addiction. Why did drug use become such a dominating force in a person's life? Counseling tries to answer that question. Without the answer there can be no long-term solution. Any treatment plan not involving counseling and behavioral therapy is destined to fail.

The benefits of group and individual behavioral therapy are twofold. First, therapy helps find the cause or causes of the drug use. Finding the cause gives drug abuse treatment a better shot at long-term success. Secondly, behavioral therapy teaches the patient how to deal with those causes. For instance, say a man has a drug problem. In order to cope with the everyday stresses of life, this man has chosen to take opiates. Behavioral therapy could help this man make better choices when dealing with the stress in his life. Simply put, through behavioral therapy, the man is taught methods other than drug use to deal with everyday stress. Those tools will also help him resist the powerful drug cravings characteristic of opiate addiction. Behavioral therapy prepares you for the battle to beat addiction and dependence. And while addiction relapse is fairly common, studies have shown that behavioral therapy dramatically improves your chances of successful, long-term recovery from opiate addiction and dependence.

The Old Standby—Methadone

Before Suboxone, one method of medicinal support for people fighting to end their opiate addiction was the addition of *methadone* to drug treatment programs. Methadone is a long-acting synthetic opiate that occupies the same receptors in the brain as opiates such as heroin, hydrocodone, and OxyContin. Methadone is prescribed in conjunction with drug abuse counseling in order to relieve withdrawal and opiate cravings during treatment for opiate abuse. Methadone has a slow onset of action with a long duration that competes with recreational drugs for receptor sites in the brain. But unlike heroin and hydrocodone, methadone is not euphoric or sedating, meaning the person can take methadone to combat withdrawal symptoms and cravings but continue to work, drive a car, and make decisions without the compromising effects of other opiates. Methadone is used in conjunction with therapy and drug abuse counseling to ease the symptoms of withdrawal and opiate cravings, making it possible for the patient to be free of recreational drugs without the uncomfortable signs of withdrawal.

In most circumstances, methadone is prescribed in methadone clinics that are part of addiction treatment programs. When combined with behavioral therapy, methadone allows drug abuses to stop taking their abused opiates and return to a more normal, stable life free of cravings and withdrawal. It has been shown to reduce addiction related deaths, criminal activity to acquire more drugs, and the contracting of HIV infection via high risk sexual behavior, including exchanging sex for money and drugs. That's not to say that methadone lacks some potential for problems. Because it is a synthetic opiate, addiction and dependence can and do occur. However, because methadone does not have the euphoria and sedating properties of other opiates, the street value and misuse potential is less than opiates like Oxy-Contin and heroin. Because of that characteristic, when used in conjunction with behavioral therapy and closely monitored prescribing programs, methadone is still a valuable tool in addiction treatment.

12

DENTAL CARE

The importance of regular medical care has been stressed throughout this text. We've learned thus far how important regular healthcare is to people living with HIV. Segments of your healthcare, such as vaccinations, regular health screenings, and adherence to your HIV medication regimen, seem to take priority among patients and providers alike. Yet, there are other areas that are just as important but seem to be all but forgotten. In this day of visit quotas and ten-minute appointments, these forgotten aspects of your health take a back seat even among HIV specialists. When time is limited and the waiting room is full, doctors have to prioritize. Unfortunately, certain aspects of your overall health are frankly left up to you. One such area is dental care. While most providers will confirm the importance of good dental care, many assign it a low priority during a medical visit. So, most often, tending to your dental health is left to you and your dentist. The truth of the matter is that dental care plays an extremely important role in the overall health of an HIV-positive person. That being the case, let's take a closer look at dental care in the HIV-positive person.

Dental Health

Good dental health, or more accurately, good oral health, is a necessary part of a long life. Experts agree that people living with HIV must maintain *"functional"* oral health in order to receive the nutrition necessary for a healthy life. What is functional oral health? Simply put, HIV-positive people must maintain a healthy mouth with a full set of healthy teeth in order to eat properly. Conversely, mouth pain, tooth pain, or missing and broken teeth interfere with eating, meaning the HIV-positive person will have a more difficult time taking in enough calories, vitamins, and nutrients to maintain a healthy diet. Functional oral health simply means maintaining a healthy mouth and healthy teeth that allow you to eat a healthy diet.

Many people take their dental health for granted until they are suffering with a toothache or painful "canker sores" that make eating an adventure in pain and torture. Few realize that besides interfering with the diet, poor oral hygiene can be a breeding ground for fungal, bacterial, and viral infections that can affect the entire body. While this is true for most anyone, people with weakened immune systems, such as people living with HIV and AIDS, are especially at risk. Mouth ulcers, gum disease, and tooth decay are all conditions that can cause serious illness elsewhere in the body if left untreated. Here are some key reasons good oral health is important to the HIV-infected person.

- Poor dental health, including loose, missing, or painful teeth, can severely impact the HIV-positive patient's ability to eat. If the patient is unable to eat, proper nutrition is impossible, weight loss is inevitable, and HIV progression is more likely.
- Health issues in the mouth can be one of the first signs of HIV infection and may identify those people with an increased probability of HIV progression. Conditions like thrush, canker sores, and herpetic lesions can be some of the first infections associated with HIV but should never be used to diagnose HIV; only an HIV test can do that.
- A weakened immune system offers little protection against infections resulting from poor oral and dental health.
- Mouth ulcers, gum ulcers, and decayed teeth act as portals that allow bacteria and other infectious organisms into the bloodstream. Dental infections can lead to heart conditions, sinus infections, and infections in the bloodstream (septicemia).
- Regular dental exams identify oral health concerns early, allowing for treatment before those problems progress to other, more serious infections.

Finding a Dentist

The first step toward good oral health is finding the right dentist for you, meaning a dentist with whom you are comfortable sharing your diagnosis. While there are dentists virtually everywhere, finding a dentist who is comfortable working with HIV-positive people can be a challenge. From a strictly medical perspective, HIV makes the management of dental issues much more difficult. Keeping your mouth and teeth healthy is more difficult for people living with HIV. Many dentists do not feel comfortable with the complexity that HIV adds to dental care. Sadly, another reason it's hard to find a dentist is fear of transmission from patient to dentist or hygienist, a fear with absolutely no basis in fact. The use of gloves and masks (universal precautions) protects the dentist and his or her assistant. Yet there are some dental professionals that prefer not to care for HIV positive people. These two factors together mean there are fewer quality dentists to care for people living with HIV.

Granted, finding a dentist to care for HIV patients can be difficult and frustrating. But they are out there; it's just a matter of finding the dentist that's right for you. Here are some tips for finding a quality dentist.

- Talk to the local HIV case management agencies. Many keep contact information for dentists that welcome HIV-positive people into their dental practice. Among the HIV community (patients and care givers), these dentists are referred to as "HIV friendly."
- Seek out recommendations from family, friends, and other HIV-positive people. Word of mouth and personal testimonials are two of the best ways to find a reliable quality dentist.
- If you are moving to a new area, speak with your current dentist. It's possible that he or she may be able to recommend a dentist in your new location. Prior to relocating, contact the HIV agencies in your new area to get the names of "HIV friendly" dentists.
- When you do find a dentist you like, make your first visit something simple—a cleaning or a consultation. By doing so you can learn about the dentist and the practice without being under the duress of a painful tooth or complicated dental procedure.

- Depending on the extent of infection (oral versus disseminated), treatment is typically amphotericin B intravenously or Sporanox (itraconazole) orally.

Angular Cheilitis ("Mouth Cracks")
- Presents as cracked and crusted skin lesions in the corners of the mouth.
- Can have a variety of causes but most often is caused by a fungal (e.g., *candida albicans*) or bacterial (e.g., *Staphylococcus aureus*) infection.
- Can mimic other mouth lesions such as those caused by the virus *herpes labialis* ("cold sores").
- Treated with topical anti-fungal (e.g., ketoconazole) or antibiotic (e.g., mupirocin) creams.

Non-Candidal Fungal Infections
- Mycoses (fungal infections) other than those caused by the fungus *Candida Albicans*.
- Less common than candida infections.
- Infection typically does not cause symptoms in those with healthy immune systems. Oral lesions as well as infection of other organs occurs in those people with weak immune systems, including people living with HIV.
- Treatment most often requires intravenous medication, the antifungal medication amphotericin B being the treatment of choice.

Viral Lesions

Herpes Labialis ("Cold Sores")
- One type of *herpes simplex* virus, *herpes labialis* presents as fluid-filled vesicles on the upper or lower lip.
- The vesicles erupt, fill with fluid, rupture, and then crust and slowly resolve. The entire cycle last about 7 to 10 days.
- Symptoms include pain, a burning sensation, and itching. Prior to eruption of the vesicles, people experience a "tingling" sensation where the lesion will appear.
- Lesions will reoccur in the same spot or spots on the lips throughout a person's lifetime.
- Diagnosis is typically made by culturing the lesions and the fluid contained in the vesicles.
- There is no cure for *herpes labialis*, but outbreaks can be shortened by using anti-viral medications such as Zovirax (acyclovir) or Valtrex (valacyclovir). Those medications can be used at a lower daily dose to help decrease the frequency of lesion outbreaks.

Herpes Zoster
- Another of the herpes virus family, herpes zoster's oral lesions are reactivated *varicella zoster* (the virus that causes chickenpox).
- Typically, herpes zoster causes fluid-filled vesicles on the skin, but oral lesions do occur.
- Initially, symptoms can mimic tooth pain.

- While herpes zoster causes skin vesicles that rupture and crust, oral lesions caused by herpes zoster are in the form of open, painful, ulcers of mouth tissue.
- The oral ulcers of herpes zoster are usually in a linear pattern along nerve tracts.
- Diagnosis is made by the appearance and distribution of the lesions.
- Like other types of herpes virus, there is no cure, but anti-viral medications like Zovirax (acyclovir) and Valtrex (valacyclovir) can limit the duration of outbreaks.

Human Papillomavirus (HPV)
- There are over 200 subtypes of HPV, some of which can cause oral lesions and oral cancers.
- HPV-related oral lesions occur most often in people with HIV-compromised immune systems.
- The subtype of HIV that causes oral lesions (HPV-16) can also cause cervical lesions in women.
- The HPV responsible for oral lesions is sexually transmitted from person to person.
- The oral warts appear as single or multiple nodules that resemble cauliflower.
- Because this HPV type is usually symptom free, diagnosis is made by biopsy.
- The lesions can be surgically removed, but relapses frequently occur.
- HPV oral lesions can progress to oral cancer if left untreated.

Cytomegalovirus (CMV)
- While it is fairly rare, oral lesions from cytomegalovirus (CMV) have been reported.
- The lesions are similar in appearance to apthous ulcers ("canker sores"), except for the necrotic (dead/black) borders of the CMV ulcer.
- CMV ulcers are diagnosed by biopsy.
- Because CMV ulcers appear in cases of systemic CMV infection, the patient should be assessed for systemic CMV infection when CMV ulcers are present.
- The ulcers will resolve with the medication Valcyte (ganciclovir), given orally or intravenously to treat the systemic CMV infection.

Oral Hairy Leukoplakia (OHL)
- OHL is caused by the Epstein-Barr virus (EBV), a virus from the herpes family of viruses.
- OHL presents as an asymptomatic, corrugated or "hairy" looking white lesion on the lateral aspects of the tongue.
- The lesion is non-movable and is more common in people with CD4 counts less than 200 cells/mm^3 of blood.
- The presence of OHL is indicative of an HIV-weakened immune system.
- Several studies indicate that people with OHL have a higher probability of progressing to an AIDS diagnosis when compared to people without OHL.
- OHL can be diagnosed by an experienced clinician simply by appearance, but a definitive diagnosis should be done with biopsy. OHL is often mistaken for thrush.

- Because OHL is asymptomatic, it typically does not require treatment.
- OHL has been proven to improve in those patients taking Zovirax (acyclovir) for a herpes outbreak.
- Diflucan (fluconazole) can be used in those patients who have "thrush" along with OHL.

BACTERIAL LESIONS

Periodontal Disease

Periodontal disease is a chronic inflammatory process, bacterial in nature, affecting the tissue and bone structures supporting the teeth. While periodontal disease can occur in anyone, regardless of HIV status, two particularly damaging types of periodontal disease are unique to people with weakened immune systems, including those people living with HIV.

Necrotizing Ulcerative Periodontitis (NUP)—This periodontal disease is considered a marker for severe immune system compromise. Formerly known as HIV periodontal disease, NUP is characterized by severe pain and bleeding, with rapid and significant bone and tissue loss. Also characteristic of this serious periodontal disease is premature tooth loss and a foul odor from the mouth. Left untreated, this periodontal condition can cause systemic infections and symptoms as well. For instance, NUP can spread bacteria to other parts of the body resulting in cardiac problems, vegetative growth on heart valves, and septicemia (blood infected with bacteria). Treatment includes extraction of badly damaged or decayed teeth; debridement of the dead and infected tissue using a solution of 10 percent povidone iodine or 0.12 percent *chlorhexidine gluconate*; and a course of oral antibiotics. Possibly the most critical part of treatment is pain control. NUP is a very painful condition so without adequate pain control, the person will not be able to eat a healthy diet. Without the proper diet and the required calories, the patient's nutritional status will not be conducive to healing of the NUP and living with HIV in general.

Linear Gingival Erythema (LFE)—LFE is commonly called "red band gingivitis" due to its characteristic red band appearance. The red band appears along the gingival (gum) line and may be accompanied by bleeding and pain. While it can extend to all parts of the gum, it primarily affects the front or anterior portions. Some experts believe there is a connection between LFE and chronic candida infections. In fact, the American Academy of Periodontology considers LFE a gingival disease of fungal origin. However, antifungal medications are not the treatment of choice. Instead, plaque debridement by a dentist, twice daily mouth rinses with a chlorhexidine solution, and meticulous oral hygiene at home are the preferred and most effective treatment.

A WORD ABOUT CHLORHEXIDINE SOLUTION

One of the most effective treatments for a variety or oral and dental infections is chlorhexidine gluconate rinses. Marketed in pharmacies and retail outlets as Peridex, chlorhexidine is an antimicrobial oral rinse that helps decrease the amount of active, infectious bacteria in the mouth. Bacteria is the culprit in many oral infections including gingivitis, a variety of gum infections, tooth decay, and halitosis ("bad breath"). While chlorhexidine is typically very safe to use, there are a few things you need to know if your doctor has prescribed chlorhexidine for you.

The typical way to use chlorhexidine is rinsing the mouth with 15ml of undiluted solution twice daily after brushing and flossing your teeth. Avoid swallowing the rinse; instead, spit the rinse out into the sink. While it sounds simple enough and without much concern for adverse effects, there are some side effects and adverse effects of which you should be aware. They include

- tooth and tongue staining;
- increased tartar buildup;
- mouth and throat irritation;
- dry mouth;
- unpleasant taste in the mouth; and
- decreased sensation of taste.

There are a few other, more serious side effects that can occur in a very small segment of the population. If you experience any of these side effects the chlorhexidine should be discontinued and you should contact your dentist or physician. These more serious side effects include

- white patches or "sores" inside your mouth on your tongue or gums;
- ulcerations on the tongue or gum line; and
- swelling of your salivary glands located just beneath the law line.

Finally, there are people who will have an allergic reaction to chlorhexidine. It is a rare occurrence, but in the event it does occur, you need to go to the nearest emergency room for evaluation and treatment. The signs of an allergic reaction include

- hives or rash;
- swelling of the lips, face, or tongue;
- swelling of the throat;
- difficulty swallowing; and
- wheezing or difficulty breathing.

Chlorhexidine gluconate is a very effective antimicrobial and can be an important addition to your daily dental care. That being said, be aware of adverse side effects and signs of allergic reaction when using chlorhexidine and if any of those adverse signs and symptoms occur, call your dentist or your physician for guidance.

OTHER ORAL MANIFESTATIONS

Apthous Ulcers (Canker Sores)

The cause or causes of apthous ulcers ("canker sores") is not well understood, but experts have identified many possibilities. These include:

- vitamin deficiencies (primarily B1, B2, and B6);
- a weakened or poorly functioning immune system;
- autoimmune inflammation;
- various disease states including HIV;

- injury to the mouth and gums from brushing or poor fitting dentures;
- emotional stress;
- highly acidic or spicy foods; and
- hormonal changes in women (e.g., more outbreaks during menstruation).

Apthous ulcers are not contagious and are not spread orally from person to person. The frequency of outbreaks can be diminished by avoiding things that may cause gum injury such as rough, sharp food that scratches the gum, vigorous brushing that results in an injury to the gums, and spicy or acidic foods.

Treatment of canker sores depends a great deal on the cause. Some examples of treatment include changing to a milder tooth paste and a softer toothbrush, using antibiotic mouth rinses (e.g., chlorhexidine), achieving pain relief from topical numbing agents, taking steroids for severe and recurrent cases, and employing antifungal medications (e.g., Nystatin solution), which can be given if the canker sores are related to a candida infection (thrush).

Xerostomia (Dry Mouth)

Xerostomia, commonly known as dry mouth, is the primary source of tooth decay in the HIV-positive person. The condition is a result of changes in the quantity and quality of saliva. There are a number of possible causes. They include:

- side effect of various medications, including some HIV medications;
- decreased saliva production by the salivary glands;
- a complication of certain illnesses, infections, and diseases, including HIV and AIDS;
- any condition that causes fluid loss and eventual dehydration, such as vomiting, diarrhea, poor fluid intake, and profound blood loss;
- a side effect of radiation therapy used to treat head and neck cancers;
- blocked salivary glands or the absence of salivary glands due to tumor growth.

Decreased saliva production can lead to other illnesses. For instance, because saliva is an important part of tooth decay prevention, xerostomia can lead to more rapid and extensive decay. Saliva is constantly rinsing the mouth of sugars left over from eating. These sugars can settle on teeth, eventually causing tooth decay. Also, saliva has antimicrobial properties, meaning it rids the mouth of harmful bacteria. Without the saliva, the unchecked bacteria can cause severe and rapid tooth decay. Experts believe that the severe tooth decay characteristic of the methamphetamine user is in large part due to xerostomia.

People with xerostomia have several complaints related to their dry mouth. Some of the most common of these complaints include:

- difficulty speaking, swallowing, chewing, or wearing dentures;
- sores under and around dentures;
- a painful tongue that sticks to the palate;
- a change in, or the absence of, taste;
- the need to drink increased amounts of water;
- cracking of the lips, tongue, and oral mucosa;
- parotid gland inflammation and swelling.

Successful treatment of xerostomia is typically accomplished by removing the cause. For instance, if it's a medication(s) causing the issue, substituting another medication may be all it takes. Sometimes changing the manner in which you take your medication can alleviate the dry mouth. Dry mouth is sometimes affected by the amount of drug in the bloodstream at any given time. In these instances, merely splitting the medication into smaller, more frequent doses may be all it takes to relieve the symptoms of dry mouth.

Sometimes the cause of xerostomia is not easily removed. In these cases, stimulating the salivary glands may be the answer. Certain chemicals, such as those containing citric acid, can stimulate the salivary glands to produce saliva. Electrical stimulation using very small electrical impulses through the skin to the salivary glands has been known to work as well. Finally, medications such as salivary substitutes and oral moisturizers may be of some benefit as well.

Kaposi's Sarcoma (KS)

During the early years of the HIV epidemic, Kaposi's sarcoma, or KS as it's called in medical circles, became the face of AIDS. All one has to do is watch the movie Philadelphia to understand the impact KS and its infamous lesions had on the HIV-infected person—physically, socially, and emotionally. While the incidence of Kaposi's has decreased dramatically since those early days, KS can still present as an oral manifestation of HIV and AIDS.

The typical KS lesion can be nodular ("lumpy"), macular (flat), or raised and ulcerated, appearing primarily but not exclusively on the roof of the mouth (the palate). The lesions range in color from red to purple, becoming darker as they age. The presentation of oral KS can range from small, flat red or purple areas along the gums (the gingiva) to large nodular lesions on the roof of the mouth. In some cases, KS lesions can get so large that they impede swallowing and speech. Often times, KS lesions are accompanied by infections such as thrush, cytomegalovirus (CMV), or a variety of herpes-type viruses (e.g., herpes zoster, or "cold sores").

In some instances, oral KS has a very distinctive appearance, making a presumptive diagnosis possible, meaning the doctor can make the diagnosis of KS simply by the appearance of the lesions. However, a definitive diagnosis can only be made via biopsy of the lesions, meaning a small sample of the lesions is taken and examined under a microscope. This is especially important in African-American and other people of color and people with darker skin tones because lesions can be missed or misdiagnosed due to the dark color of the oral mucosa in these people.

Treatment of oral KS lesions can be localized or systemic however, most patients need systemic treatment for adequate KS treatment.

Localized—as the name suggests, localized KS treatment attacks the lesion itself. Radiation therapy directly to the lesion is the most common treatment. Beam radiation is targeted to the lesion, reducing its size over the course of several treatments. Depending on the size and location of the lesion, radiation therapy is typically one to two times a week for four to six weeks. Radiation therapy to the oral cavity can produce many unpleasant side effects, including inflammation and burns to the oral mucosa, as well as an overgrowth of fungal and herpetic infections. Newer radiation therapy application tools have been developed to minimize radiation absorption by healthy mucosa and therefore less unpleasant side effects. That being said, it's still important to limit radiation therapy to those oral lesions producing symptoms (e.g., pain or bleeding) or that are impeding swallowing, eating, or speech. Other types of localized treatment include topical creams that impede KS growth, freezing with liquid nitrogen, or chemotherapy drugs injected directly into the KS lesion. Despite best efforts, re-growth of the KS lesion will often occur within four to six months after treatment.

Systemic—This form of treatment is reserved for KS that is growing rapidly or is life threatening. Similar to cancer, systemic treatment consists of chemotherapy medications given in pill form or intravenously, infused directly into a vein. Chemotherapy drugs are *cytotoxic*, meaning they kill cells—in this case the intended targets are the KS cells. When exposed to the cytotoxic properties of chemotherapy, the KS lesion rapidly reduces in size. KS treatment can be a single chemotherapy agent or a combination of two or more. Unfortunately, chemotherapy has many side effects, some of which are very unpleasant. Chemotherapy kills healthy cells as well as KS cells, resulting in adverse effects such as hair loss, nausea, and abnormally low blood counts. Because of these side effects, chemotherapy is reserved for only the most aggressive or rapidly growing KS.

Because Kaposi's sarcoma is viral in nature, anti-viral medications are sometimes used to treat the lesions. Depending on the type of KS lesion, the state of the patient's immune system, and the presence or absence of other illness, the first line antiviral medications for KS are the patient's HIV medication regimen. Optimal control of a person's HIV infection is an integral part of successful KS treatment. Controlling HIV replication results in successful KS treatment. However, in people with lower CD4 counts or with KS lesions that are more aggressive or invasive, antiretroviral therapy is rarely enough to get the KS under control. In these cases, addition antiviral medication is needed.

Interferon is an antiviral medication that is used along with antiretroviral medication to treat more complicated KS. Used alone, high doses of Interferon are needed to be effective. However, high-dose Interferon causes significant toxicity and side effects. However, by using certain HIV medications in conjunction with Interferon the Interferon dose can be decreased and as a result the toxic side effects decrease as well. Caution when choosing the antiretroviral medications must be used because the combination of Interferon and some HIV medications can cause side effects and toxicities of their own.

Treatment of KS has variable success. As odd as it sounds, sometimes starting an HIV medication regimen can actually lead to KS lesions. As the medication control the HIV and the CD4 count begins to climb, patients can actually have a recurrence of their treated KS due to a condition known as immune system reconstitution syndrome, a condition we discussed in an earlier chapter. That being said, since the advent of HIV medications, the incidence of KS has gone down and the prognosis has improved. While oral KS is seldom fatal, pain, cosmetic changes and possible airway and esophageal obstruction justify aggressive treatment. Most times, peripheral KS can be successfully treated with radiation, but in the case or oral lesions, severe side effects, such as burns and inflammation to the oral mucosa, make intravenous chemotherapy the better choice in a majority of cases.

Oral Hygiene and Health Maintenance

It has been estimated that upwards of 90 percent of all people living with HIV will present with at least one oral manifestation of the disease during the course of their infection.

Several studies have demonstrated that 40 to 50 percent of all HIV-infected people have some type of fungal, bacterial, or viral infection of the oral cavity early in the course of their HIV. The ability to differentiate one manifestation from another and manage these manifestations is the key to the overall health of the HIV patient. Maintaining the health of the mouth and teeth is the best way to prevent most oral manifestations of HIV. In addition to the effects periodontal infections have on the overall health of an HIV-infected person, there are studies that suggest the presence of periodontal disease and inflammation in HIV-negative people can actually increase their risk of HIV infection via oral transmission. The importance of oral health in the positive and negative person can't be overstated. That being said, let's take a look at some oral hygiene and oral health tips.

Healthy Dentures Healthy Mouth

As we have learned, one of the most common oral manifestations of HIV is the fungal infection *Candida albicans,* more commonly known as thrush. People are generally very good about taking the medications prescribed to treat thrush because the fungus can be painful, can alter taste, and can affect swallowing. However, the one thing they tend to overlook is the possibility candida can grow on the surface of their dentures as well. It's important to rid your dentures of candida and other infectious organisms to prevent reinfection every time you put them into your mouth. This is best accomplished by cleaning the dentures once a day and soaking them overnight in a 1:1 solution of chlorhexidine (a solution with equal parts water and chlorhexidine). The brand names PerioGard Oral Rinse or Peridex are examples of oral rinses that are effective means of reducing the risk of infection caused by dirty dentures.

HIV Medication Regimens

We know that HIV medications suppress HIV and therefore help preserve the immune system. But a paper published in 2004 points out that in addition to suppressing the HIV virus, initiation of highly active antiretroviral therapy (HAART) decreases the incidence of the oral manifestations of HIV. But as is the case in HIV suppression, HAART works best when the regimen is adhered to as prescribed each and every day. By controlling HIV viral replication, the body's immune system has a chance to rebuild and strengthen. The stronger the immune system, the lower the chance of HIV-related oral infections.

Maintaining Good Dental Health

Keeping your mouth healthy is a very important part of preventing the oral manifestations of HIV. Luckily, the things the individual can do are relatively easy, and most are inexpensive as well. Better to get in the habit of using these inexpensive techniques each day than to wait until there is an issue and the cost of repairing the problem increases dramatically. Let's review some of these good oral hygiene techniques.

Brush Your Teeth Twice a Day
Use either a manual or electric toothbrush, but make sure the bristles of the toothbrush are soft. Trauma to the gums from aggressive brushing or a hard bristle toothbrush can lead

to many of the oral manifestations you are trying to prevent. The head of the toothbrush should also be small enough to get to the hard-to-reach places in the back of the mouth. Some recommend you not rinse your mouth with water immediately after brushing because it dilutes and rinses away the fluoride from the toothpaste, diminishing its preventative effects. And remember, brush your tongue gently when brushing your teeth to decrease the build-up of sugars, food particles, or infectious organisms that can lead to thrush, tooth decay, and other periodontal infections.

Floss Your Teeth Daily

Flossing is one thing that most people neglect, but, in fact, it is probably the best way to prevent tooth decay and dental problems. Flossing helps remove plaque that builds up between teeth in places brushing can't access. It also removes food particles that can help cause decay. Dentists recommend you floss before brushing at bedtime so your teeth feel clean when you go to bed. Flossing has become easier with the advent of dental flossers— small disposable handles with floss at one end that makes flossing less cumbersome.

Regular Dental Exams and Cleanings

The one prevention means that can be pricey is regular dental exams and cleanings. If dental insurance is not available, the cost of seeing a dentist and hygienist can be steep. However, most commercial and government funded dental insurances do provide for these basic services at least once a year, some even twice each year. A dentist will examine not only your teeth for tooth decay, but your oral tissue as well. The dentist will look for any lesions, infections, or areas of inflammation that could signal that a serious HIV-related problem is brewing. The hygienist will do a very thorough cleaning of your teeth, much more thorough than you can do using a toothbrush and floss. Ideally, people should get a dental exam and cleaning at least every six months. However, people with a higher risk of oral disease should schedule these more than twice a year. Unfortunately, if insurance is an issue, this could be difficult. Talk with your HIV agency or case manager. Many states offer a dental assistance program for HIV patients who qualify. Many local communities have publicly funded community dental clinics for those people without the means to pay for a private dentist. Finally, check out the local universities in your area. Their dental schools often offer dental services at a very decreased cost, usually based on your ability to pay. These services are usually performed by dental students under the supervision of certified dentists who instruct at the dental school.

Antimicrobial Mouth Rinses

Antimicrobial mouth rinses, such as Listerine, PerioGard Oral Rinse or Peridex, can provide some additional prevention from the bacteria that can cause some of the most common oral conditions. However, using such a rinse does not replace the need to see a dentist regularly, and in many cases will not do much to prevent some of the more complex and serious manifestations of HIV. In addition to antimicrobial rinses, there are fluoride rinses that can help prevent tooth decay when used as directed.

KNOW YOUR MOUTH

We stress to anyone living with HIV to learn about their body and what is normal for them, so that when a change does occur it's identified early and is reported to the physician as soon as possible. The same is true for your mouth. Examine your mouth on a regular basis. Keep an eye out for lesions, ulcerated areas, bleeding, loose teeth, etc., and report these changes to your HIV specialist or dentist right away. If you develop pain (tooth pain, jaw pain, headaches, or tenderness of the oral tissue), report it to your physician and dentist as well. Early detection can be the difference between successful treatment or a long, hard road of dental and oral problems.

STOP SMOKING AND TOBACCO USE

Many people don't realize that smoking and tobacco use can be a major contributor to oral and dental disease. Tobacco use greatly increases your risk of oral cancers, gum disease, and tooth decay. Plus, smoking can slow down healing after oral procedures, and from oral diseases and infections. Smoking cessation is understandably one of the hardest things there is to do. But smoking isn't the only unhealthy use of tobacco. Chewing tobacco, "dipping," and the use of tobacco pouches inside your lip have been proven to greatly increase a person's risk or oral and neck cancers. Such cancers are extremely invasive and require very invasive surgical procedures to treat the cancerous lesions. In addition, chemotherapy and/or radiation therapy is also needed to make certain the cancerous lesions do not recur. Consult your HIV specialist or case manager, who can refer you to smoking cessation and tobacco cessation programs in your area that can help you kick the tobacco habit.

Summary

Oral health and your overall health are more closely related than you may have originally thought. Clues to one's overall health can be gained by assessing the health of the mouth, teeth, and oral mucosa. In the HIV-positive person, oral health is extremely important, but, unfortunately, is an area that seems to have a low priority with patients and even some physicians. Virtually all HIV patients will have some sort of oral manifestation sometime in the course of their infection. Therefore, it's very important to maintain the health of the mouth, teeth, and oral mucosa, just as it's important to maintain the health of the immune system. Make certain you see a dentist at least once a year, preferably twice each year; make certain you follow your dentist's advice and perform regular brushing and flossing; and finally, if you have any pain, lesions, loose teeth, or other abnormality in your mouth, notify your HIV physician and/or dentist right away. By maintaining good oral health, you will improve your overall health as well.

13

EXERCISE AND NUTRITION

Nutrition

There's the old saying "You are what you eat." In other words, your health and well-being is largely dependent upon the types of food you eat. Eating lean meats, whole grains, and fish is a lot better for you than fast food, potato chips, and candy. The more nutritious the foods you eat the better you will feel. And in the case of people living with a chronic disease such as HIV, fighting that disease requires a higher number of calories, vitamins, and minerals. Unfortunately, as is the case with good dental care, people often place a lower priority on good nutrition. In actuality, good nutrition should be given the highest priority.

Studies show that nutritional status is a strong predictor of survival and functional status in people living with HIV. In other words, HIV-positive people who are struggling with poor nutrition will also struggle with their HIV. Nutritional interventions—those interventions that can improve nutrition—can have a very positive impact on mortality, morbidity, and the quality of life of those people living with HIV. For instance, nutritional counseling from a registered dietician has been proven to decrease hospitalizations and trips to the emergency room. Simply put, your body needs proper nutrition in order to heal and to maintain good health while living with HIV. Let's take a closer look at nutrition and diet and the role they play in the life of people living with HIV.

Barriers to Good Nutrition

Most everyone loves to eat, but eating just any old food isn't good enough. A healthy diet is one that has the right amount of fats, carbohydrates, proteins, and calories that meet a person's dietary needs. But when it comes to calories, more is less, meaning if you take in more calories than you need, the excess is stored as fats. Too much fat and you become overweight, a condition that can make treating any chronic disease, including HIV, much more difficult. In addition, diseases such as diabetes and heart disease emerge as a result of being overweight, further complicating your HIV treatment. The proper number of calories and types of vitamins and minerals can significantly enhance your health and ability to fight your HIV. But, unfortunately, many people find there are barriers to eating right—barriers that interfere with a proper diet. Let's look at some of those barriers.

POOR HEALTH AND NOT FEELING WELL

If you are living with HIV, the reality is that there are times you just don't feel well. Nausea caused by opportunistic infections, HIV medications, or by HIV itself makes it very difficult to eat a proper diet. Vomiting, abdominal pain, or diarrhea can leave you with little or no appetite, making it difficult to eat a nutritious meal, which in turn makes it unlikely you will get the calories and nutrients you require each day. Losing your appetite can happen on occasion, and it typically will return in a couple of days. Keep in mind that as long as you are drinking the proper amount and type of fluids each day, a decreased appetite for a short period of time is nothing to worry about. However, if your appetite doesn't improve after three to four days, or you are losing weight as a result of not eating, you should contact your doctor right away.

While poor health can make it difficult to eat a nutritious meal, the symptoms that accompany your HIV can make it difficult to prepare one as well. Standing at your kitchen counter to prepare your breakfast, lunch, or dinner can be made difficult by the fatigue and weakness that sometimes accompanies HIV. Nausea and vomiting can make handling or smelling foods undesirable. Typically, nutritious meals do require more preparation than do those foods offering little in the way of nutrients. Meals that require minimal preparation time and effort are usually those with the least amount of nutrients. In most cases this means processed foods such as "TV dinners," boxed meals, or the worst case scenario—fast food. While these foods provide calories, they offer little else in the way of nutrients. In fact, these types of food provide excessive amounts of fat, sugars, salt, and artificial ingredients that do little to improve the nutritional status of the HIV-positive person.

ORAL LESIONS, MOUTH PAIN OR TOOTH PAIN

As we discussed in previous chapters of this book, oral manifestations of HIV are common occurrences for most people living with HIV. Oral lesions, ulcers, mouth pain or infections common to HIV can interfere with eating and drinking, and, in turn, with proper nutrition. Poor dental hygiene will eventually cause tooth decay, painful dental caries (cavities), and broken or loose teeth, all of which make it difficult to eat. Viral infections such as herpes, fungal infections such as thrush (candidiasis or yeast), and bacterial infections such as periodontitis (infection of the gum tissue) cause mild to severe pain that makes eating difficult to impossible, sometimes affecting appetite as well. If you can't eat, you can't maintain proper nutrition. Therefore, maintaining optimal dental health is essential to good nutrition.

FINANCIAL RESOURCES

When money is tight, people find ways to cut costs and save a few dollars. Preparing healthy meals at home can be too expensive for someone on a fixed income or who has limited financial resources. Unfortunately, fast food is affordable for most but not a good source of nutrition. But for people with a limited income, foods high in nutrients may be too expensive for their budget, meaning fast food is the remaining option. Luckily, there are publicly funded programs, such as the food stamp program, that help people buy nutritious food and thereby decrease the amount of fast food in their diet. Many HIV treatment programs employ dieticians that can assist low income families in planning nutritious meals using foods that fit into a limited budget. There are local community agencies that sponsor food banks, collecting donations of food and money from the community and making it available free of charge to those people in need. However, because they rely on donations, the availability of these resources is limited. Food supplies are rationed to insure as many families as possible get something, meaning the food they receive may not go far in terms of feeding a family.

Being Homeless

For those people who are homeless, buying and storing food is impossible. There are homeless shelters and soup kitchens that try to provide at least one healthy meal each day, but, as is the case with food banks, funding is very limited. Along with limited funds, shelters are often very tight on physical space, decreasing the number of people that can be accommodated each day. Sadly, because of limited funding, limited food inventory, and the growing number of homeless people they need to feed, agencies may limit individuals to one meal each day, or, in extreme circumstances, may only offer meals on holidays like Christmas and Thanksgiving. In addition to the limited availability of food, there is a high incidence of alcoholism and drug use among the homeless. When these individuals have money they typically use it to buy alcohol or drugs, forgoing nutrition in order to satisfy their addiction.

Drug and Alcohol Addiction

As was mentioned in the previous section, living with an alcohol or drug addiction can severely impact a person's ability and desire to eat healthy food and follow a healthy diet. In fact, drug or alcohol addiction can cause very poor eating habits and in turn poor diet can make addiction recovery more difficult, increasing the incidence of relapse. Recovery and withdrawal from drugs or alcohol can also impact the amount of nutrients and vitamins in the body. The vomiting and diarrhea common in withdrawal will cause vitamin deficiencies as well as electrolyte imbalances. Simply put, addiction and nutrition are entwined, meaning one will most definitely impact the other. People who are addicted will choose a drink or a drug "fix" over a meal most of the time. When addicted, a person's desire to eat and feelings of hunger are often suppressed in favor of drug or alcohol cravings. During recovery the hunger pains and food cravings return but people will often mistake them for drug and alcohol cravings, resulting in relapses. By improving eating habits during recovery, the risk of relapses declines. For those not in recovery, every effort should be made to make certain people are eating healthy foods and taking in plenty of water, vitamins, and minerals. The following will help:

- encourage regular mealtimes each day;
- eat foods low in fat and high in proteins, complex carbohydrates (sugars), and dietary fiber;
- and make an effort to take at least a multivitamin or vitamin and mineral supplement each day.

Addiction, be it to alcohol, illegal drugs, or prescription drugs, can have a serious negative impact on diet and nutrition, making HIV treatment all the more difficult. Get treatment for your addiction and in the process your nutritional status will improve as well.

POOR MOBILITY OR TRANSPORTATION

Depending on the overall health and the living situation of the individual, acquiring food of any kind can be a challenge. If their medical status impedes their mobility, or they are without reliable transportation, getting to the grocery store to purchase food is difficult or impossible. Being confined to their home, they must rely on others to bring them the food they need. For those whose mobility is limited, preparing meals may be difficult. For instance, standing at the counter or at the stove for hours can be difficult for those with fatigue, back pain, or weakness due to the compromised medical condition. But help is available if you know where to look. In many communities there are agencies that provide volunteers who shop and deliver groceries for those who are unable to do so for themselves. Some grocery stores or private businesses offer food shopping and delivery services for a fee. Services like Meals on Wheels will bring food to the individual; however, most often it is limited to once daily or a couple times a week. There are even clubs that will prepare ingredients for multiple meals and ship them to the individual, who can then prepare and freeze them for future use. Granted, such services can be costly in some instances, but can be a good option for people who have some financial means. Finally, the ideal solution would be a neighbor, family member, or loved one coming to the home to help plan and prepare a meal. This solution has the added benefit of having someone that provides support, companionship, and love to the person stuck at home.

The Nutritional Impact of HIV

We know that HIV impacts every aspect of your health and body. The HIV program I work in has a slogan that goes something like this: *"Because we realize HIV impacts your life in so many ways."* And certainly nutritional status is one of those ways. We've shown that diet and nutrition can have a great deal of impact on your health and how well you live with HIV. However, the inverse is also true: your disease impacts your nutrition in a number of ways. The impact HIV has on nutrition is classified into three categories.

INADEQUATE INTAKE

In any disease state, including HIV, the human body needs increased amounts of calories and nutrients to fight their disease and to heal completely. One would think by just eating, your body's nutrient requirements would be met. But HIV and conditions associated with the virus makes that easier said than done. HIV increases the body's metabolic needs, meaning nutrients such as protein and carbohydrates are being used at an accelerated rate. The body's energy requirements are also increased, meaning the number of calories the body needs to produce that energy increases as well. But keep in mind the quality of the calories taken in is as important as the number of calories taken in each day. The body needs calories that are made up of quality proteins, fats, and carbohydrates that satisfy the body's many nutritional needs during this increased metabolic state. For instance, you can increase your calories by eating either potato chips or baked fish, but it's the baked fish that will offer you the best kind of calories—those complete with the proper nutrients, vitamins, and minerals that are required for the body to fight your disease. Potato chips and foods like them provide what are called "empty calories"—those calories that offer very little in terms of nutrition.

There are many causes for inadequate intake of nutrients in the HIV-positive person. The most common causes are nausea and vomiting, common side effects of many HIV medications. Altered taste and poor appetite can also affect nutrient intake and can be a medication side effect as well. Associated illnesses, like HIV wasting or opportunistic infections, specifically those of the gastrointestinal (GI) tract, also make it very difficult to take in the quantity and quality of essential nutrients needed for a healthy life.

Poor Absorption of Nutrients

You can take in all the nutrients you want, but without the proper absorption of those nutrients they'll do you no good at all. In the absence of HIV, opportunistic infections, or other disease states, absorption is a natural process of utilizing the food we eat by absorbing the nutrients contained in that food. However, in the presence of HIV, absorption is often compromised, most often caused by infections of the GI tract or damage to the GI tract by HIV itself. Normally, nutrients are absorbed through the walls of the intestines. But infections or damage to the absorptive surfaces of the gastric mucosa interferes with the normal absorption of nutrients, vitamins, and minerals. Diarrhea and increased gastric motility (movement) through the intestinal tract can also interfere with the body's ability to absorb nutrients. For absorption to occur, the digesting food and gastric acid mixture must have contact with the walls of the intestinal tract. But if that mixture is moving too fast through the GI tract, there is not enough time for proper absorption to occur, and most of the nutrients are lost in the form of diarrhea. If the surfaces of the mucosa are damaged or compromised by infection or disease, proper absorption can't occur and again, nutrients are excreted along with the bodily waste.

Altered Metabolism of Nutrients

Metabolism is defined as the sum total of all the chemical and physical processes occurring in a living organism. It's all the metabolic processes that use food and oxygen we take in to produce the energy and basic materials needed for life processes. In a healthy body, metabolism is a finely tuned process of converting what we take in each day into the energy, proteins, fats and carbohydrates we need for life processes. Metabolism is also responsible for the breakdown and excretion of waste products, medication by-products, and harmful substances that may enter the body. HIV can alter metabolism and the way in which the body processes, utilizes, stores, and excretes the nutrients we take in each day. Other factors, including immune system dysfunction, medication side effects, opportunistic infections, and hormonal changes, can also alter metabolism. Conditions commonly associated with HIV, including poorly controlled blood sugar, lipodystrophy, and elevated cholesterol and triglyceride levels, are all evidence of the disruptive effects HIV can have on metabolism.

What Is a Good Diet?

Whether you are watching television or reading the newspaper, you are bound to come across the terms "proper nutrition" and "a good diet" more than once. But what constitutes proper nutrition and a good diet? A simple definition of proper nutrition and a good diet could go something like: "*a diet that provides all the daily required vitamins and minerals with the right balance of calories, fats, carbohydrates (sugars), and protein.*" Pardon the pun, but that's a mouthful. Luckily, there are established standards and guidelines for what we are calling a good diet. Let's look at the different aspects of a good diet and proper nutrition.

CALORIES

The calorie is a unit of measure used to quantify energy. Specifically, the calorie is a unit of measure for both stored energy and the energy contained in foods. When discussing diet (calories eaten) and exercise (calories burned) we are actually discussing *kilocalories*; the term calorie is used as a short version of the more accurate term kilocalories. The scientific definition of a kilocalorie is *the amount of heat needed to raise the temperature of one kilogram of water one degree Celsius at sea level*. But that definition really does little for you when trying to put together a healthy diet. A better definition may be that a calorie measures *the amount of energy contained in the foods we eat*. For instance, the six-ounce steak you ate for dinner provides energy in the form of calories, energy that is used to fuel the body's processes. So where do we find these calories, and are some calories healthier than others? In fact, there are calories that are better for you than others. For example, 100 calories from a candy bar are not as healthy as 100 calories from baked fish. To find the healthy calories and develop a healthy diet we first have to understand where calories are found. Let's examine the three sources of calories in our diet.

Carbohydrates

Carbohydrates are the body's primary source of energy, providing four calories for every gram of carbohydrates. Most carbohydrates in the diet are naturally occurring, found in such foods as fruits, vegetables, legumes, and grains. Depending on the size of the molecule, carbohydrates can be complex or simple. The small-molecule carbohydrates are in the form of simple sugars—namely, glucose and fructose. Honey, fresh fruit, and dairy products contain these simple sugars. Because of their small molecular size, they can be broken down for energy very quickly. However, their energy lasts only a short time. Under certain circumstances, carbohydrates in the form of simple sugars can chain together and form large, complex carbohydrates in the form of starch or fiber. These complex carbohydrates can also be broken down for energy relatively quickly but last longer than do the simple sugars. Examples of complex carbohydrates include breads, grains, vegetables, and pasta. People often interchange the words carbohydrates and sugars, using them to mean the same thing. But actually sugars are only one of three types of carbohydrates, the others being starch and fiber.

> *Sugar*—The simplest form of carbohydrates. Sugar occurs naturally in many foods, including fruits, vegetables, milk and milk products. Some specific types of sugars include fruit sugar (fructose), table sugar (sucrose) and milk sugar (lactose). Added sugar is also in the form of simple sugars. A healthy diet includes the right amount of sugar and minimal added sugar. While we need sugar to survive, excess sugar in the diet can cause a myriad of issues including weight gain and hyperglycemia (high blood sugar).

> *Starch*—A complex carbohydrate, made of many sugar units bonded together. Starch occurs naturally in vegetables, grains, and cooked dry beans and peas. Some starch is

digested rapidly and elevates blood sugar a great deal. Others are slowly digested and have a lesser effect on blood sugar. There are even some starches the body can't digest at all that have no effect on the blood sugar.

Fiber—Also a complex carbohydrate, fiber occurs naturally in fruits, vegetables, whole grains, and cooked dry beans and peas. There are two primary types of fiber: soluble, meaning it dissolves in water, and insoluble, which does not dissolve in water. Soluble fiber helps regulate sugar absorption by binding with fatty acids and slowing the rate of stomach emptying. Insoluble fiber promotes regular bowel movements and speeds the elimination of toxic waste.

Fats

Fats are complex molecules comprised of substances called *fatty acids*. There are many kinds of fats; some are manufactured by the body when excess calories are ingested and others are found in the foods we eat at each meal. Fat is essential to many bodily functions. For instance, fats are necessary because there are vitamins in the body that are only fat soluble, meaning they need fats to be absorbed and utilized by the body.

When energy is needed and there is a shortage of carbohydrates, fats are broken down into fatty acids, and they, in turn, are burned for energy. Fats are a major source of energy for the body, released slowly but efficiently. Because they are such an efficient source of energy, the body stores its excess calories as fat beneath the skin (subcutaneous), in certain organs such as the liver, and within the walls of blood vessels. There are nine calories stored in every gram of fat. This is more than twice the amount of calories as the same amount of proteins or carbohydrates. Because there are certain fatty acids the body can't manufacture, fats must be taken in as part of a healthy diet. However, fat need only be taken in to a certain extent. Excessive fats in the diet get deposited throughout the body and contribute to such health conditions as obesity, high blood pressure, diabetes, and heart and vascular disease.

There are two types of dietary fat, those that are healthy and those that are potentially harmful. The potentially harmful fats are of two types:

- *Saturated Fats*—mostly from red meats, poultry, and dairy products, these fats cause elevated cholesterol, increase your risk of heart disease, and increase your risk of Type II Diabetes.

- *Trans Fats*—most of these are made from oils during a food manufacturing process known as hydrogenation. These trans fats can raise the unhealthy cholesterol in your blood and can greatly increase your risk of heart and vascular disease.

On the other hand, there are three types of healthy fats, and they are mostly unsaturated:

- *Monosaturated Fatty Acids*—these types are found in a variety of foods and oils. Eating these types of fats can help lower blood cholesterol and can help insulin better control blood sugar. Research has shown these fats can decrease your risk of heart disease.

- *Polyunsaturated Fatty Acids*—these fats are found mostly in plant-based food and oils. Eating foods rich in polyunsaturated fatty acids will decrease cholesterol and your risk of heart disease.

- *Omega-3 Fatty Acids*—this type of polyunsaturated fat is found as fish oil and can decrease blood cholesterol and the risk of heart and vascular disease.

Proteins

Proteins are compounds consisting of long, complex chains of amino acids joined together by *peptide bonds*, chemical bonds that occur between two amino acids. A healthy human body needs amino acids to function properly. Proteins are involved in controlling the metabolism of cells, controlling the structure and movement of cells and larger structures and coordinating the response of cells to internal and external factors. Amino acids are found in plant-based foods (e.g., vegetables) and animal-based foods (e.g., beef), meaning you don't have to eat animal foods (beef, chicken, pork, etc.) in order to get the required amino acids. There are three groups of amino acids:

- *Essential Amino Acids*—they can't be made by the human body; therefore, essential amino acids must be part of our diet. All the day's required amino acids do not have to be taken in at one meal. In fact, it's better to spread them out over the course of the day.
- *Nonessential Amino Acids*—these amino acids are manufactured by the body from the essential amino acids in our diets and by the normal breakdown of proteins.
- *Conditional Amino Acids*—not essential to the functioning of the body, these amino acids are primarily needed in times of stress and illness.

Because protein molecules are so large, the energy in protein is released slowly and lasts longer than carbohydrates or fats. Proteins are the building blocks of the human body, providing substances needed to manufacture skin, muscles, and bone. Every gram of protein in the diet stores four calories of energy available for use by the body. However, excess proteins are not stored in the body. Proteins are broken down into amino acids that are immediately used by the body. Those excess amino acids that are not used within a certain amount of time are sent to the liver where they are reconfigured to glucose and used for energy or reconfigured and stored as fat.

VITAMINS

Another part of a good diet and proper nutrition, vitamins are small molecules that your body needs in minute quantities in order to carry out body processes and chemical reactions. Vitamins act as catalysts—those compounds that "kick start" or initiate chemical reactions in the body. Like the match that starts the fire, vitamins start chemical reactions and, in some cases, speed up reactions necessary for life. There are two types of vitamins, fat soluble and water soluble.

- *Fat Soluble*—these vitamins are stored in the liver and are not excreted from the body. Because they are not excreted they do not need to be replaced each day. However, they can be taken in excess and accumulate toxic levels. These vitamins also need fat to be absorbed by the body. The fat soluble vitamins are A, D, E and K.
- *Water Soluble*—these vitamins are very soluble and are not stored in the body, meaning they need to be replenished each day. Because they are not stored there is little chance of taking toxic levels. These vitamins require water to be absorbed. Because they are so

soluble, they can be lost during cooking so care must be taking when preparing foods that contain these vitamins. The water soluble vitamins are the B-complexes and C.

Vitamins aren't manufactured by the body in sufficient amounts so they must be taken in with the foods we eat, the sunlight warming our skin, and vitamin supplements taken each day (e.g., once-a-day multivitamin). There are thirteen different vitamins that are considered essential to a healthy life. These vitamins are absolutely necessary if the body is to function properly. Let's look at some of these essential vitamins.

Vitamin A (Retinol)

Vitamin A, also known as Retinol, is one of four fat soluble vitamins. This essential vitamin is produced in the stomach by the enzymatic breakdown of beta-carotene, a naturally occurring nutrient found in plants and vegetables. The vitamin A produced in the stomach in turn produces the substance retinal, which is used by the rods and cones of the eye to sense light. It's this fact that has spawned the belief that eating carrots (a source of beta-carotene) is good for your eyes. In fact, this is more accurate than you may think. Your body can't make retinal without Vitamin A, and you can't see without retinal, so sources of vitamin A such as carrots are good for your eyesight. Because it's a fat soluble vitamin, it's possible to take in too much vitamin A. Because it is fat soluble you can take too much vitamin A. Toxicity of vitamin A is almost always due to excessive amounts of vitamin A supplement.

Daily Requirement: Men—900 micrograms (mcg); Women—700 mcg

Vitamin B (B-complex)

The B vitamins are actually a collection of eight water soluble vitamins that are referred to as the *B complex vitamins*. Because they are water soluble, toxicity of the B-complex vitamins is very seldom a concern. The B complex vitamins perform many functions, including the breakdown of carbohydrates for energy, the breakdown of proteins and fats for normal nervous system function, and the maintenance of muscle function and tone in the stomach and intestinal tract. The B complex vitamins include:

- B1—thiamine—important in nervous system and muscle function.

  Daily Requirement: Men—1.2 mg; Women—1.1 mg

- B2—riboflavin—helps to produce energy and acts as an antioxidant, ridding the body of damaging free radicals.

  Daily Requirement: Men—1.3 mg; Women—1.1 mg

- B3—niacin—helps the functioning of the nerves, skin, and digestive system

  Daily Requirement: Men—16 mg; Women—14 mg

- B5—pantothenic acid—critical in the manufacturing of red blood cells and sex and stress-related hormones.

  Daily Requirement: Men and Women—5 mcg

- B6—pyridoxine—helps manufacture neurotransmitters, hormones that control mood and sleep, and necessary for normal brain function.

  Daily Requirement: Men and Women—19–50 years old—1.3 mg; 50+ years—1.5 mg

- B9—folic acid—involved with brain function and mental health and emotional health

  Daily Requirement: Men and Women—400 mcg

- B12—cyanocobalamin—maintains healthy nerve cells, the production of DNA and RNA, and the production of red blood cells.

  Daily Requirement: Men and Women—2.4 mcg

- H—biotin—helps metabolize carbohydrates, fats, and amino acids, recommended for healthy skin and hair.

  Daily Requirement: Men and Women—14–18 years old—25mcg; 18+ years—30 mcg

Vitamin C (Ascorbic Acid)

Also known as ascorbic acid, vitamin C is the most well known but least understood of all the vitamins. A very important vitamin, it's responsible for the production of collagen, an important part of skin, tendons, ligaments, cartilage, and blood vessels. Vitamin C is also necessary for healthy bones, teeth, and gums. In addition, the vitamin also acts as a strong antioxidant (substances that protect from free radicals, the damaging effects of oxygen); it controls and helps limit infections; and it treats diseases such as anemia. A vitamin C deficiency results in the disease known as scurvy. There has been some conjecture that large daily doses of vitamin C will prevent the common cold. Unfortunately, that theory has never panned out. Studies have shown that while the doses of vitamin C found in a once-a-day vitamin may ease the symptoms of a cold, there is no proof that much larger doses will prevent a cold from occurring.

Daily Requirement: Men—90 milligrams (mg); Women—75 mg

Vitamin D

The body stores vitamin D and makes vitamin D when the skin is exposed to sunlight. This fat soluble vitamin is important in the absorption and retention of calcium and phosphorus, both essential minerals found in healthy bones and teeth. Very few foods have significant quantities of vitamin D. Milk and breakfast cereals, both fortified with vitamin D, and some types of fish are the best dietary sources of the vitamin. Unlike other vitamins, the body does produce some vitamin D naturally. When the sunlight's ultraviolet rays strike the skin, a photochemical reaction occurs, producing vitamin D. Technically, vitamin D is considered a hormone because of its regulatory role in the absorption and excretion of calcium. There is also evidence that vitamin D strengthens the immune system, helps balance mood and emotional health, and even prevents some types of cancer. As was mentioned earlier, few foods provide vitamin D unless the food has been vitamin enriched during the manufacturing process. Therefore, in order to get the daily required amounts of vitamin D, having some time in the sunlight and taking a once-a-day multivitamin is recommended.

Daily Requirement: Men and Women—15 mg

Vitamin E

As one of the fat soluble vitamins, vitamin E acts as a powerful antioxidant that protects cell membranes from the damage caused by oxidation. The vitamin also increases the availability of vitamin A by inhibiting its intestinal oxidation. When vitamin A is in the intestinal tract, its structure is changed and destroyed by coming in contact with oxygen molecules (oxidation). Vitamin E inhibits this process, making more vitamin A available for body processes. Finally, vitamin E helps the body utilize vitamin K, a vitamin important in the blood clotting process.

Vitamin E is found in foods derived from plants, such as wheat germ and whole grains. Other foods, such as nuts, peanut butter, and vegetable oils, are also good sources of vitamin E. Early studies suggest that vitamin E helps decrease the risk of cardiac disease by slowing the oxidation of bad cholesterol (LDL). Oxidation of LDL produces the fatty plaques that contribute to arterial narrowing and the formation of blood clots, both of which lead to heart attacks. However, there is some recent evidence that caution is warranted when suggesting vitamin E in those cardiac patients taking drugs to lower their cholesterol. The combination of the two has been shown to inhibit the anti-inflammatory action of cholesterol-lowering drugs, which actually increases the risk of heart disease in those patients. Experts continue to suggest vitamin E be taken by those patients not prescribed cholesterol-lowering drugs. It must be noted that in order for vitamin E to have arterial benefits (benefits to your blood vessels), it must be taken along with vitamin C.

Daily Requirement: Men and Women—15 mg

Vitamin K

Another of the fat soluble vitamins, vitamin K is necessary for normal blood clotting and the production of proteins needed for plasma, bone and kidney formation. In addition, its antioxidant properties protect the skin from the negative effects of oxidation. The primary sources of vitamin K are leafy green vegetables, such as kale, cabbage, and broccoli, which together provide about half of the dietary requirement. The remainder of necessary vitamin K comes from such things as wheat bran, cereals, certain fruits, dairy products, and eggs. While healthy adults typically have plenty of vitamin K, infants and especially newborns commonly have deficiencies. In fact, vitamin K is routinely given to newborns to protect against blood clotting difficulties that occur with vitamin K deficiencies.

Daily Requirement: Men—120 mcg   Women—90 mcg

MINERALS

As important as vitamins are to a healthy body, they can do very little without the catalytic actions of minerals. Like vitamins, minerals are substances needed in very small amounts in order for the body to function properly. Outside of the body or by themselves, minerals do very little. But in the body they function as catalysts, meaning they help initiate biological reactions—reactions that are necessary for life. Examples of these reactions include such processes as transmission of nervous impulses, proper muscle function, and the utilization of nutrients in the foods we eat.

Many people equate vitamins and minerals, but in actuality they are quite different. While the two do function together, there is one very important difference. Vitamins are organic, meaning they contain carbon atoms. Minerals, on the other hand, are inorganic, meaning they contain no carbon atoms. There are some vitamins that can be produced in the body. However, the absence of carbon atoms means the body is unable to produce minerals naturally. Instead, essential minerals come from a healthy diet and dietary supplements, such as once-a-day multivitamins. Some of the minerals in highest abundance in the body include:

- *Calcium*—found in such foods as dairy products, kale, broccoli, cabbage, and a variety of whole grains.

  Daily Requirement: Adults 19–50 years old—1000 mg; 50+ years—1200 mg

- *Phosphorus*—found in food sources such as yeast, wheat germ, soy, hard cheeses, eggs, poultry, and fish.

  Daily requirement: Adults—700 mg

- *Potassium*—found in foods such as bananas, potatoes, orange juice, spinach, tomatoes, and lima beans.

  Daily Requirement: Adults—4700 mg

- *Sodium*—found in just about all foods to some degree; major sources include bread, rolls, and processed foods (e.g., deli meat and canned soup).

  Daily Requirement: Adults—2300 mg

- *Iron*—found in such foods as red meats (e.g., beef and liver), poultry, seafood, spinach, beans, peas, nuts, and raisins.

  Daily Requirement: Men 19–50 years old—8 mg; Women 19–50 years—18 mg; Adults 50+—8 mg

- *Magnesium*—found primarily in leafy green vegetables, nuts, and whole grains.

  Daily Requirement: Men 19–50 years old—400 mg; Women 19–50 years—310 mg; Men 50+—420 mg; Women 50+—320 mg

In total there are literally hundreds of minerals in various quantities found throughout the body, but of those, twenty-five are considered essential to a healthy life. These twenty-five minerals are divided into two main categories:

Macrominerals

These minerals are required by the body in amounts greater than or equal to 100mg per day. Some examples of macrominerals include calcium, magnesium, sodium, potassium, phosphorus and chlorine. These minerals are found in virtually every cell in the body and are essential to critical bodily functions, such as muscle contraction, heart function, and bone growth. The body maintains mineral levels in a very small normal range because normal mineral levels are so important to the functioning of the body. For instance, the potassium level in the blood can only vary from 4.5 to 5.5 millimoles per liter (mmol/l). Anything outside that very small range can have very detrimental effects. Granted, dietary causes of mineral deficiency are rare, but keep in mind that insufficient or excessive quantities of certain minerals, such as potassium, can cause severe disruption in the functioning of the human body, even death. For that reason, HIV specialists monitor the level of these essential minerals using frequent blood tests (e.g., electrolytes) and urine tests (e.g., urinalysis).

Microminerals (Trace Minerals)

Also known as trace minerals or micronutrients, these are chemical elements needed by the body in quantities less than 100mg per day. Examples include elements such as iron, cobalt, chromium, copper, iodine, manganese, selenium, zinc, and molybdenum. Despite being used in such minute quantities, trace minerals perform many important roles and functions. Trace minerals are necessary for oxygen transport throughout the body; the uptake of nutrients, including vitamins and other minerals; proper hormone and enzyme function; and, finally, the breakdown of nutrients to produce energy.

It's important to note that mineral deficiencies are more critical to the functioning of the body than are most vitamin deficiencies. That being the case, if there is a mineral deficiency, a physician should address the issue. In addition, since different minerals are store in different organs, the signs or symptoms of mineral deficiency will vary a great deal. That being said, it's important to know that trace minerals, even though they are needed in just small quantities, can become toxic if supplements are taken in excess. Therefore, any mineral deficiencies should be corrected by a physician using prescription mineral replacement.

A Word About Oxidation

When most people think about oxidation, the first thing that comes to mind is the rust that forms on the fenders of an old car. Years of moisture on exposed metal causes a layer of rust to form. If left untreated, rust can eat its way through a car's bumper or door in no time. But oxidation is not limited to the body of a car. In fact, oxidation can do great harm to the human body as well. Technically speaking, oxidation is the process by which substances interact with oxygen, causing that substance to lose electrons. Those lost electrons cause the release of reactive substances known as free radicals. Circulating free radicals make their way through the body looking for an electron to replace the one they lost. They steal electrons from other substances, creating even more free radicals in the process. The cycle continues over and over, stressing and damaging cells throughout the body. The natural aging process is an example of the damaging effects of accumulating free radicals and oxidation. The process will continue and free radicals will accumulate in the body unless something interrupts the cycle. That's where antioxidants come into play.

Obviously, we are all going to age over time. However, certain foods, vitamins, and minerals act as antioxidants, slowing the damage done by oxidation. Antioxidants like vitamin C and E donate an electron to the circulating free radicals. Because the antioxidant is chemically stable with or without the electron, donating the electron to the free radical does not create another free radical, meaning the free radicals don't accumulate and the body's aging process slows. For instance, certain compounds found in dark chocolate and red wine are known to have antioxidant properties, meaning they can donate an electron to the damaging free radicals, eliminating them and the damage they cause the body. Many antioxidants are often identified in food by their distinctive colors. For example, the deep red of cherries and tomatoes, the orange of carrots, the yellow of corn, mangos, and saffron, and the blue-purple of blueberries, blackberries, and grapes are all examples of antioxidants. Finally, vitamin E has long been considered to be a vitamin that can ward off the aging process. Obviously, we will all age, despite vitamin E and other antioxidants. But the inclusion of antioxidants in our diet can help our bodies stay healthier longer and may just slow the aging process.

How Much of These Nutrients Do We Need?

Now that we know what is included in a healthy diet, it's important for us to know how much of these things we need in order to stay healthy. You have probably heard the expression "too much of a good thing." That goes for nutrition as well. You need plenty of calories, fats, proteins, vitamins and minerals to stay healthy. However, excessive amounts of any of these things will damage your health.

Vitamins, Minerals, and HIV

Studies indicate that people living with HIV have a greater risk of developing vitamin and mineral deficiencies than those people without the virus. And, in fact, the recommended daily requirements of vitamins and minerals are greater in people living with HIV compared to those who are HIV-negative. In fact, a U.S. study suggested that people living with HIV may need six to twenty-five times the recommended daily requirement of some vitamins and minerals. For example, because of certain HIV medications, vitamin D deficiency in HIV-positive people is common. A study published in 2008 reported almost one-third of HIV-positive people have some degree of vitamin D deficiency. Furthermore, nutrient deficiencies will increase the probability that HIV will progress to AIDS. Because of the increased risk inherent to HIV-infected people, experts agree that people living with HIV should, at minimum, take a multivitamin, complete with essential minerals, once each day to reduce the risk of vitamin and mineral deficiencies.

The Role of Antioxidants in HIV

Earlier in this chapter we discussed oxidation and the role antioxidants play in staying healthy. As a review, antioxidants are vitamins, minerals, and other nutrients found in foods or produced by the body that protect cells from circulating reactive substances called free radicals. Free radicals are released as a byproduct of oxidation, the interaction of oxygen and other compounds within the body. Circulating free radicals can stress and damage cells throughout the body.

Typically, the body maintains a balance between free radicals and the antioxidants that take care of them. But chronic infections, such as HIV, can throw that balance off, creating a greater number of free radicals—too many, in fact, for the body to handle. Exposure to such things as toxic chemicals or cigarette smoke can also add to the number of circulating free radicals. This free radical imbalance is sometimes referred to as *oxidative stress*—in other words, stress placed on the cells of the body due to increased numbers of circulating free radicals. Boosting the body's antioxidants will help handle the oxidative stress and slow the damaging effects of oxidation. Certain vitamins and minerals act as antioxidants, boosting the body's natural defenses against the deleterious effects of free radicals and oxidative stress.

Get Help with Your Nutrition

For those people living with HIV, there are so many issues that need attention. Medications need to be taken on time each and every day. Regular visits to your HIV specialist need to be scheduled and kept. There are possible issues with your employer, your finances, and your relationships. There are times you will feel sad, times you will feel happy, times you will feel alone, and times you will feel anxious. Finally, there are concerns of prejudice, stereotypes, and mistreatment. With so much on your mind, and additional stresses being added all the time, something has to give and often times that something is nutrition. Like all of us, there are times when eating a healthy diet is not the number one concern in our day. Sometimes it's just easier to grab a burger and fries. But as we have learned that is probably not the best thing for us to do. There is help available and whether you admit it or not the fact is you are going to need help and guidance to get your diet and nutritional state into the best shape it can be. You are going to need a dietician.

The Role of the Dietician

The management of HIV is a very complex and difficult task for provider and patient alike. With the advent of new medications and treatments, people are living longer and, as a result, need expertise in all areas of HIV care over the course of their lives. With the emergence of metabolic problems such as elevated cholesterol and triglycerides, lipodystrophy, and blood sugar dysfunction, nutritional expertise is needed now more than ever. A registered dietician can provide that expertise.

Experts agree that it has become evident over the course of the epidemic that all people living with HIV should have access to a registered dietician—ideally, one with expertise in HIV and AIDS as well as nutrition. In fact, nutrition and proper diet are so important to the HIV-positive person that experts recommend that HIV care programs employ a registered dietician or have a dietician available for referral—again, one with an expertise in HIV and AIDS. The roles of the dietician would include such things as nutrition screenings, counseling, education, and medical referral, to name just a few. Let's take a closer look at ways a dietician can help people living with HIV and AIDS.

SCREENING/REFERRAL/ASSESSMENT

Obviously, before any nutritional issues can be addressed they have to be identified. A thorough nutrition screening is necessary to identify any problems or deficiencies. The screening should include a complete medical and nutrition history; body measurements that include *body fat composition* (percentage of total body weight that is fat) and *body mass index* (BMI— a comparison of body weight to height); and a complete set of blood tests, including cholesterol and triglyceride levels, electrolytes, blood counts, and kidney and liver function. Keep in mind that a nutrition screening should be done as soon as possible after entrance into HIV care, and any time that the clinical picture suggests that there is a nutrition problem. Depending on the nutritional needs and risks of the HIV-positive person, the American Dietetic Association classifies nutrition risk in one of three categories.

- **High Risk**—people with two or more medical conditions in addition to HIV or those having a weight loss of greater than 10 percent of their body weight over four to six months should be seen by a dietician within one week of their entrance into HIV care.

- *Moderate Risk*—people suffering from chronic conditions such as chronic nausea, vomiting, and diarrhea, or those having signs of lipodystrophy, should been seen no later than one month after entry into HIV care.
- *Low Risk*—people without signs or symptoms of poor nutrition should be seen by a dietician at least once for an initial screening, and then again only as needed.

Once an issue has been identified, the patient should have a complete examination to assess how the identified nutritional issue is affecting overall health. This exam should include an evaluation of physical appearance and function. Does the patient look thin; is the skin dry and cracked; is there weakness or muscle atrophy; is the patient overweight or underweight when compared to height and body type; how much of the body's composition is fat; and finally, what is the waist and abdominal girth? All these factors are important in assessing the nutritional status of the HIV-positive person.

One other area that must be evaluated is the need for special dietary considerations. Are there issues that may affect the person's ability to eat, such as poor dental health, mouth pain, jaw pain, or absence of teeth altogether? Other considerations include assessment of the person's eating habits; what foods does the person like or dislike; is there any alteration in taste or smell that may interfere with eating; is the person taking vitamins or supplements; and finally, are there cultural requirements, financial factors, or problems with living arrangements (i.e. homelessness) that may affect nutrition or the ability to take in nutrients.

TREATMENT AND INTERVENTIONS

The key to avoiding nutritional deficiencies in the HIV-positive person is initiating nutritional interventions soon after the diagnosis of HIV is made. Early access to nutritional care can help prevent malnutrition, lipodystrophy, and AIDS wasting syndrome. Preventing problems with nutrition starts with education. One of the primary roles of the dietician is to provide basic nutritional education to the HIV-positive patient, thereby providing that person with the tools to improve their nutritional status. Nutrition awareness and education allows people to identify problems early and take steps to avoid and correct problems in their diet.

In the first decade of the HIV epidemic the only nutritional concerns were weight loss, wasting syndrome, and malnutrition due to nausea, vomiting, and overall poor health. But in 2016 with excellent medication regimens, undetectable viral loads, and overall good health, obesity, high blood sugar, and cholesterol issues are now a concern as well. That being said, dieticians can also make certain people aren't overeating, eating the wrong things, or living on diets high in fats and carbohydrates. While there are still patients that have to deal with weight loss and poor appetite, wasting is no longer the only issue facing the HIV-positive person today.

Besides education, the dietician can refer patients to medical providers in order to treat the underlying cause of any nutritional deficiencies, abnormally elevated blood sugar, or issues with high cholesterol that may be present. For instance, if there is pain from an infected tooth preventing a patient from eating, the dietician can refer the person to a dentist who will treat the infection, making it possible for the patient to eat again. If there are financial issues preventing the patient from getting enough food, a referral to case management or social services can be made to help the patient obtain food via food banks, mobile meal programs, or food stamp programs. A medical referral can be made to evaluate and treat the cause or causes of diarrhea, vomiting, or other medical problems that may be interfering with proper nutrition. Finally, the dietician can refer patients with blood sugar and cholesterol issues to a specialist in those fields in hopes of getting blood sugar and cholesterol under better control. In the case of the overweight patient, a referral to a weight loss specialist or, in extreme cases, a bariatric surgeon can be made to help intervene in a patient's battle with obesity.

A Few Words About Metabolic Syndrome

In this day of longer lives and better medication regimens, there is a condition or syndrome that is becoming more common among the general public and the HIV-positive person as well. *Metabolic Syndrome* is a collection of risk factors that raises your risk of heart disease. Thirty years ago the thought of someone with HIV having any of the risk factors included in metabolic syndrome was unheard of. But as is the case in the general population, these risk factors are becoming more of a problem in the HIV positive population as well. There is a collection of five risk factors included in metabolic syndrome. If you have three of the five, you are considered to have metabolic syndrome and your risk of coronary artery disease is increased. The five risk factors are:

1. A large waistline, often referred to as "central adiposity" is a collection of fat in the area of the stomach or abdomen.

2. An elevated triglyceride level or you are taking a prescription medication to lower triglycerides and cholesterol.

3. An abnormally low HDL (high density lipids/"good cholesterol") because HDLs help rid the blood vessels of cholesterol that would otherwise build up on the walls of the vessel, resulting in diminished blood flow and eventually occlusion.

4. You have an elevated blood pressure or you take prescription medication to control your blood pressure.

5. You have an elevated fasting blood sugar or you are on a prescription medication to help control your blood sugar.

Remember, if you have three of the five risk factors you are considered to have metabolic syndrome. But don't wait for three risk factors to occur. Speak with the HIV dietician before you have three of these risk factors to avoid the coronary artery risk altogether.

Nutritional Counseling

Countless studies have proven that nutrition counseling from a registered dietician greatly improves outcomes and facilitates healthy dietary habits for those people living with HIV. Nutrition counseling can provide the patient with methods that will help overcome barriers to good nutrition. These methods can be explored in a cooperative effort between the dietician and the person living with HIV. Part of nutritional counseling and education may include topics such as alternative therapies, naturopathic treatments, holistic medicine, and "fad" diets. A dietician can also teach you how to read the food nutrition label that is on the food your purchase at the grocery story. Understanding these labels can help you choose food that is perfect for your needs. Making the HIV-positive person aware of the pros and cons of their diet can insure that patients have the tools necessary to make informed decisions regarding their nutritional status.

The importance of good nutrition and timely nutritional interventions can't be over-stated. Proper nutrition, adequate nutrient intake, elimination of nutritional deficiencies, and eliminating the risks of being overweight and developing metabolic syndrome are essential to a healthy life with HIV.

Much of what we must do to stay healthy involves choices. People choose to start smok-ing or choose to have that second bowl of ice cream. Making the right choices can mean the difference between being sick and being healthy. The importance of one such choice is often underestimated—the choice to exercise each day. We all know the importance of regular exercise but all of us have come up with reasons why today is not a good day to go to the gym. For people living with a chronic illness, regular exercise is especially important. Exer-cising even twenty minutes every other day can improve your body's ability to fight infection, can improve heart function, and can help maintain an optimal body weight. Let's take a look at exercise and how it plays a role in living healthy with HIV.

The Role of Exercise in HIV

It's no secret; whether you have HIV, diabetes, asthma, or don't have a chronic illness at all, exercise is beneficial to your overall health. In fact, you really can't be your healthiest without having exercise as part of your life. Keeping your body in tip-top shape can only be accomplished if you are physically active. The human body is like no other machine. A car will eventually break down with daily use: its tires wear down; the brakes wear down; even the paint fades and becomes scratched. If you want your car to last longer, put it in the garage and drive it sparingly. The human body, unlike your car, will break down with inactivity. If you lay in bed for a few days, you will become weak, stiff, and very fatigued. Unlike other machines, the human body needs to be active in order to stay healthy. Without exercise, your body will break down, and you will not be as healthy as you could be. While these facts are true for each one of us, exercise is especially beneficial for people living with chronic illnesses such as HIV. There are several advantages and benefits to regular exercise. Here are just a few:

- Improved muscle mass, strength, and endurance.
- Improved heart and lung function.
- Increased energy levels throughout the day.
- Reduced stress and enhanced sense of well-being.
- Strengthened immune system, including boosted CD4 counts.
- Increased bone strength.
- Decreased cholesterol and triglycerides.
- Better weight control and decreased fat accumulation.
- Improved metabolism and blood sugar use and control.
- Improved sleep.

So, given its benefits, it's obvious we should include a program of regular exercise in our daily lives. However, there can be risks when starting an exercise program. Everybody can benefit from some degree of regular exercise—as long as the exercise program is geared to the person's physical abilities and takes into account their physical and emotional limitations. For instance, running ten miles each day will benefit a professional athlete, but it would probably do great harm to a 75-year-old grandmother. Lifting weights each day is a good way to build strength unless you are recovering from a dislocated shoulder. Exercise programs must take into consideration past injuries, health problems, current physical condition, and current medical conditions in order to be beneficial. Here are some factors to consider before starting any exercise program.

- Exercising beyond your physical abilities or limitations can actually be harmful. Before starting any exercise program, have a complete physical exam by your physician. Ask for specific recommendations regarding the level of exercise that is right for you. If you have access to a dietician or personal trainer, ask for their recommendations as well. Start slow, building strength and endurance before moving to the next level of difficulty. For instance, start by running a half mile each day, increasing to one mile each day only after being able to run the half mile comfortably. When weightlifting, start at lighter weights or fewer repetitions and move up as you get stronger.

- When we exercise, we lose bodily fluids in the form of sweat and the water vapor we exhale with every breath. If our body fluid losses exceed what we are taking in, eventually our bodies will be depleted of fluid, a condition called *dehydration*. Dehydration can be a very serious condition, especially in the elderly, young children, and people with chronic illnesses including HIV. If dehydration does occur, it is imperative that it be corrected or exercise performance will decline rapidly. You will also start to feel lousy, feeling dizzy, light-headed, headache, rapid heart rate, and fatigue. In extreme cases of dehydration, oral fluids can't replace what has been lost fast enough. In those cases, intravenous fluids are given, most often requiring a trip to the emergency room. Keep in mind that in order to avoid dehydration, the person exercising should drink water or electrolyte replacement fluids before, during, and after exercise to replenish what has been lost. Keep in mind that fluid replacement must be in the form of water or electrolyte replacement drinks like Pedialyte. Caffeinated beverages like soda or tea will actually make dehydration worse and should be avoided.

- Regular exercise will help you lose weight. Excess body fat will be the first to go, but people who have very little body fat will lose lean body mass (protein in the form of muscle) instead. If you are overweight, losing excess fat will make you healthier. By decreasing your daily calorie intake, exercise will help you shed the pounds. However, if you have very little body fat, losing muscle mass can be a problem. Therefore, if you choose to exercise and wish to maintain or build muscle, you must increase your caloric intake to match the increased caloric requirements of exercise. In addition, a diet with the proper amounts of fats, carbohydrates, and especially proteins must be taken in to address the increased needs caused by exercising. If you are trying to build muscle, the amount of protein in the diet must increase so there are protein resources to create more muscle.

- As careful as we are or try to be, exercise can lead to injuries. Before exercising make certain you warm up your muscles by stretching and flexing those muscles that you are about to exercise. If you are going to run, make certain your leg muscles are loose, stretched, and ready to take the punishment of running. To avoid injuries during your exercise, make certain you are performing the exercises correctly. For instance, if you are lifting weights, make sure you are using proper body mechanics to avoid pulled muscles, torn tendons, and muscle strains and sprains. If your exercise regimen employs exercise equipment, learn how to operate the equipment properly and safely before starting your exercise program. Heard of the phrase "*No pain no gain*"? Ignore that phrase and not the pain you are having. Pain is a sign that injury has occurred or may occur if exercise continues. Ignoring the signs of pain can cause or worsen injuries. After you are done with your exercising or running, make certain you have a "cool down" period, a period of less strenuous stretching and flexing to help flush the lactic acid from your muscles. Lactic acid is a byproduct formed in the muscles as oxygen in those muscles starts to decrease. A cool down helps replace the lactic acid with freshly oxygenated blood, just what the weary muscles need after exercise. If you do sustain an injury, see your doctor and suspend your exercise program until your injury is completely assessed, treated, and healed.

- Give your body a chance to recover. During exercise, muscle fibers stretch and tear. The muscle fibers must be given a chance to heal before taxing them again. By exercising every other day instead of every day, your muscles are given a chance to recover and heal. If you prefer to exercise every day, change the type of exercise you do each day. For instance, do aerobic exercises (e.g., running) on odd numbered days and weight training on even numbered days. Make sure you incorporate one day of rest each week in order to allow your body to fully recover.

Exercise Tips and Suggestions

Once you obtain medical clearance from your doctor and you understand how to exercise safely, you can begin your exercise program. But before you begin, take a look at these tips and suggestions that will make your exercise program safer and much more beneficial.

KNOW YOUR LIMITATIONS

Just because exercise is good for you doesn't mean more exercise is better. In fact, exercising more than your body is able to tolerate can be harmful. Remember the adage "Everything in moderation." The same holds true for exercise. Start slowly, three times per week, for instance, allowing your body to build up strength and endurance. As your strength and endurance improve, increase the amount of exercise and the difficulty of the exercises you are doing. Even this smallest amount of exercise will have an impact on your overall health. You will build muscle, lose excess weight, and even help control your cholesterol and triglycerides in your blood. The best part about exercising is you will have more energy and feel better in the process. Keep in mind that your progress may be slow or you may find it hard to exercise due to fatigue, lack of motivation, physical injury, or a medical issue. Take it slow, be patient, and do only what your body allows. Getting into the habit of exercising is the biggest challenge. Once it becomes a part of your day you will find that getting motivated will become much easier. Remember, any exercise, even 15 minutes a day is better than none at all.

Proper Diet Is Key

As we discussed earlier in this chapter, proper diet and healthy eating are an important part of staying healthy. If you exercise regularly, a proper diet is especially important. Keep in mind your diet must be adjusted according to the goal of your exercise program. If you are trying to lose weight and burn excess fat, then decreasing your calorie, carbohydrate, and fat intake is necessary. However, if you are trying to build muscle and lean body mass, then a diet with increased calories and protein is necessary. Keep in mind that if you are exercising to maintain your body weight or tone your muscles, your calorie intake must be about the same as the number of calories burned while exercising.

Not just any calories will do. The calories you take in must be "good calories"—calories that are part of a nutritious diet. For instance, a person can increase their calorie intake by eating nothing but potato chips every day. However, those calories are nothing but "empty calories," meaning they are calories that have no nutritional value and will do nothing but add to your fat stores. Instead, a person would be better served by increasing their calories by eating fish or lean meats, foods that will help build lean body mass.

Drink Plenty of Fluids to Avoid Dehydration

Another important aspect of any exercise program is proper fluid intake. During exercise, your body loses large quantities of bodily fluids due to perspiration (sweat), exhalation of water vapor, and body temperature regulation. Exercise generates body heat that must be dissipated in order to maintain proper body temperature. Body temperature is largely regulated by perspiring (sweating). Exertion causes sweat to form on the surface of the skin. As the sweat evaporates, it takes excess heat away from the body, and in doing so restores the body's normal temperature. It's hard to believe that the amount of water lost through sweating is enough to cause dehydration. But it certainly is, and therefore must be replaced by drinking the proper amount and type of fluid. If fluid is not replaced, the bloodstream and cells throughout the body become fluid depleted. In addition, fluid depletion also causes electrolyte (mineral) imbalances. These imbalances can affect muscle, nerve, and heart function. The importance of good hydration while exercising can't be stressed enough. When doing any physically taxing activity, it is extremely important to replace bodily fluids in order to avoid dehydration. It's extremely important to recognize the signs and symptoms of dehydration, and know what to do if you do become dehydrated. The symptoms of dehydration include:

- dry skin, tongue, or other mucous membranes;
- extreme thirst;
- poor skin turgor (doesn't spring back when stretched);
- dark, concentrated urine; smaller amounts of urine; urinating less often;

- headache, lightheadedness, or dizziness, especially when changing position; and
- low blood pressure with high heart rate, again especially after changing positions.

Mild dehydration may be nothing more than an uncomfortable inconvenience. If left untreated, however, it can become a serious, potentially fatal condition. So when you feel the signs and symptoms of dehydration coming on, it's important not to ignore them. Fluid replacement is of utmost importance, but treating dehydration is more than just drinking water. Granted, drinking water will replace the fluids you have lost, but there is still the matter of electrolyte imbalances common in dehydration. Electrolyte solutions such as Pedialyte can be used to replace both fluids and electrolytes. Eating fresh fruits such as oranges and bananas, or drinking Gatorade is also a good way to replenish the minerals lost during exercise. Be careful to avoid energy drinks, soda, or other caffeinated beverages. Caffeine can actually make dehydration worse.

The best way to treat dehydration is to avoid it altogether. Water or electrolyte solutions should be taken before, during and after exercise or physical exertion to keep up with fluids lost during exercise. Avoiding dehydration will make exercise less difficult and will help you avoid potential problems afterward.

Enjoy Your Exercise Program

I'll be the first to admit that as much as I tout the benefits of exercise, it's not always fun and entertaining. In fact, exercise can be downright unpleasant. It's the unpleasantness that makes it so hard to continue your exercise program. So it makes sense to choose a type of exercise or a program of exercise that you will enjoy. For instance, it makes little sense to include jogging in your exercise program if you hate to jog. If you don't care for weightlifting, choose another means of building and toning muscle. If you like what you're doing it will be much easier to stick to your regimen. If you like rollerblading, add that to your exercise program. If swimming is more your cup of tea, jump in feet first (pardon the pun). You have to like what you're doing in order to stick with the program.

Another reason why people can't seem to stick to their exercise program is boredom. People get tired of doing the same thing day in and day out, regardless of how much they typically enjoy the activity. You may love to rollerblade, but if you have to do that an hour each day every day as part of your regular exercise program you can count on becoming bored eventually. Variety is the spice of life it is said. The same holds true for exercise. If you get bored, you will find it harder to stick to the program. If you find it's becoming harder to find the ambition and motivation to exercise, try changing up your routine a bit. Instead of rollerblading on Wednesdays, ride your bike. If you're tired of jogging every other day, join an aerobics class instead. Boredom can destroy your motivation no matter how intent you are on getting healthier. Motivation is the key to any exercise program, and variety will keep you motivated while making exercise more fun.

Summary

Done properly and within the limitations of your body and your health, exercise will increase strength, reduce stress levels, improve the health of your immune system, help control cholesterol and triglyceride levels, maintain an optimal body weight, and improve metabolism, endurance and cardiac health. Exercise in some form should be a part of everyone's day, even as little as thirty minutes every other day. But remember, before starting any program of exercise, consult your doctor. He or she can help you design a program of exercise that will be right for you.

14

LIVING WITH HIV

It's time to bring it all together. For thirteen chapters we discussed everything from HIV prevention to HIV diagnosis and beyond. We have talked about medications, opportunistic infections, exercise and nutrition. But the purpose of this text is to make living with HIV easier. Day to day life with HIV can be a challenge, but hopefully this text will make that challenge less imposing. Our last chapter is called "Living with HIV," and that's exactly what we are going to discuss. This last chapter offers information that will help you handle the practical side of HIV, those issues most everyone faces but that are made more difficult because of an HIV diagnosis. The first topic we will cover is the special concerns of women living with HIV.

The Special Needs of Women Living with HIV

Like all chronic diseases, HIV can make life more complicated at times. No longer considered a terminal illness, HIV will, however, change your life. Experts agree that while HIV will impact the lives of all who are infected, women have a unique set of issues that must be dealt with. From opportunistic infections to social issues, the impact of HIV on the life of a woman is very different than its impact on a man. For example, everyone living with HIV must understand and be concerned with medications, opportunistic infections, and safer sex. But women have those concerns and more. For instance, an HIV-positive woman of child bearing age has to be aware of the risks some HIV medicines pose if she were to get pregnant. Her male counterparts just don't need to worry about such things. The topic of safer sex and condoms takes on a whole different meaning when we speak of women. A man with a condom in his wallet for that "special occasion" is praised as being a "player." However, in some parts of the world a woman merely suggesting safer sex and condom use may be subjected to abuse, both verbal and physical. A woman living with HIV has additional issues she must be aware of and must deal with in order to have a healthy life with HIV. We are going to discuss a couple of those issues here.

PREGNANCY AND HIV

At the outset of the epidemic, life after an HIV diagnosis was so short and so difficult that starting a family was out of the question. But as new, very effective HIV medications have come to market, life spans have become longer and life styles are now not much different than someone living without HIV. Today, having a family while living with HIV is not only possible, it occurs all the time. This is great news for couples having one or both partners infected with HIV. Planning and starting a family, however, is something that should not be taken lightly by anyone, HIV-positive or HIV-negative. But for HIV-positive couples there are additional considerations that must be addressed before getting pregnant. Let's look at some of the issues facing HIV-positive couples who want to start a family.

Who Is the Positive Partner?

How couples approach starting a family depends largely on which partner is positive. There are unique issues to consider, depending on who is positive—the male or female member of the couple. Anytime serodiscordant partners (one positive and one negative partner) have sex, there is concern over HIV transmission from the positive partner to the negative. Typically, the answer is a simple one: safer sex—namely, using latex condoms during each sexual encounter. After all, condoms have been proven to be an extremely effective barrier to HIV transmission. Unfortunately, condoms have also been proven to be an effective barrier to pregnancy as well. So obviously, if the goal is pregnancy, latex condoms are not an option. The degree of HIV transmission risk depends primarily on which partner is positive and the HV viral load of that person. Let's look at a couple of different scenarios and what methods can be used to get pregnant, while at the same time minimizing the risk to the negative partner.

Positive Mother/Negative Father—The first possible scenario involves couples whose positive partner is the mother-to-be. Statistics have shown that the risk of HIV transmission from a woman to a man is far less than the risk of transmission from a man to a woman. In fact, a woman's risk of being infected by a man during sex is approximately eighteen times greater than a man's risk of being infected by a woman according to one study. In cases where the woman has an undetectable HIV viral load, the risk to negative father is even less. But as low as the risk of transmission is, the risk is still there, and, in fact, transmission from women to men does occur. In fact, in a study published in 2005, female to male transmission carried a 1 to 159 risk, significant in medical terms. But there are ways to decrease that risk while still providing the opportunity for pregnancy.

- Outside of condom use, the best way to decrease the risk of HIV infection is to minimize the negative partner's exposure to active virus. By reducing the positive partner's HIV viral load, the negative partner's exposure to HIV is reduced and therefore the risk of infection is also reduced. This is accomplished by the use of HIV medications with the goal of suppressing HIV to an undetectable level. Keep in mind that while an undetectable viral load does reduce the risk of HIV transmission, it does not eliminate that risk entirely.
- The foreskin has a high concentration of CD4 cells providing HIV a very target rich environment in which to attach to CD4 cells and begin viral replication. Men who have been circumcised have a decreased risk of HIV infection because the foreskin and its high concentration of CD4 cells have been removed. Making certain the male partner is circumcised can decrease the risk of HIV infection during unprotected sex.
- It's also possible to reduce the risk of infection by treating the HIV-negative man with a post-exposure prophylaxis (PEP) regimen. In cases of accidental exposure or needle

sticks in the workplace, HIV medication regimens are prescribed in order to reduce the risk of infection. An early study published in 1997 demonstrated that even using a post-exposure regimen of zidovudine (Retrovir, AZT) alone decreased HIV transmission by 79 percent. But these days we use multi-drug PEP for better effectiveness. The CDC guidelines released in 2016 recommends Truvada (tenofovir + emtricitabine) plus either Isentress (raltegravir) of Tivicay (dolutegravir). If indicated, PEP should be given as soon as possible after the exposure but must be given less than 72 hours after exposure to be effective. PEP is taken for a period of four weeks after exposure—or in this case, four weeks after unprotected sex with a positive female partner hoping to become pregnant.

- The safest means of getting pregnant when the male is negative and the female is positive is *artificial insemination*. No actual intercourse and therefore no actual exposure to HIV takes place. The sperm of the male is collected and artificially placed in the female in hopes of fertilizing the woman's egg. Sometimes it is referred to as the "turkey baster" method because the sperm is inserted into the woman's vagina using a large syringe that resembles a turkey baster. While this method is the safest it's very expensive, making it an unrealistic option for many couples.

Positive Father/Negative Mother—This scenario involves a positive man and a negative mother-to-be. As we mentioned in the previous section, the risk of HIV transmission from a man to a woman is much greater than from a woman to a man. But even in this scenario, there are ways to reduce the risk and allow these couples the opportunity to start a family.

- As is the case with a positive female, the risk of HIV transmission from a positive male partner to a negative female partner can be reduced by the use of HIV medications. Using HIV medications to suppress the virus to undetectable levels will reduce the risk of transmission to the negative partner significantly. Once again, even with an undetectable viral load, the HIV transmission risk is not eliminated entirely. However, the risk is diminished enough that many couples trying to start a family the natural way are willing to accept that risk in exchange for the possibility of having a baby.

- Another option that is getting some attention is a procedure called *sperm washing*. Sperm washing is a technique that was first developed in Milan, Italy. The concept of sperm washing rests on the premise that HIV resides mainly in the seminal fluid (the thin liquid portion of the ejaculate) of an HIV-positive male. Sperm washing concentrates and separates the fertilizing sperm from the infectious seminal fluid. During ovulation, the woman is artificially inseminated with the concentrated sperm. Without the infectious seminal fluid, the theory is that the risk of the woman being infected with HIV is greatly reduced. According to a 2012 study, over 3000 sperm washing procedures were done and there were no HIV seroconversions in the women undergoing insemination and no children tested positive for HIV infection. However, the same study indicates that sperm washing offers no additional protection when compared to unprotected sex if the following conditions exist.
    - The man is taking an effective antiretroviral regimen and adheres to his regimen;
    - he and his female partner only have unprotected sex during the woman's ovulation period;

- the man has an HIV viral load of less than 50 copies; and
- there are no sexually transmitted infections in the man or woman.

While it appears sperm washing is an effective option, potential barriers do exist. Few, if any, medical insurance plans will cover sperm washing, and, unfortunately, the procedure is very expensive. Besides cost, the procedure is not widely available. It may be necessary to travel considerable distances to a facility offering the procedure, adding to the already expensive price tag. Finally, sperm washing does decrease the chance the artificial insemination will result in pregnancy

- The third option actually involves a third person. Specifically, the HIV-negative mother-to-be is artificially inseminated with donated sperm from an HIV-negative man. In most cases the sperm is obtained from an anonymous donor by way of a sperm bank. The couple does not know the donor of the sperm, and the donor does not know where his sperm was used. In some circumstances, a known donor can be used to impregnate the negative woman. For instance, a brother of the positive male partner may agree to donate the sperm that will be used to artificially inseminate the negative female partner or wife. The donor is sometimes referred to as a *surrogate*, meaning a substitute or stand-in. Keep in mind that there is widespread controversy surrounding artificial insemination. There have been cases of surrogates taking legal action in order to obtain visitation and parental rights after the baby is born. There also can be religious objections or ethical questions surrounding its use. Some see the procedure as unnatural or "tampering" with God's plan, while others view it as a gift that science has provided, allowing women who have trouble becoming pregnant to experience the joy of having children.

- Another option used to decrease the HIV transmission risk is post-exposure prophylaxis (PEP). Just as people who have been accidentally exposed to HIV take PEP to reduce the risk of infection, women can take PEP after having unprotected sex in an attempt to get pregnant. Caution must be used when prescribing PEP because there are HIV medications that can cause harm to an unborn child.

- Pre-exposure prophylaxis (PrEP) is growing in popularity among HIV-negative men and women who are considered at high risk for HIV-infection (e.g., men who have sex with men). The medication used in PrEP is Truvada (tenofovir + emtricitabine) that is taken once daily. For PrEP to be effective it must be taken each day without missing even a single dose. The Centers for Disease Control (CDC) recommends the PrEP be started one month before conception is attempted and should continue for one month after each conception attempt. Because the effects PrEP may have on the unborn fetus after conception are not entirely known, the PrEP is discontinued after conception is confirmed.

Positive Mother/Positive Father—You may think that because both partners in this scenario are HIV-positive there is nothing to consider. Actually, there are a couple of issues that have to be addressed. First, keep in mind that even though both partners are positive, the issue of HIV re-infection must be considered. If you recall, earlier in this text we discussed HIV re-infection. To summarize, an HIV-positive person can be re-infected with another strain of HIV when having unprotected sex with his or her HIV-positive partner. This can make treating the HIV in the re-infected partner much more difficult. So when trying to start a family, the couple with two positive partners should only have unprotected sex during the female's time of ovulation—that time when the female is most likely to get pregnant. During other times of the month, and after conception has occurred, the couple with two positive partners should return to using condoms to prevent HIV re-infection.

The other consideration is that once conception has occurred it is absolutely imperative that the pregnant partner get into prenatal care as soon as possible. The positive mother will be placed on an HIV regimen suitable for a pregnant woman and her unborn child if she wasn't already on such a regimen. After delivery the mom may stay on her current medication regimen or may return to the regimen she was on prior to getting pregnant. But to re-emphasize, once pregnant, the mother-to-be must get into prenatal care as soon as possible for the health of her and her baby.

Other Risk Reduction Methods for Discordant Couples Trying to Have a Baby

Along with the options we have just discussed, there are other risk reduction methods that will make it possible for discordant couples to start the family they have been dreaming of while at the same time keeping each partner as safe and healthy as possible.

- Prior to starting a family, both partners should be tested for sexually transmitted infections (STIs). Any active STIs should be treated prior to getting pregnant. Because the presence of STIs can increase the risk of HIV transmission to the negative partner, any STIs should be treated as soon as possible.
- Couples should only have unprotected sex during the woman's most fertile time of the month (during ovulation) when the chance of pregnancy is highest. While ovulation varies from woman to woman, it is typically about ten to fourteen days after your menstrual period ends. Safer sex methods should be used during the rest of the month and after conception (pregnancy) occurs.
- Couples should avoid "dry sex" (sex with little or no lubrication). Friction can cause small tears or irritation to the vaginal tissue, which opens portals that allow HIV to enter the bloodstream. Also avoid the use of any lubricating products that could irritate the mucosa of the vagina for the same reason; tissue irritation increases the risk of HIV infection.

Preventing Mother-to-Child HIV Transmission

HIV can spread from a woman to her baby in two ways—during pregnancy and delivery, and during breastfeeding. Without interventions, *vertical transmission* (transmission from an infected pregnant woman to her unborn child) is very efficient—about one in four births. Exposure to the infected blood and amniotic fluid while in the uterus or during a vaginal delivery is the route by which HIV enters the baby's bloodstream. The longer the baby is exposed to these fluids the higher the risk of infection. But there are methods used today that have succeeded in virtually eliminating the risk of vertical transmission.

- An HIV medication regimen safe for the unborn child is given to the mother during pregnancy and during delivery in hopes of bringing her HIV viral load to an undetectable level. The lower the viral load the lower the risk of transmission.

- Typically, in those women with detectable viral loads, the child is delivered using a Caesarean section (C-section), thereby reducing the amount of time the baby is exposed to the fluids of delivery. For those women with undetectable viral loads, vaginal delivery is sometimes considered.
- After delivery, an HIV medication is prescribed for the newborn. Typically, treatment consists of the drug *zidovudine* (Retrovir, AZT) that begins six to twelve hours after delivery and continues four to six weeks after delivery.

Another route of HIV infection in newborns is breastfeeding. In fact, breastfeeding carries an extremely high risk of transmission—somewhere between 25 and 30 percent. Because of the high risk, HIV-positive mothers are cautioned not to breast feed or manually express breast milk to feed their baby when clean water and baby formula are readily available. In parts of the world where clean water and alternatives to breast milk are readily available, this is not a problem. However, in less developed areas of the world such as sub-Saharan Africa, breastfeeding may be the only option. Scientists are researching ways to reduce the risk of HIV infection from breastfeeding. Recent studies suggest that placing the newborn on daily Viramune (nevirapine) after delivery provides protection against HIV transmission during breastfeeding. While the recommendation is still to avoid breastfeeding when possible, research is making breastfeeding safer in those circumstances where it is the only option.

Final Considerations for Discordant Couples Trying to Get Pregnant

Before taking that big step and getting pregnant, there are a few items discordant couples need to consider. While these issues should not deter efforts to become parents, couples must understand the potential barriers and risks associated with pregnancy.

- Realizing that trying to start a family can put the negative partner at risk and can affect sexual spontaneity, sexual drive, and the ability to conceive. Experts believe that stress related to concerns of HIV infection can affect a woman's likelihood to conceive or a partner's desire to have sex at all.
- With today's very effective HIV medication regimens, people are living near normal to normal lifespans. That being said, it is possible that the positive partner will at some point in their life have health-related issues that could impact his or her ability to parent a child. Discordant couples often let this possibility influence their decision to have a family. There are no guarantees in life for anyone, HIV positive or negative, so why let the possibility of illness stop you from having a family?
- Despite measures that minimize the risk of having an HIV-infected baby, there is still the very remote possibility that the newborn could be HIV-infected. The stress of that possibility can cause relationship issues and diminish the desire to start a family.
- Depending on available resources, not all measures that reduce the HIV risk to negative partners will be available. For instance, sperm washing and artificial insemination reduce transmission risk, but because these methods are not covered by most insurance, they may not be available to couples with limited resources.

WOMEN STAYING HEALTHY

HIV-positive people face many issues that can in some way jeopardize their health. From medication side effects to AIDS-related weight loss, people with HIV are at risk for a variety of conditions, illnesses and infections. However, HIV-positive women face all these issues and more; issues only women face each and every day. In fact, there is evidence that women are more vulnerable to HIV and the conditions that accompany the virus. So why is that the case?

Physical Differences

The incidence of heterosexual transmission in the United States has been on the rise since 1985. In 2010 about 18 percent of new cases were heterosexually transmitted. By 2014 that figure jumped to 24 percent. The rate of heterosexual transmission varies greatly depending on geographic location but experts agree when considering worldwide HIV infections, a majority are a result of heterosexual transmission. Unfortunately, it's women who bear the greatest risk—due in large part to the female anatomy. The vagina is lined with very fragile and highly vascular mucosal tissue. Women are especially susceptible to heterosexual transmission because that mucosal lining offers a large surface area that can be exposed to HIV-infected seminal fluid during unprotected sex. In addition, because vaginal tissue is so fragile, small tears can form during intercourse, creating portals of entry that allow HIV to reach the bloodstream. These factors are what make infection from men to women easier than from women to men.

Gender Inequities

Especially in developing countries, prevailing gender inequities lead to higher-risk behaviors. For instance, in many cultures women are not free to refuse sex or to insist on safer sex. In fact, in some parts of the world women are subjected to violence or rape by merely suggesting condom use. Many cultures assume women are prostitutes or are promiscuous for simply having a condom in their possession or for suggesting the use of safer sex practices. And as unbelievable as it may sound, in some parts of the world possession of condoms by women is actually a criminal offense.

Sexually active women are not the only women at risk in some parts of the world. In some cultures, having sex with a virgin—even a virgin child—is thought to exorcise demons and spirits. As a result, female children are being HIV infected by adult men because the men are trying to rid themselves of "demons." In these cultures, and societies, men assume a position of power and control over women, minimizing the amount of input women have when deciding whether or not to use safer sex practices. In addition, women have less access to employment and education. Often, the sex trade is the only option for women trying to earn money to feed their children. And, sadly, sexual violence against women is very high in some areas, exposing these women to high-risk behaviors and sexually transmitted infections from multiple partners, all without their consent.

Increased Risk of Illness

Women have an increased risk of reproductive illnesses, including vaginal yeast infections, pelvic inflammatory disease (PID), and cervical cancer, as a result of Human Papillomavirus (HPV) infection. It's the risk of cervical cancer from HPV that makes the HPV vaccine an important part of a woman's health maintenance program. Unfortunately, in developing parts of the world this important preventative vaccine is not readily available as it is in the United States and other developed countries. Another important fact is that the presence of sexually transmitted diseases significantly increases the risk of HIV infection, especially in women.

No Resources/No Insurance

Sadly, even in developed countries women often have lower incomes than men or work in jobs that offer minimal benefits. As a result, they have less access to affordable medical insurance and therefore HIV care. Without a means to pay for healthcare or medications, women are more likely to postpone trips to their doctors, or will not fill their HIV medication prescriptions. With the emergence of the Affordable Care Act ("Obamacare") women have greater access to insurance even if they have lower or no income. However, women have more issues with lack of transportation than do men, meaning they will often miss appointments with their HIV specialist or gynecologist. And, as we know, without regular healthcare it's difficult to maintain your health.

Family First

Women have been known to sacrifice their own healthcare in order to care for their family, especially their children. For instance, in situations of limited resources, mothers may stop their medications so they can afford the medicines for their children. And it's not uncommon for a mother to forgo her own doctor's appointment in order to get her child to theirs. Such conflicts pose a serious danger for an HIV-positive woman, whose health depends on regular care and adherence to a medication regimen. It's not uncommon for a woman who does not adhere to her medication regimen to agree to take her HIV medications while pregnant in order to protect her own child. Unfortunately, she will stop the drugs after the baby has been born. But for nine months she adhered to her regimen and as a result was able to get her virus under control, if only for a short time.

Opportunistic Infections Unique to HIV-Positive Women

As we learned in an earlier chapter, being infected with HIV places you at risk for a variety of associated conditions and illnesses. While women are subject to the same group of conditions as men, there are some conditions and diseases that are unique to women. These conditions jeopardize a woman's health and in some cases can jeopardize a woman's life. Let's look at several of those conditions that can be a serious threat to a woman's health.

Pelvic Inflammatory Disease (PID)

Pelvic Inflammatory Disease (PID) is actually a group of infections that affect the female reproductive system—specifically, the vagina, cervix, uterus, fallopian tubes and ovaries. While chlamydia and gonorrhea are the common infectious organisms, various other organisms can lead to PID, including tuberculosis and various bacterial infections. The difference between PID in HIV-positive women and HIV-negative women is not well documented, but there have been studies that attempt to identify the differences. One such study found that HIV-positive women were more likely to require surgical intervention as a result of PID— necessary because of damage caused by the infection. Also, HIV-infected women were more likely to develop an abscess (pocket of infection) as a result of PID. Thankfully, the study also showed that HIV-positive women responded to antibiotics just as well as their HIV-negative counterparts. While this study, and ones like it, did show PID can be aggressive in HIV-positive women, whether it needs to be treated more aggressively in HIV-infected women is still unclear.

The classic signs and symptoms of PID include severe abdominal pain, pelvic pain, vaginal discharge, and fever. Oddly, in women living with HIV, PID can often be silent, exhibiting no signs or symptoms at all. However, even in the absence of symptoms, PID in the HIV-positive woman can advance quickly, leading to the formation of fallopian tube abscesses. These abscesses, if left untreated, can result in sterility or, in severe cases, can be fatal.

Treatment of PID consists of antibiotics, either oral or intravenous (given directly into a vein), depending on the severity of the infection. In fact, severe infections may require hospitalization and both oral and intravenous antibiotics.

TABLE 12. PELVIC INFLAMMATORY DISEASE

Signs and Symptoms
- Some women have no symptoms at all
- Severe abdominal pain
- Pelvic pain
- Vaginal discharge
- Fever

Treatment
- Treatment varies depending on severity of the infection.
- Antibiotics are given orally or intravenously, depending again on the severity of infection.
- Severe infections may require both oral and intravenous antibiotics and hospitalization.

Vaginal Yeast Infections

We have seen that oral yeast infections ("thrush") are very common in men and women living with HIV. Another type of yeast infection, the vaginal yeast infection, is common in HIV-positive and -negative women alike. And while this type of fungal infection is easily treated in negative women, the infection can be more frequent, more severe and much more difficult to treat in HIV-positive women. In fact, chronic and frequent vaginal yeast infections can be an early sign of HIV.

Symptoms of chronic yeast infections include thick white to yellow vaginal discharge; foul odor, pain, burning, and/or itching of the vaginal area; and white or gray patches on the vagina. Once again, these symptoms are difficult to effectively treat in HIV-positive women, and with each recurrence the symptoms often become more severe and can become resistant to traditional antifungal medications.

HIV-negative women can usually treat their vaginal yeast infections with as little as a single dose of prescription-strength oral antifungal medication. In fact, some yeast infections in negative women can be treated with as little as an over-the-counter antifungal cream. Positive women, on the other hand, struggle with frequent, recurrent vaginal yeast infections that seldom are able to be treated with a single-dose medication or an over-the-counter cream. Depending on the severity of the infection, the treatment of choice is typically oral antifungal medications taken over a three- to ten-day period. However, in cases of severe or recurrent infections, it may take multiple courses of antifungal medication to completely resolve a yeast infection in an HIV-positive woman.

The best way to treat a yeast infection is to prevent it from occurring in the first place. There are simple things you can do to reduce the frequency and severity of yeast infections. These include eating yogurt that contains activated bacterial cultures in order to replenish "good bacteria" that wards off fungal infections. In addition, decreasing the amount of sugar in your diet makes a less hospitable environment for the growth of candida. Both of these simple steps make it harder for vaginal yeast to grow and flourish. One thing to keep in mind is that yeast infections can be passed between sexual partners, so sex should be avoided during active yeast infections.

TABLE 13. VAGINAL YEAST INFECTION

Signs and Symptoms
- Caused by a fungal infection
- Thick white or yellow vaginal discharge
- Foul vaginal odor
- Vaginal pain, burning or itching
- White or gray patches on and around the vagina

Treatment
- Treatment varies, depending on severity of the infection, and is typically oral or topical.
- In HIV-negative women treatment can be as little as one dose of medication.
- Treatment is typically a 3 to 10-day course of antifungal medications.
- HIV-positive women may need multiple course of antifungal medication to completely resolve the infection.

Bacterial Vaginosis

While somewhat similar to vaginal yeast infections, bacterial vaginosis differs in that it is caused by a bacterium, while yeast infections are caused by a fungus. Spread during unsafe sex, vaginosis is characterized by foul smelling, frothy vaginal discharge. There are available treatments for bacterial vaginosis; however, treatment for HIV-positive women sometimes requires a longer course of medication. In HIV-negative women treatment with the antibiotic metronidazole (Flagyl), taken twice a day for seven days, usually clears the infection. However, HIV-positive women sometimes need to take a second course of antibiotic to completely clear the infection. For those women who have a hard time taking oral medications, there are topical antibiotic creams that can be used. However, this type of treatment typically is not effective for HIV-positive women. One thing to keep in mind is that since vaginosis can be sexually transmitted to other women, female sexual partners of women with vaginosis must be treated as well. Also, sexual toys such as vibrators or dildos should not be shared and should be washed thoroughly between uses.

TABLE 14. BACTERIAL VAGINOSIS

Signs and Symptoms
- Caused by a bacterial infection
- Foul vaginal odor

- Frothy vaginal discharge
- Infection is sexually transmitted from one woman to another, so partners of women with the infection should be treated as well
- Sex toys should not be shared, especially when symptoms are present

Treatment

- Treatment for HIV-positive women requires a longer course than that for HIV-negative women.
- Treatment is administered typically twice a day for 7 days using the medication metronidazole (Flagyl).
- HIV-positive women usually need a second course of treatment to completely resolve infection.
- Topical antibiotics may be used in some cases.

Trichomoniasis

One final type of vaginal infection common in HIV-positive women is called trichomoniasis. This vaginal infection is caused by protozoa, a large group of one-cell microscopic organisms that can cause infection in people living with HIV. This infection is characterized by a large amount of thick, green or yellow vaginal discharge, accompanied by pain, soreness, and severe vaginal itching. In women with normal immune systems, about 95 percent of these infections can be successfully treated with a single two-gram dose of the antibiotic metronidazole (Flagyl). On the other hand, women with weakened immune systems, including those with HIV, typically need to be treated for seven days with a twice-daily dose (375 milligrams) of metronidazole (Flagyl) to clear the infection. Like bacterial vaginosis, all sex partners should be treated to prevent recurrence and to stop the spread of trichomoniasis to other people.

TABLE 15. TRICHOMONIASIS

Signs and Symptoms

- Caused by a single-cell organism known as a protozoan
- Characterized by a large amount of thick, green or yellow vaginal discharge
- Vaginal pain, soreness, and itching

Treatment

- In women with a normal immune system, 95 percent can be treated with a single 2-gram dose of metronidazole.
- Women with HIV need to be treated with seven days of twice-daily metronidazole.
- All sex partners should be treated to prevent recurrence and the spread of trichomoniasis to others.

HEALTH SCREENING—THE IMPORTANCE OF PAP TESTS

The *Papanikolaou test*, more commonly known as the *Pap test* or *Pap smear*, is an important health screening tool for all women, HIV-positive and -negative alike. Specifically, the Pap test is the best screening tool available for the early detection of cervical cancer. For HIV-positive women the importance of regular Pap tests can't be overstated. In fact, HIV and gynecology experts alike agree that teaching women about the importance of Pap tests should be part of every HIV education program. Positive women must understand the importance of the Pap test as an essential part of a complete health screening program.

TABLE 16. CERVICAL CANCER SCREENING GUIDELINES— HIV-NEGATIVE WOMAN

When should a woman start having Pap tests?
3 years after first episode of intercourse but no later than the age of 21 years.

How often should conventional Pap tests be done?
Initially should be done once per year. Can be done every 2–3 years for women older than 30 who have had 3 negative tests.

How often should thin prep Pap tests be done?
Initially should be done once per year. Can be done every 2–3 years for women older than 30 who have had 3 negative tests.

How often if HPV testing is used?
Every 3 years of HPV and the cell cytology is negative.

When should a woman stop having Pap tests?
Women older than 70 years with 3 recent and consecutive tests, and no positive tests in the last 10 years.

Should women who are post–total hysterectomy have Pap tests?
Discontinue if hysterectomy was for benign reasons and no history of high grade CIN lesions.

What Is a Pap Test?

Gynecologists, doctors that specialize in the treatment of female reproductive diseases, use the Pap test to examine cells of the cervix. The cervix is the most distal part of the uterus and is located at the point where the uterus and vagina come together. Gynecologists examine cells of the cervix for changes that may indicate cancer or precancerous conditions. Because cells of the cervix are prone to cancerous and precancerous changes, frequent examination of these cells is indicated. And because HIV-positive women are at an increased risk for cervical cancer, Pap tests every six to twelve months are absolutely essential. Typically, the first two Pap tests will be done six months apart. If both are negative, the HIV-positive woman can then have a Pap test every twelve months. If either of the first two are positive for an abnormality, then the HIV-positive woman must have her Pap tests every six months.

By using the Pap test and examining cervical cells regularly, gynecologists are able to detect any cellular changes early, allowing steps to be taken to treat those cells before they become cancerous or before any cancer spreads to other parts of the body. Early detection of cancer and precancerous cells allows for earlier treatment, proven to translate to a better prognosis for the woman.

How Is a Pap Test Done?

A Pap test is typically done as part of a routine pelvic exam. The gynecologist does a visual examination of the external parts of the female reproductive system—namely, the external anatomy of the vagina—looking for lesions, genital warts, or other abnormalities. To examine the inside of the vagina, an instrument called a *speculum* is inserted and opened slowly, spreading the entrance of the vagina, allowing the gynecologist to see the vaginal walls and cervix. Again, the gynecologist is looking for lesions, vaginal discharge, irritation, masses, or bleeding. After the visual examination of the vagina and cervix, a Pap test is done.

Examining the cells of the cervix requires a sample be sent to the lab. To collect the cells, a mascara-like brush known as a *cytobrush* is inserted into the vagina and wiped against the cervix. When the swab comes in contact with the cervix, cells adhere to the brush. The brush is then placed in a container of special liquid that washes the cells off the brush and into the solution. Once in the lab, specially trained lab technologists examine the cell-rich liquid under a microscope, looking to identify any changes in cellular structure, changes that may indicate the early stages of cervical cancer. If cancerous or precancerous cells or cellular changes are identified, the results are reported to the physician, and further follow-up and more frequent Pap tests will be necessary.

What Do the Results of the Pap Test Mean?

Typically, most HIV-negative women will have a normal Pap test, meaning the cells collected from the cervix show no signs of structural change. If this is the case, nothing more has to be done except schedule your next Pap test, typically for one year later. However, HIV-positive women have a higher incidence of abnormal Pap tests. In other words, the cells collected during the Pap test show some degree of structural change. These changes are classified in one of several categories based on the type and degree of structural changes that are present, using a system of classification called the Bethesda System. These classifications are:

- **Mild, Moderate, or Severe Dysplasia (abnormal growth)**—These cells have undergone changes, but those changes are not yet cancerous. They can also be referred to as *"atypia squamous cells of undetermined significance"* (ASC-US). However, these cells may become cancerous if left untreated or are not monitored regularly. More frequent monitoring, in the form of more frequent Pap tests are required, and may eventually lead to invasive treatment. Changes classified as ASC-US can also be caused by inflammation or infection, including HPV. Depending on how extensive these changes are, your doctor will do another Pap test in six months. There are cells in this group that while the changes are of undetermined significance, the changes can be high-grade epithelial changes that carry a higher risk for progression to cancer. These cells are classified as ASC-H.
- **Squamous Intraepithelial Lesion (SIL)**—These are abnormal cells found only on the surface of the cervix often caused by HPV infection. The cellular changes can range from low-grade (LSIL) to high-grade (HSIL) and can indicate the presence of cancer as well as HPV.
- **Cervical Intraepithelial Neoplasm (CIN)**—This is another way to describe abnormal cells on the surface of the cervix. The cells that have undergone the most severe changes are those that can be cancerous or become cancerous over time if left untreated. Depending on how much of the cervix contains these types of cells, they are classified as CIN 1, CIN 2, or the most extensive, CIN 3.
- **Carcinoma In-Situ**—This describes cells that have changed and become cancerous. They only affect the surface layers, but left untreated can migrate deeper into the cervical tissue, resulting in cervical cancer. You may see these results referred to as HSIL or CIN 3. Left untreated, cervical cancer can be fatal.
- **Cervical Cancer**—These results indicate that cancer has already migrated deep into the cervix. This result will require further, more invasive testing, chemotherapy treatment, radiation therapy, and/or possibly surgery to remove the areas of cancer.

TABLE 17. WHAT DO YOUR PAP RESULTS MEAN?

Atypia Squamous Cells of Undetermined Significance (ASCUS)
(Mild, moderate or severe dysplasia)
- These cells have begun to undergo abnormal changes, but those changes are not yet considered cancerous.
- These changes can become cancerous if ignored.
- More frequent monitoring is indicated, typically every 6 months.
- These changes are typically due to inflammation or infection.

Squamous Intraepithelial Lesion (SIL)
(Low-grade/LSIL to high grade/HSIL)
- These abnormal cells are found only on the surface of the cervix.
- The degree of abnormality ranges from low grade (LSIL) to high grade (HSIL).
- This can indicate the presence of cancer.

Cervical Intraepithelial Neoplasm (CIN)
(Ranges from CIN 1 to CIN 3)
- CIN 1—One-third of the surface of the cervix has abnormal cells (mildly abnormal cells).
- CIN 2—Two-thirds of the surface of the cervix has abnormal cells (moderately abnormal cells).
- CIN 3—The entire surface of the cervix has abnormal cells (severely abnormal cells); sometimes called *carcinoma in situ.*

Carcinoma in situ
(HSIL or CIN 3)
- Sometimes referred to as HSIL or CIN 3.
- Left untreated, carcinoma in situ can be fatal.

Cervical Cancer
- These results indicate a condition where cancerous cells have already migrated deep into the cervix.
- This requires more invasive testing (biopsy), chemotherapy treatment, radiation therapy, and possibly surgery to remove the cancerous areas.

HPV AND CERVICAL CANCER IN HIV-POSITIVE WOMEN

In an earlier chapter we learned that Human Papillomavirus (HPV) is a very common sexually transmitted virus. About 45 percent of all 20- to 24-year-olds have HPV infection. But as common as it is in the general population, it is even more common in HIV-positive women. One study indicated that greater than 85 percent of HIV-positive women have cervical HPV infection. And while the typical HIV-negative woman has an immune system strong enough to fight off many HPV complications, most HIV-positive women tend to have weakened immune systems and have more persistent HPV. In other words, HIV-positive women are more likely to develop abnormal cellular changes of the cervix, which in turn can progress to cancer much faster. Even after treatment, the rate of recurrence in HIV-positive women is higher than in the general population. Because HPV tends to be more aggressive in HIV-positive women, and because the risk of cervical cancer as a result of HPV infection is high, regularly scheduled Pap tests are an absolute must.

Our Final Lap

Medical issues associated with HIV are numerous. Vaginal yeast infections, genital herpes, lymphoma and invasive cervical cancer are only a few of the medical complications associated with the disease. But there are other non-medical issues that accompany HIV that can make life difficult for positive men and women alike. Social issues, including prejudice, discrimination, and isolation, are common. Practical issues, such as traveling with prescription medications or restricted travel due to an HIV diagnosis, can make life very complicated for any positive person whose job or recreation includes travel. Finally, deciding who will care for your children or make your financial decisions if you are unable to make them yourself can wear heavily on the emotional state of people living with HIV. We conclude our educational journey through this text with information that will help you deal with the practical side of HIV. The following issues are among the most common that affect your day to day life when living with HIV.

Legal/Ethical Issues Faced by HIV-Positive People

As this text has demonstrated, HIV infection presents a variety of challenges for those infected. Some are medical in nature—the dangers of opportunistic infections, for instance. Some are psychological, such as the emotional challenges resulting from an HIV diagnosis. And finally, some issues can be social in nature—dating for the first time after diagnosis, to name just one. All these challenges can make for a complicated and sometimes difficult life. And if those issues weren't enough, legal and ethical issues seem to crop up fairly often in the lives of many HIV-positive people: being fired unjustly, denied an apartment, or losing medical insurance have all been known to occur as an indirect result of HIV. So what are some of the most common issues, and what can be done to make them more manageable?

DISCRIMINATION AND PREJUDICE

Since the earliest days of the epidemic, people living with HIV and AIDS have been subjected to discrimination and prejudice at almost every turn. By misunderstanding the true nature of HIV, those without the disease become afraid—afraid of that which they don't understand. Their fear is directed outward toward those suffering the ill effects of the virus, adding to the issues HIV introduces into day-to-day life. Simply put, instead of helping those living with the disease, the fearful and ignorant turn away, creating an atmosphere of prejudice, isolation, and discrimination for those trying to live a healthy and normal life in the face of some pretty big odds.

Don't for a minute believe this sort of ignorance and insensitivity is unique to the lay person. When the epidemic first emerged, experts identified groups of people they felt were at increased risk of acquiring the new infection. Gay men were one such group. So high was the risk that experts referred to the new infectious disease as *"GRID,"* meaning "gay-related immunodeficiency," insinuating that being gay somehow was responsible for HIV. Some even referred to the new infection as *"gay cancer."* In response to these labels, lay people passed judgment upon gay men, suggesting they were the true cause of HIV and its rapid spread.

Thankfully, those labels were abandoned many years ago, replaced with the terms HIV and AIDS. However, the public perception that HIV and being gay go hand in hand is, for the most part, alive and well. Realizing people still associate homosexuality with HIV and AIDS, infected people fear they will become the target of hatred and prejudice. They fear more than anything that their diagnosis will somehow become public knowledge, which could lead to mistreatment, discrimination, or in some cases violence and physical harm. And their fears are not unfounded. People have lost jobs, their insurance, and their homes as a result of their HIV status. Sure, there are "official" reasons behind these occurrences, but we all know that an HIV diagnosis plays an "unofficial" role. But fortunately, legislators have recognized the struggles some HIV-positive people have to endure just to feed their family or put a roof over their head. Legal measures have been taken to protect HIV-positive people from the mistreatment of others. Understanding the legal resources you have at your disposal is an important way to protect yourself from the fear and ignorance of others.

The Americans with Disabilities Act (ADA)

Fortunately, experts in the field of HIV, as well as enlightened members of our government, have recognized the issues faced by HIV-infected people and have taken steps to protect them. One such step is voting to designate HIV and AIDS as a disability. By doing so, HIV-positive people are able to benefit from the protective umbrella of the *Americans with Disabilities Act* (ADA). The ADA provides civil rights protection to people living with disabilities. Persons living with HIV, whether they are symptomatic or not, are considered to have a disability that significantly impairs their daily lives. Because of this fact they are protected by the ADA.

The legal precedence for this decision involves the case of an asymptomatic HIV-positive woman whose dentist refused to fill her decayed tooth, claiming the woman needed to have the procedure done at a hospital because of risks associated with her HIV. The woman disagreed, believing that the dentist's decision was based on fear for himself and not on what was best for her as his patient. She felt being forced to take on the extra cost of a hospital visit was unjust. So she filed a lawsuit against the dentist, citing the ADA as the basis of her civil complaint. The dentist contended that because the woman was asymptomatic she should not be protected by the ADA. In other words, the dentist felt that because the woman was not symptomatic she could not be considered disabled and therefore could not be protected by the ADA. The courts disagreed, and from that point forward, HIV-positive people, symptomatic and asymptomatic alike, have been protected by the ADA.

In addition to protecting the civil rights of the disabled, the ADA also guarantees equal opportunity for employment; equal access to state and local government services, transportation, and telecommunications; and equal access to public accommodations such as hotels, hospitals, restaurants, and housing.

Public Accommodations—The ADA assures that people with disabilities, including people living with HIV, have access to public accommodations. In other words, people can't be deprived of such things as employment, housing, access to health care, or admission to restaurants or hotels due to their disability. In addition, reasonable accommodations must be made for those people with disabilities, allowing them to access these public services. Reasonable accommodations are defined as, but not limited to:

- making employee facilities usable by those employees with disabilities; for example, installing amplified telephones for those employees that are hard of hearing;
- job and schedule restructuring or reassignment to a position better suited to the person and his or her disability;
- acquiring or modifying equipment, devices, policies, or training material in an effort to accommodate the disabled employee;
- providing qualified readers or interpreters for those employees who are unable to read or who speak a language other than English.

For example, public places must have wheelchair accessible restroom facilities for those people confined to a wheelchair. The ADA also prevents doctors, hospitals, and dentists from categorically refusing to treat HIV-positive patients due to "public health concerns." The exception to that rule is that doctors can refuse to treat patients outside of their specialty, meaning for instance that a general medicine physician can refuse to treat a person's HIV because infectious disease is not their specialty. However, the refusing physician is legally and ethically required to refer such patients to a specialist—in the case of our example, an HIV specialist.

Employment—Part of the protection offered through the ADA is the right to equal employment opportunities. The ADA protects people with disabilities from being discriminated against in the workplace. For instance, the ADA prohibits employers from refusing to hire a person living with HIV because the employer fears a future illness with negatively impact the person's ability to work. In fact, having a diagnosis of HIV without complications is never a valid reason to deny employment. Furthermore, an employer can't require a medical exam before making a job offer. However, an employer can make an offer contingent upon passing a medical exam if a medical exam is required by all people in that job category.

Keep in mind that if you request accommodations under the umbrella of the ADA, your medical condition may come into question, which may jeopardize your confidentiality. While you are not obligated in any way to disclose your HIV status, you may have to do so if you are asking for accommodations under the ADA. You will be required to prove your disability in order to access the benefits and protections offered by the ADA, which will require you to divulge your diagnosis. Your employer must be aware of your HIV diagnosis in order to make "reasonable accommodations" surrounding your job. Once your employer is aware of your disability, he or she is obligated to make "reasonable accommodations" that allow you to perform your job. For example, if you have peripheral neuropathy in your hands that makes it difficult to use a mouse, your employer must provide you with a special type of mouse designed to minimize the symptoms of neuropathy (e.g., a trackball).

Insurance—The ADA prevents employers from denying insurance coverage to disabled employees or from charging increased insurance premiums based on a disability. In fact, the ADA prohibits employers from entering into contracts with any insurance company that discriminates based on a disability. Even with the Affordable Care Act ("Obamacare"), preexisting conditions do play a role in your care. While coverage cannot be denied, insurance premiums can be raised to reflect the additional risk of illness resulting from preexisting conditions. Make certain you are upfront about any preexisting conditions you may have. Eventually, insurance companies will find out if there is a preexisting condition that was not declared, and once the preexistence of the condition is discovered, your coverage could be jeopardized.

Ways to Fight Discrimination

If you feel you are being discriminated against due to your HIV diagnosis, there are avenues you can pursue to fight for your rights and for equal and fair treatment. Your first step is to contact the U.S. Department of Justice to file a complaint, either at the website ADA.gov, by mail, or by fax. Keep in mind you must file your complaint within 180 days of the alleged discrimination. Another thing to keep in mind when taking on your fight is that your diagnosis and medical history will most likely come into the public light. In fact, every aspect of your work record, attendance history and private life in general may come into question. Any privacy you had will probably be lost to some degree. Depending on whom you name in your complaint, it could be a very stressful fight. Regardless, discrimination needs to be fought, and the ADA is there to protect you.

Legal Assistance—As we all know, hiring an attorney can be costly. Unless you have a very good job, hiring a private lawyer to assist with your legal issues will be difficult. However, most large cities have lawyers and law practices that assist people on fixed incomes or with limited resources. To find these law practices or individual lawyers, contact the State Bar Association in your state. You can find their telephone number in your local directory or search the internet for the Bar Association in your state.

One more thing to keep in mind when seeking an attorney is to find a lawyer familiar with issues associated with HIV. For example, find an attorney that is experienced in the ADA and what it offers HIV-infected people. Just as you would choose a doctor specializing in broken bones to fix your broken leg, you should choose a lawyer that specializes in HIV issues. And while it may be expensive, there are government and private funds available to offset some of the cost. Many times, if you have a case, an attorney will represent you with the understanding that their fee will be paid out of the final financial settlement, if there is one. You may even come across a lawyer that will donate their time ("pro bono"), depending on your case and situation. Obviously, there are limits to this sort of benevolence and you should never expect it of any law practice. When you find an attorney to represent you, make sure they outline their fee schedules and requirements at your first visit.

ADVANCE DIRECTIVES

Whether we are healthy or sick, we all think about our own mortality from time to time. Most of us fear death to some degree, so much so, in fact, that we push it aside and choose to think about it another day. Like so much of our life, our death and circumstances surrounding that death are out of our control. However, there are ways to regain some control over certain aspects of our death and how it impacts survivors. *Advance directives* are legal documents that allow us to maintain some control over end-of-life issues in hopes of making our death as "good" as possible and to minimize the impact our death has on survivors. Advance directives allow us to make our end-of-life wishes known ahead of time in case we are unable to do so later. While it is very important to have an advance directive in place, there are a few questions you should first consider before having your attorney draw up the papers.

- Who would you like to make your personal decisions in the event you are unable to make them for yourself?
- If you become unconscious, become senile, or are diagnosed with a terminal illness that will likely end your life within six months, do you want to be placed on life-prolonging measures such as mechanical breathing machines (ventilators), drugs, feeding tubes, or resuscitation (CPR)?
- What type of medications are you willing to take, and to what extent would you like to be treated, if you suffer a stroke or other catastrophic event that makes you totally dependent on others for your daily care?
- What sort of physical, mental, and social abilities do you consider essential for a good quality of life?
- Do you want to receive all treatments recommended by your physicians and other members of your treatment team?
- Do you want doctors, nurses, etc. to perform heroic measures (CPR, breathing tube, and breathing machine) to save your life at all costs?

Is an Attorney Necessary to Write Your Advance Directives?

You can use an attorney if you wish to prepare your advance directives, but it's not necessary. If you choose not to use an attorney, there are a few things you want to make certain of prior to signing any documents. First, make certain that you discuss your intent with the person you name on the advance directive prior to drawing up the document. Make certain they will be able to make difficult decisions in the event you become incompetent, unconscious, or terminally ill. Second, remember that your advance directive needs to have a witness signature along with your signature. The law prohibits a family member, the person you name in the directive, your attorney, or any member of your health care team to act as a witness for your advance directives.

Durable Power of Attorney—The unpleasant reality of any chronic disease, HIV included, is that eventually illness may make it difficult or impossible for you to make rational decisions regarding your health care, finances, or legal issues. There is a legal document that can benefit those people who are unable to make decisions due to illness. A *durable power of attorney* is a document that legally gives another person the power to make personal decisions for you in the event you are unable to make them yourself. In other words, it is a document that allows someone to speak on your behalf in times when you are unable to speak for yourself. When you ("the principal") sign a durable power of attorney, another person ("the agent") will have the legal right to make decisions for you. Typically, the powers are broad, covering just about any decision or act that you make regarding your personal affairs. One exception is that the power of attorney does not give the agent the right to change or revoke your will. While some durable powers of attorney take effect or remain in effect regardless of the principal's mental status, those related to health care issues typically include clauses stating that the power of attorney only takes effect in the event the principal becomes mentally incapacitated.

LIVING WILLS

A living will is one of the most widely known advance directives. Simply put, a living will allows you to refuse medical treatment in the case of terminal illness. For instance, a person dying of cancer can have a living will that states he or she does not want to have any heroic life-saving procedures. For example, a living will can state you do not want to be placed on a breathing machine in order to prolong life. In other words, a living will permits the terminally ill—a person whose death is expected in six months or less—to legally refuse any life support measures. While the living will is useful in the face of terminal illness, there are situations where a durable power of attorney is better suited.

- Living wills are not valid in all states. Check with your state to see if living wills have legal standing where you live.
- Living wills are valid only in the case of terminal illness. A durable power of attorney applies to any illness.
- Living wills only allow you to refuse treatment, whereas a durable power of attorney allows you to accept, refuse, or withdraw different forms of treatment.
- Unlike the durable power of attorney, a living will does not allow you to appoint a person to make decisions for you when you become unable to make those decisions for yourself.

STANDBY GUARDIANSHIP ORDER

Most of us don't cherish the thought of having someone care for our children. But what happens if an illness makes you temporarily unable to care for them yourself? Most people would want to choose who cares for their children in that situation. A *standby guardianship order* is a legal document that allows you to designate who will care for your children if you are unable. The document assigns temporary legal guardianship to the person or persons of your choice, and only takes effect in the event you become unable to care for the children on your own. The document typically has to be renewed every sixty days. There are permanent guardianship orders that will assign permanent decision-making rights to the person of your choice, and in the process sacrifice your own parental and guardianship rights. A permanent guardianship order is typically only used in the case of your permanent incapacitation or death. In times of temporary incapacitation, a standby guardianship order is sufficient.

TRAVELING WITH HIV

Since the tragedy of 9/11 and the growing number of terrorist crimes against innocent people, security measures associated with travel are tighter than ever before. More stringent policies regarding what can be carried onto an airplane, cruise ship, or train have made traveling with prescription medications much more difficult. Also, the stigma associated with an HIV diagnosis can make travel outside the United States complicated. While most people have very little difficulty traveling with HIV, those who do are usually not properly prepared for the issues related to their diagnosis and traveling abroad. Let's look at some traveling tips that will make your vacation carefree.

Traveling with Prescription Medication

Throughout this text it has been repeatedly stressed that taking your medicines each and every day is important if you are to stay healthy and your HIV medications are to be effective. Even missing one or two days' worth of doses can ultimately lead to viral mutation, eventually necessitating a medication change. So when you are traveling it's important to make sure your medications travel with you. Here are some ideas that will make traveling with your medications much easier.

Anticipate What You Will Need—Before leaving on your trip, assess how much medication you have on hand and how much you will need while on vacation. If it looks as if you may run out of medications before returning home, have your doctor call in refills that you can pick up before you leave. If your insurance company says it is too soon for refills, talk with your doctor; he or she can request an exception, explaining to the insurance company that you will be away from home when it will be time for refills. If possible, keep an extra supply of medications with you in case you are away from home longer than expected.

Keep Your Pharmacy Information with You—Make certain you carry your pharmacy information with you while traveling. It is a good idea to have the pharmacy name, telephone number, and fax number in your purse or wallet. That way, if you run out of medications while away from home, a pharmacy near where you are vacationing can contact your local pharmacy to transfer prescription information, allowing you to get a refill while you're away. It's also a good idea to find a pharmacy near where you'll be staying while away from home. If you use a large pharmacy chain, find an outlet near your vacation spot. That will make transferring prescriptions much easier in the event you will need to fill your prescriptions away from home.

Known Your Physician's Office Number/Have Your Insurance Information—Make certain you carry your doctor's name, office number, and fax number with you while away from home. Keep a copy of this information in your wallet or purse, and another copy with your luggage. In the event you or a pharmacy needs to call for new prescriptions, having the information on hand will make getting refills much easier. Have your insurance information on hand as well in order to pay for any prescriptions you get refilled while away from home.

Keep Your Medications with You—If you are traveling by air, train, or bus, make certain you have your medications in your carry-on luggage, not in the bags you have checked and stowed in the luggage compartment. First, having them in your carry-on luggage allows access to them if you need to take a dose while en route to your destination. Second, your checked baggage can be lost or tampered with, meaning your medications could be lost as well. Keep in mind that security measures on airplanes limit the amount of liquid you can carry on your person to about three ounces. Check with your airline well in advance of your departure date to get specific rules and limitations regarding liquid medication rules. If your dose and type of medication allows, switch to tablet or capsule form while travelling, and then switch back to liquid if you prefer upon your return.

Store Your Medication Properly—When at all possible, keep your prescription medications in the bottle you received from the pharmacy. Make sure you keep the bottle's label in place as well. The prescription information contained on the label will help you prove the medications you are carrying are your prescriptions. Taking medications out of prescription bottles will delay your time through security. If you have them, keep your medicines in their original stock bottles you received from the pharmacy. Most HIV medications are packaged in stock bottles of a 30-day supply, making it easier for the pharmacy to dispense your medications. Certain medications—specifically, soft gel capsules—require special handling and storage. If they get too warm, they will melt and stick together. Do not leave them in your car, near a heat source, in the sunlight, or anywhere else where they can get too warm. Ideally they should be refrigerated, so request a hotel room with a small refrigerator if available. If the hotel does not have refrigerators in the room, bring a small cooler or use the room's ice bucket to keep them cool. Place the prescription bottle in a plastic bag and place the plastic bag on ice, keeping the medication cool but not so cold that it freezes. Finally, if your hotel room has a safe, store your medications there while you are out for the day; having medications out in the open is sometimes a temptation to theft.

Needles and Syringes—If you have been prescribed injectable medication, such as insulin or the HIV medication Fuzeon, the medication and syringes must be carried together in order to be allowed in your carry-on. Do not take the syringes out of their sterile packaging; syringes not in packaging may be confiscated or at the very least will slow your time through security. Once again, make certain you keep labels on all injectable prescription medication to make it easier for security to identify the medications as belonging to you.

You Are Entitled to Privacy—If airport security feels they need to question you regarding your medications, or for any reason during the screening process, you are entitled to privacy and confidentiality. It is within your rights to request that the questioning be done in a private area.

Special Travel Considerations

Traveling with an HIV diagnosis presents problems that few others experience. We discussed special measures that can make travel with medications less problematic, but there are other issues outside of those surrounding your HIV regimen. There are special considerations that must be taken into account in order to travel safely when living with an HIV diagnosis. Depending on your destination, there can be health concerns associated with your travel. Water-borne illnesses, infectious diseases, or other epidemics can present a risk to anyone with a weakened immune system, HIV-positive people included. But there are steps that can be taken to minimize the risk.

Before You Travel

- Speak with your doctor about any possible health risks associated with your destination. For instance, are you traveling to a part of the world where you may be at increased risk for hepatitis A? Is malaria a problem where you are vacationing? Is the water safe to drink? Large hospitals or university clinics typically have travel clinics that specialize in preparing you for travel to places outside the U.S. Depending on your destination, you may require certain vaccinations to protect you from illnesses common to the area you're visiting. To make certain your body has time to respond to any vaccinations you may require, visit a travel clinic a few months before your departure.
- Depending on the area you are heading to, *"traveler's diarrhea"* may be a problem. Traveler's diarrhea is a condition that results from ingesting food or water contaminated with diarrhea-causing microbes. Usually it's an affliction that occurs when you travel from areas of good sanitation to poor. Your doctor can prescribe an antibiotic you can carry with you to start taking at the first sign of diarrhea.
- Insect-borne illnesses such as malaria may be present at your destination. Take plenty of insect repellent with you when traveling. Also, make sure you sleep under mosquito

netting in those areas where mosquitoes are known to carry diseases that may put you at risk for illness.

- If you are leaving the United States, check with the countries you are visiting before your trip to see if that country has any special health requirements or rules pertaining to HIV. Be aware that some countries require vaccinations that are unsafe for people with HIV (e.g., live vaccines). If that is the case, you will need a letter from your doctor explaining why you are unable to take that particular vaccine.

- Check with your medical insurance to learn the extent of coverage if you are traveling out of the country or out of the network area. Take proof of insurance with you, regardless of where you travel.

While Away from Home

- If you are traveling out of the United States, be aware that the quality of water may not be what you are accustomed to. In fact, it may be very poor. In some cases, there are parasites and bacteria in the water that make it unsafe to drink. In these areas drink only commercially bottled water. Rinse your toothbrush and your mouth with the same bottled water to avoid exposure to parasites or bacteria that may be in the local drinking water. The same precautions are advised if you are camping in the wild and get your water from streams or ponds. Do not eat raw fruit or vegetables you have not cleaned and peeled yourself. Do not drink local tap water; do not drink any mixed drinks made with tap water; and do not use ice made from tap water.

- Avoid foods from local street vendors. Eat only those foods deemed safe, including those that are steaming hot, those you have cleaned and peeled yourself, and water that you have brought to a rolling boil for at least a full minute.

- Tuberculosis (TB) is a common disease outside of the United States. If you must go to a hospital or clinic while you are traveling, avoid people with productive coughs, fevers, or other signs of respiratory illness. Use only clinics or medical facilities that are clean and use sterile equipment.

- In many parts of the world, domesticated farm animals such as cows and chickens are left to roam free. Do not swim in any water or walk any beach you suspect may be contaminated with animal droppings or waste. Never drink or swallow water while you are swimming, and avoid opening your eyes under the water.

Where to Go to Learn More

So now that you have come to the end of this text, where do you go from here to learn even more about your illness? If you are like most people you will turn to the Internet for more information. Why wouldn't you? The Internet is full of information about any topic you can fathom, including HIV. Yet, you have to use the information you glean from the Internet with caution. Some of it is excellent; some of it is a bunch of bunk. The key is being able to sort out the good from the bad, the current from the obsolete, the true from the false. As amazing as the Internet is there are pros and cons having it available at your fingertips.

Pros of the Internet

- The information is available 24 hours a day, 7 days a week.
- Outside of the cost of your Internet connection, a majority of the information you can access is free of charge.
- The individual web pages can be updated as often as necessary; a newspaper is updated once a day; a magazine or journal once a month.
- Publishers of newspapers and magazines also have online sites that include the contents of their publications.
- The Internet is available in your home and while you are on the road.

Cons to the Internet

- Anybody with the right software can create and publish a webpage.
- The validity and accuracy of the content found on a webpage is often difficult to confirm.
- The expertise of the person or person who publish information can be suspect.
- A webpage that is available today may be different or gone altogether tomorrow.
- The content you find on the internet may be out of date.
- It's very difficult to efficiently sort through the vast amount of information in a timely manner.

So with all the pros and cons it's important to know how to use the Internet in a manner that provides you with the most expert, accurate, and current HIV information available. Let's take a look at some tips that will help you when you use the Internet; if done correctly, researching the web can be a valuable tool that will help you learn even more about your disease. Here's what you need to know.

- *Use a Strong Search Engine*—The first step when using the web is finding the information you are looking for among the millions of web pages available at the click of your mouse. A strong search engine is the key to finding what you are looking for and they narrowing down your choices to what suits you best. Search engines like Google, Bing, and Yahoo will help narrow down your choices and guide you right to what you are looking for in your quest for more information.
- *Be Specific with Your Search Terms*—Once you choose a search engine, make sure you plug in the right search terms. The more specific your search terms the more specific and accurate the information will be that is returned in your search. Searching the term "HIV" will produce millions of selections, old and new, good and bad, accurate and not so accurate. By using specific terms like "new HIV regimens in 2017" you will retrieve items closer to what you are trying to find.
- *Use Dates in Your Search*—Because there is so much information on the web, when you search you will get information published yesterday or ten years ago. Keep in mind that when it comes to HIV information, anything older than a couple years is probably outdated. Using the year (e.g., "2017") or a year range (e.g., "2015–2017") will limit your search results to those year qualifiers. However, even if you use a year in your search, check and double check the content to make certain it is indeed current.

- ***Stick to Reputable Sites***—As mentioned before, anyone from anywhere can post content to the web. Some sources of information are more reputable and reliable than others. For instance, obtaining HIV information from the Centers for Disease Control (CDC) webpage is more likely to be accurate and current than information from a site thrown together in someone's basement one afternoon. In addition, the more reputable sites have the resources and the staff to maintain very current and accurate information. Sites like the CDC site are updated and renewed regularly by authors that have the expertise necessary to provide useful HIV information. But note, just because a site is large and well known does not mean that it is a source of useful information. For instance, there are sites on the web that allow anyone to contribute content, content that often goes unchecked and is not verified as accurate and current.

- ***Stick to Sites That Are Right for You***—Make certain the sites you choose provide information that is appropriate for your level of understanding. For instance, if you are newly diagnosed and want to know about your diagnosis and how it will affect your life you won't choose a site that discusses the molecule and cellular physiology of HIV, at least not yet.

- ***Beware of Fraud***—Remember the adage "If it sounds too good to be true it usually is." Be alert and very skeptical of any site that claims it offers a cure or a miraculous HIV treatment. Also, any site that asks for money or personal information before providing the information should be accessed using great caution.

The Internet is possibly the most obvious and amazing benefit of this age of technology. It provides the users with information on an infinite number of topics, including HIV and AIDS. Used properly, it will enhance your knowledge base and help you live a healthier life. But as was mentioned earlier, be careful that the information you obtain is current, accurate, and from reputable sources.

HIV Prevention, Diagnosis and Beyond

Our journey from HIV prevention to diagnosis and beyond has come to a close. It's my wish that this text will help you cope with your illness, help you understand your disease, and finally, help you live with HIV. This text is complete, but your journey with HIV continues. If I could give you one piece of advice, I would say learn everything you can about your disease. Knowledge is power, so learn all you can and take control of your disease; in doing so you will take control of your life.

Live healthy...

BIBLIOGRAPHY

Acria Staff. (2012). HIV Treatment Education: Community Perspectives. *ACRIA Update* 11(4), 1–20.

AIDS 101: Guide to HIV Basics. (1998). San Francisco AIDS Foundation.

AIDS.gov. (2009, August 23). Do You Have to Tell? https://www.aids.gov/hiv-aids-basics/just-diagnosed-with-hiv-aids/talking-about-your-status/do-you-have-to-tell/index.html.

AIDS.gov. (2011, August 8). Immune System 101. U.S. Department of Health and Human Services, https://www.aids.gov/hiv-aids-basics/just-diagnosed-with-hiv-aids/hiv-in-your-body/immune-system-101/.

AIDS.gov. (2014, December 2). HIV in the United States: At a Glance. https://www.aids.gov/hiv-aids-basics/hiv-aids-101/statistics/index.html.

AIDS.org Staff. (2005). Why Should I Be Tested: The Benefits of Knowing. http://www.sfaf.org/aids101/hiv_testing.html.

AIDSinfo.nih.gov. (2015, August 17). Preventing Mother-to-Child Transmission of HIV During Childbirth. https://aidsinfo.nih.gov/education-materials/fact-sheets/24/70/preventing-mother-to-child-transmission-of-hiv-during-childbirth.

AIDSinfonet.org. (2014, February 24). Fact Sheet 129: Tropism Tests. http://aidsinfonet.org/uploaded/fact sheets/18_eng_129.pdf.

AIDSinfo.com. (2015, March 26). The HIV Life Cycle. https://aidsinfo.nih.gov/education-materials/fact-sheets/19/73/the-hiv-life-cycle.

AIDSmap.com. (2012, July 1). Resources/Booklets: Viral Load. http://www.aidsmap.com/Viral-load/page/1327496/.

AIDSmap.com. (2015). HIV & Testing, p. 24. http://www.aidsmap.com/p24-antigen/page/1322964/.

AIDSmap.com. (2015). HIV & Testing: HIV RNA. http://www.aidsmap.com/HIV-RNA/page/1322967/.

AIDSmap.com. (2015). HIV Transmission & Testing: Breastfeeding. http://www.aidsmap.com/Breastfeeding/page/1321393/.

AIDSmap.com. (2015). HIV Transmission & Testing: Risk of Infection. http://www.aidsmap.com/Risk-of-infection/page/1324549/.

AIDSmeds.com. (2013, January 23). Undetectable Viral Load Essentially Eliminates Transmission Risk in Straight Couples. http://aidsmeds.com/articles/heterosexual_transmission_1667_23387.shtml.

Altman, L.K. (1981, July 3). Rare Cancer Seen in 41 Homosexuals. *The New York Times.*

Ammann, A. (2006, March 2006; cited 2008, March 3). Counseling HIV-Infected Patients Who Want to Have Children. http://www.womenchildrenhiv.org/wchiv?page=tp-02-01.

Anderson, R.N., and B.L Smith. (2005). Deaths: Leading Causes for 2002. *National Vital Statistics Report*, 53(17).

Anil, S.N., R.G. Nair, V.T. Beena, and T. Vijuyakumar. (1995). Dental Professionals' Attitude and Knowledge Towards HIV Infection and AIDS: An Indian Perspective. *Community Dentistry and Oral Epidemiology*, 23(3), 187–188.

Arhel, N. (2010). Revisiting HIV-1 Uncoating. *Retrovirology*, 1–10.

Arquin, P.M., P.E. Kozarsky, and C. Reed, eds. CDC Health Information for International Travel 2008. (2008). Chapter 4: Prevention of Infectious Diseases—Travelers Diarrhea. Atlanta: Centers for Disease Control, 648.

Atif, M.S. (2006). Low CD4+ Nadir Is an Independent Predictor of Lower HIV-Specific Immune Responses in Chronically HIV-1 Infected Subjects Receiving Highly Active Antiretroviral Therapy. *The Journal of Infectious Disease* 194, 661–665.

Bailes, E., F. Gao, F. Bibollet-Ruche, V. Courgnaud, M. Peeters, P. Marx, and P. Sharp. (2003). Hybrid Origin of SIV in Chimpanzees. *Science* 1713.

Ball, S. (2002). Diarrhea in a Patient with AIDS. *AIDS Reader* 12(9), 1–5.

Barankin, B. (2007, June). Answer: Can You Identify This Condition? *Canadian Family Physician* 53(6), 1022–1023.

Barnabus, R., and C. Celum. (2012, April). Infectious Co-Factors in HIV-1 Transmission Herpes Simplex Virus Type-2 and HIV-1: New Insights and Interventions. *Current HIV Research* 10(3), 228–237.

Barry, A.M., J.G. Kahn, S.D. Pinkerton, et al. (1999). Postexposure Prophylaxis Following HIV Exposure. *Journal of the American Medical Association* 281(14), 1269.

Bartlett, J. (2012). HIV Treatment as Prevention: Models, Data, and Questions: Towards Evidence-Based Decision-Making. *PLoS Medicine*, 1–8.

Bartlett, J.G., and R.D. Moore. (1998). Improving HIV Therapy. *Scientific American* 279(1), 84–87, 89.

Berger, F. (2014, February 24). Diet and Substance Use Recovery. https://www.nlm.nih.gov/medlineplus/ency/article/002149.htm.

Biel-Cunningham, S. The Importance of Dental Care. (November/December 2004). *Survival News.*

Blancou, P., J. Vartanian, C. Christopherson, N. Chenciner, C. Basilico, S. Kwok, and S. Wain-Hobson. (2001). Polio Vaccine Samples Not Linked to AIDS. *Nature*, 1045–1046.

Boonstra, H. (2003). U.S. AIDS Policy: Priority on Treatment, Conservatives' Approach to Prevention. *The Guttmacher Report on Public Policy*, 1–3.

Bryg, R. (2006). High Cholesterol: Cholesterol Basics. *Cholesterol Management Guide.* Cleveland: Cleveland Clinic Foundation.

Buchaman, M.J.W, and L. Kent. (1998). What Makes Cryptococcus a Pathogen? *Emerging Infectious Diseases* 4(1), 71–83.

Cairns, G. (2014, January 6). Life Expectancy Now Considerably Exceeds the Average in Some People with HIV in the U.S. http://www.aidsmap.com/Life-expectancy-now-considerably-exceeds-the-average-in-some-people-with-HIV-in-the-US/page/2816267/.

Callahan, R. (2016, January 10). Needle Exchange Leaders Cheer Relaxed Federal Funding Ban. *USA Today.*

Carter, M. (2008, December 5). High Prevalence of Vitamin D Deficiency in Patients with HIV. http://www.aidsmap.com/High-prevalence-of-vitamin-D-deficiency-in-patients-with-HIV/page/1432671/.

Carter, N. (1994). Support Groups: Places of Healing. *HIV/AIDS*, Focus Paper #23.

Castro, K.G. (1992). 1993 Revised Classification System for HIV Infection and Expanded Surveillance Case Definition for AIDS Among Adolescents and Adults. *CDC Mortality and Morbidity Weekly Report* 44 (No. RR-17).

Centers for Disease Control and Prevention. (1998). Recommendations for Prevention and Control of Hepatitis C Virus (HCV) Infection and HCV Related Chronic Disease. *Morbidity and Mortality Weekly Report* 47 (No. RR-19), 1–54.

Centers for Disease Control and Prevention. (2010). HIV Transmission Through Transfusion: Missouri and Colorado, 2008. *Morbidity and Mortality Weekly Report (MMWR)*, 1335–1339.

Centers for Disease Control and Prevention. (2011, August). Estimates of New HIV Infections in the United States, 2006–2009. http://www.cdc.gov/nchhstp/newsroom/docs/HIV-Infections-2006-2009.pdf.

Centers for Disease Control and Prevention. (2013, February 23). Diagnoses of HIV Infection in the United States and Dependent Areas, 2013. CDC HIV Surveillance Report, vol. 25: http://www.cdc.gov/hiv/library/reports/surveillance/2013/surveillance_Report_vol_25.html.

Centers for Disease Control and Prevention. (2013, April 15). Prevention Benefits of HIV Treatment. http://www.cdc.gov/hiv/prevention/research/tap/.

Centers for Disease Control and Prevention. (2014, July 1). HIV Transmission Risk. http://www.cdc.gov/hiv/policies/law/risk.html.

Centers for Disease Control and Prevention. (2015, June 4). State HIV Testing Laws: Consent and Counseling Requirements. http://www.cdc.gov/hiv/policies/law/states/testing.html.

Centers for Disease Control and Prevention. (2015, August 13). State Laboratory Reporting Laws: Viral Load and CD4 Requirements. http://www.cdc.gov/hiv/policies/law/states/reporting.html.

Centers for Disease Control and Prevention. (2015, August 20). Cervical Cancer Statistics. http://www.cdc.gov/cancer/cervical/statistics/index.htm.

Centers for Disease Control and Prevention. (2016). Updated Guidelines for Antiretroviral Postexposure Prophylaxis after Sexual, Injection Drug Use, or Other Nonoccupational Exposures to HIV, United States, 2016. http://www.cdc.gov/hiv/pdf/programresources/cdc-hiv-npep-guidelines.pdf.

Centers for Disease Control and Prevention. (2016, May 28). Provider Information Sheet: PrEP During Conception, Pregnancy, and Breastfeeding. From National Center for HIV/AIDS,Viral Hepatitis, STD, and TB Prevention, http://www.cdc.gov/hiv/pdf/PrEP_GL_Clinician_Factsheet_Pregnancy_English.pdf.

Chander, G., B. Lau, and R. Moore. (2006). Hazardous Alcohol Use: A Risk Factor for Non-Adherence and Lack of Suppression in HIV Infection. *JAIDS: Journal of Acquired Immunodeficiency Syndromes* 43(4), 411–417.

Chitnis, A., D. Rawls, and J. Moore. (2000). Origin of HIV Type 1 in Colonial French Equatorial Africa? *AIDS Research and Human Retroviruses*, 5–8.

Cichocki, M. (2014, June 19). HIV and Sinus Infections. http://aids.about.com/cs/conditions/a/sinus.htm.

Cichocki, M. (2014, June 26). Integrase Inhibitors. http://aids.about.com/od/generalinformation/a/integrasein.htm.

Cichocki, M. (2015, November 2). Vitamin D Deficiency and Its Connection to HIV. http://aids.about.com/od/nutrition/a/vitamin_d.htm.

Cichocki, M.W. (2004, January; cited 2007, August 3). Bacterial Opportunistic Infections. http://aids.about.com/cs/conditions/a/bacterialoi.htm.

Clavel, F. (2004). Mechanisms of HIV Resistance: A Drug Primer. *The PRN Notebook* 9(1), 3–7.

Cleveland Clinic Foundation. (2012, February 28). Oral Human Papilloma Virus (HPV) Infection. http://my.clevelandclinic.org/health/diseases_conditions/hic_oral_human_papilloma_virus_hpv_infection.

Collins, S. (2012). Risk of HIV Reinfection May Be Similar to Risk of Initial HIV Infection. Conference on Retroviruses and Opportunistic Infections, Seattle.

Cornforth, T. (2003, December 7; cited 2007, November 18). Abnormal Pap Smears. http://womenshealth.about.com/cs/papsmears/a/abnormalpaps.htm.

Cowley, G. (2014, April 23). The Day They Discovered the AIDS Virus. http://www.msnbc.com/msnbc/the-day-they-discovered-the-aids-virus.

Cunha, J. P. (2015, May 5). Peridex Side Effects Center. http://www.rxlist.com/peridex-side-effects-drug-center.htm.

Davenport, T. (2007, March 28; cited 2007, December 19). How to Prevent Gum Disease. http://dentistry.about.com/od/toothmouthconditions/ht/preventing.htm.

Davis, C. (2015, November 29). Sinus Infection (Sinusitis). http://www.medicinenet.com/sinusitis/article.htm.

Department of Health and Human Services. (2015, August 6). Recommendations for Use of Antiretroviral Drugs in Pregnant HIV-1-Infected Women for Maternal Health and Interventions to Reduce Perinatal HIV Transmission in the United States. https://aidsinfo.nih.gov/guidelines/html/3/perinatal-guidelines/187/infant-antiretroviral-prophylaxis.

Dolson, L. (2016, February 21). What You Need to Know About Complex Carbohydrates. https://www.verywell.com/what-you-need-to-know-about-complex-carbohydrates-2242228.

Drainoni, M.L. (2003). *Reports and Studies: Substance Abuse and HIV*. H.A. Bureau, ed. Health Resources Services Administration (HRSA).

Evans, D. (2008, April 1). Spring Awakening: HIV, Allergies and Sinusitis. http://www.aidsmeds.com/articles/hiv_allergies_sinuses_2042_14336.shtml.

Eversole, L.R, A.S. Leider, P.L. Jacobson, and E.P. Shaber. (1983). Oral Kaposi's Sarcoma Associated with Acquired Immunodeficiency Syndrome Among Homosexual Males. *Journal of American Dentistry Association* 107(2), 248–253.

Fact Sheet Number 802: Exercise and HIV. (2008, April 14; cited 2008, January 18). New Mexico AIDSInfonet Fact Sheets.

Ferri, J. *There Is Hope: Learning to Live with HIV*, 2d ed. HIV Coalition, 1998.

Fischbach, F. *A Manual of Laboratory and Diagnostic Tests*, 7th. ed. Philadelphia: Lippincott, Williams and Wilkins, 2004.

Foster, L. (2009, April 10). How Mental Illness and Addiction Influence Each Other. http://www.everydayhealth.com/addiction/mental-illness-and-addiction.aspx.

Fox, M. (2002, November 26). Study: AIDS Prevention Saved Up to 1.5 Million. http://www.thebody.com/content/treat/art18742.html.

Fudala, P.J., et al. (2003). Office Base Treatment of Opiate Addiction with a Sublingual Tablet Formulation of Buprenorphine and Naloxone. *New England Journal of Medicine* 349(10), 949–958.

Functional Foods Fact Sheet: Antioxidants. (2006, March.). Fact Sheets 2006. http://www.ific.org/publications/factsheets/antioxidantfs.cfm.

Gallo, R. C., and L. Montagnier. (2003). The Discovery of HIV as the Cause of AIDS. *The New England Journal of Medicine*, 2283–2285.

Garcia-Ditta, A. (2014, December 10). Is 2015 the Year for Legalized Clean Needle Exchange? *San Antonio Current*.

Gaynes, B., B. Pence, J. Atashili, J. O'Donnell, D. Kats, and P. Ndumbe. (2012). Prevalence and Predictors of Major Depression in HIV-Infected Patients on Antiretroviral Therapy in Bamenda, a Semi-Urban Center in Cameroon. *PLoS One* 7(7), 1–8.

Gilead Sciences. (2015). Genvoya. Foster City, CA: Gilead Sciences.

Giovedoni, L., C. Hui-Ling, V. Hodara, L. Chu, L. Parodi, L. Smith, and D. Sodora. (2013, February). Impact of Mucosal Inflammation on Oral Simian Immunodeficiency Virus Transmission. *Journal of Virology* 87(3), 1750–1758.

Gottlieb, M. Pneumocystis Pneumonia in Los Angeles. (1981). *CDC Mortality and Morbidity Weekly Report* 30, 250–252.

Grodeck, B. (2007). *The First Year—HIV: An Essential Guide for the Newly Diagnosed*, 2d ed. New York: Perseus.

Guaraldi, G., N. Squillace, C. Stentarelli, G. Orlando, R. D'Amico, G. Ligabue, and F. Patella. (2008). Nonalcoholic Fatty Liver Disease in HIV-Infected Patients Referred to a Metabolic Clinic: Prevalence, Characteristics, and Predictors. *Clinical Infectious Diseases* 47(2), 250–257.

Hader, S.L, D.K. Smith, J.S. Moore, and S. D. Holmberg. (2001). HIV Infection in Women in the United States. *Journal of the American Medical Association* 285(9), 1186–1192.

Harvard Health Publications. (2016, March 14). Understanding Addiction. Harvard Mental Health Letter, http://www.helpguide.org/harvard/how-addiction-hijacks-the-brain.htm#what.

Health Resources and Services Administration. (2014, October 1). About the Ryan White HIV/AIDS Program. http://hab.hrsa.gov/abouthab/aboutprogram.html.

Hearps, A., V. Greengrass, J. Hoy, and S. & Crowe. (2009, December 6). An HIV-1 Integrase Genotype Assay for the Detection of Drug Resistance Mutations. *Sex Health*, 305–309.

Highleyman, L. (2014, March 6). HIV Attachment Inhibitor BMS-663068 Shows Good Safety and Efficacy in Phase 2b Study. http://www.aidsmap.com/HIV-attachment-inhibitor-BMS-663068-shows-good-safety-and-efficacy-in-phase-2b-study/page/2833447/.

Hilton, B. (1990). AIDS Week—Reagan: Better Late Than Never? *San Francisco Sunday Examiner and Chronicle*, p. A4.

Hinman, A. (1998, February 3; cited 2006, August 8). Researchers Trace First HIV Case to 1959 in the Belgian Congo. http://www.cnn.com/HEALTH/9802/03/earliest.aids/.

The HIV/AIDS Program: Ryan White Parts A–F. (2008), http://hab.hrsa.gov/aboutus.htm.

HIV Medicine Association. (2010). Qualifications for Physicians Who Manage the Longitudinal HIV Treatment of Patients with HIV. Arlington, VA.: Infectious Diseases Society of America.

HIV Newsline Staff. (1998; cited 2008, April 5). The Most Common Opportunistic Infections in Women with HIV. *HIV Newsline*. http://www.thebody.com/content/art12622.html.

HIV Resource Services Association. (2014, April). Necrotizing Ulcerative Periodontitis and Gingivitis. http://www.aidsetc.org/guide/necrotizing-ulcerative-periodontitis-and-gingivitis.

Hoofnagle, J. (2007). Viral Hepatitis. In L. Goldman and D. Ausiello, *Cecil Medicine*, 23rd ed., Chapter 151. Philadelphia: Saunders Elsevier.

Hooper, E. (1999). *The River*. Boston: Little Brown.

Horsburgh, R. (2000, July). Antiretroviral Therapy Reduces Risk of Bacterial Pneumonia. *American Journal of Respiratory Critical Care Medicine*.

Hutter, G., D. Nowak, M. Mossner, S. Ganepola, A. Mubig, K. Allers, and E. Thiel. (2009). Long-Term Control of HIV by CCR5 Delta32/Delta32 Stem-Cell Transplantation. *The New England Journal of Medicine*, 692–698.

Hwijin, K., and A. Perelson. (2006, October 13). Viral and Latent Reservoir Persistence in HIV-1–Infected Patients on Therapy. http://journals.plos.org/ploscompbiol/article?id=10.1371/journal.pcbi.0020135.

Ingraham, C. (2015, March 31). Politicians Need to Get Over Their Squeamishness About Needle Exchange Programs. *Washington Post*.

Institute, T. S. (2015, February 18). Scientists Announce Anti–HIV Agent So Powerful It Can Work in a Vaccine. *Science Daily*, http://www.sciencedaily.com/releases/2015/02/150218073059.htm.

International and American Association for Dental Research. (2009, April 12). Can Periodontal Disease Act as a Risk Factor for HIV-1? *Science Daily*, https://www.sciencedaily.com/releases/2009/04/090403080727.htm.

Johanson, D. (2007). *A Practical Guide to Nutrition for People Living with HIV*, 2d ed. Canadian AIDS Treatment Information Exchange (CATIE).

Kania, D., T. Truong, A. Montoya, N. Nagot, P. Van de Perre, and E. Tuaillon. (2015). Performances of Fourth Generation HIV Antigen/Antibody Assays on Filter Paper for Detection of Early HIV Infections. *Journal of Clinical Virology*, 92–97.

Kennedy, I., and S. Williams. (2000). Occupational Exposure to HIV and Post-Exposure Prophylaxis in Healthcare Workers. *Occupational Medicine* 50(6), 387–391.

Krist, A.H., and A. Crawford-Faucher. (2002). Management of Newborns Exposed to Maternal HIV Infection. *American Family Physician* 65(10), 2049–2058.

Krist, M.D., and H. Alex. (2001). Obstetrics Care in Patients with HIV Disease. *American Family Physician*.

Krugman, P. (2013, May 26). The Obamacare Shock. *The New York Times*, A17.

Kumar, P. (2013). Long Term Non-Progressor (LTNP) HIV Infection. *Indian Journal of Medical Research*, 291–293.

Kusmer, K. (1990). Farewell to the Young Symbol of Courage. *Washington Post*, C1.

Lab Tests Online. (2001–2005; cited 2008, May 3). http://www.labtestsonline.org/understanding/analytes/viral_load/test.html.

Lawson-Ayayi, S. (2005).Avascular Necrosis in HIV-Infected Patients: A Case-Control Study from the Aquitane Cohort, 1997–2002 France. *Clinical Infectious Disease* 40(8), 1188–1193.

Lee, D. Canker Sores (Apthous Ulcers). (2005, October 6; cited 2007, November 7). http://www.medicinenet.com/canker_sores/article.htm.

Leece, P., C. Kendall, C. Touchie, K. Pottie, J. Angel, and J. Jaffey. (2010). Cervical Cancer Screening Among HIV-Positive Women. *Canadian Family Physician*, 425–431.

Levin, J. (2013). HIV Controllers Have Inflammation & ART Should Be Considered, Study Investigators Say. 20th Conference on Retroviruses and Opportunistic Infections, Atlanta.

Linnemeyer, P.A. (1993, November; cited 2008, October 11). The Immune System: An Overview. http://www.thebody.com/content/art1788.html.

Lipodystrophy. (2002, June). Cited Fact Sheet 39. http://www.aidsmap.com/en/docs/pdf/fs39.pdf.

Liszewski, W., A. Ananth, L. Ploch, and N. Rogers. (2014). Anal Pap Smears and Anal Cancer: What Dermatologists Should Know. *Journal of the American Academy of Dermatology*, 985–992.

Live Science Staff. (2011, June 6). 30 Years Later: AIDS by the Numbers. http://www.livescience.com/35732-aids-statistics-thirty-years.html.

Lurie, P. (1998, December). Does Needle Exchange Work? http://caps.ucsf.edu/uploads/pubs/FS/pdf/nepFS.pdf.

Lynch, D. (2014, November 12). Hairy Leukoplakia Treatment and Management. http://emedicine.medscape.com/article/279269-treatment.

Ma, J. D., K.C. Lee, and G.M. Kuo. (2010). HLA-B*5701 Testing to Predict Abacavir Hypersensitivity. *PLoS Currents*, 1203.

Magee, E. (2014, May 24). Vitamin D Deficiency. http://www.webmd.com/diet/guide/vitamin-d-deficiency.

Margolies, L., and B. Goeren. (2009). Anal Cancer, HIV and Gay/Bisexual Men. *Gay Men's Health Crisis—Treatment Issues*, 1–2.

Marks, J. (2015, July 21). Fatty Liver (Nonalcoholic Fatty Liver Disease/Nonalcoholic Steatohepatitis). http://www.medicinenet.com/fatty_liver/article.htm.

Marsh, L.A. (2005). Comparison of Pharmacological Treatment for Opioid Dependent Adolescents: A Randomized Control Trial. *Archives of General Psychiatry* 62(10), 1157–1164.

Matafsi, M., L. Skoura, and D. Sakellari. (2010). HIV Infection and Periodontal Diseases: An Overview of the Post–HAART Era. *Oral Diseases*, 1–13.

Mayo Clinic. (2014, January 2). Cryptosporidium Infection. http://www.mayoclinic.org/diseases-conditions/cryptosporidium/basics/prevention/con-20030375.

Mayo Clinic. (2014, May 2). Carbohydrates: How Carbs Fit Into a Healthy Diet. http://www.mayoclinic.org/healthy-lifestyle/nutrition-and-healthy-eating/in-depth/carbohydrates/art-20045705/.

Mayo Clinic. (2016, February 2). Dietary Fats: Know Which Types to Choose. http://www.mayoclinic.org/healthy-lifestyle/nutrition-and-healthy-eating/in-depth/fat/art-20045550.

Mayo Clinic Staff. (2014, December 5). Drug Addiction: Risk Factors. http://www.mayoclinic.org/diseases-conditions/drug-addiction/basics/risk-factors/CON-20020970.

Mayo Clinic Staff. (2015, March 21). Avascular Necrosis. http://www.mayoclinic.org/diseases-conditions/avascular-necrosis/basics/tests-diagnosis/con-20025517.

McEwan, M. (2008, September 30). *Pneumocystis Jirovecii Pneumonia*. http://en.wikipedia.org/wiki/Pneumocystis_pneumonia.

Mehta, N., & Pinsky, M. (2014, October 10). Drug Induced Hepatotoxicity. Retrieved from Medscape: http://emedicine.medscape.com/article/169814-overview#a2

Mehta, P., M. Nelson, A. Brand, and F. Boag. (2013, January). Avascular Necrosis in HIV. *Rheumatology International* 33(1), 235–238.

Meyer, J. H. (2006, November 1). Elevated Monoamine Oxidase A Levels in the Brain. *Archives of General Psychiatry* 63(11), 1209–1216.

Minnich, R. (2005). Pep on the Down Low. Poz.

Mirken, B. (2001). HIV Testing 101. *AIDS Treatment News*, 374.

National Association of People with AIDS. (2008). Types of HIV Tests. http://www.thebody.com/content/art6876.html.

National Institute on Drug Abuse. (2010, August 1). Drugs, Brains, and Behavior: The Science of Addiction. https://www.drugabuse.gov/publications/drugs-brains-behavior-science-addiction/preface.

National Institutes of Health. (2015, November 6). What Is Metabolic Syndrome? National Heart, Lung, and Blood Institute, http://www.nhlbi.nih.gov/health/health-topics/topics/ms/.

National Institutes of Health. (2016, May 25). Strengthening Knowledge and Understanding of Dietary Supplements. Retrieved from National Institutes of Health—Office of Dietary Supplements, https://ods.od.nih.gov/factsheets/list-all/.

National Kidney Foundation. (2015, December 13). How Your Kidneys Work. https://www.kidney.org/kidneydisease/howkidneyswrk.

National Treatment Improvement Evaluation Study (NTIES): Highlights. (1997). U.S. Department of Health and Human Services, Substance Abuse and Mental Health Services Administration, pp. 241–242.

Nauert, R. Why Mental Illness and Addiction Occur Together. (2007; cited 2007, December 3). *Psych Central News*, http://psychcentral.com/news/2007/12/03/why-mental-illness-and-addiction-occur-together/1602.html.

Nerad, J., M. Romeyn, E. Silverman, et al. (2003). General Nutrition Management in Patients Infected with Human Immunodeficiency Virus. *Clinical Infectious Disease* 36(Supplement 2), 552–562.

Nissapatorn, V., and N. Sawangjaroen. (2011). Parasitic Infections in HIV Infected Individuals: Diagnostic & Therapeutic Challenges. *Indian Journal of Medical Research* 134(6), 878–897.

Nolan, A., W. McIntosh, B. Allam, and P. Lamey. (1991, September). Recurrent Apthous Ulceration: Vitamin B1, B2 and B6 Status and Response to Replacement Therapy. *Journal of Oral Pathology & Medicine* 20(8), 389–391.

Office on Women's Health. (2012, July 16). Birth Control Methods Fact Sheet. http://www.womenshealth.gov/publications/our-publications/fact-sheet/birth-control-methods.html#b.

Padiun, N. HIV and Heterosexual Gender Gap—Man to Woman Transmission More Likely Than Woman to Man. (1991, October 5; cited 2008, July 28). http://findarticles.com/p/articles/mi_m1200/is_n14_v140/ai_11489577.

Palmer, M. (2004). *Dr. Melissa Palmer's Guide to Hepatitis and Liver Disease: What You Need to Know.* New York: Penguin Putnam.

Parish, C., K. Siegel, M. Pereyra, T. Liguori, and L. Metsch. (2015, September 4). Barriers and Facilitators to Dental Care Among HIV-Infected Adults. *Special Care in Dentistry* 35(6), 294–302.

Parisi, S., M. Cruciani, R. Scaggianti, C. Boldrin, S. Andreis, F. Dal Bello and G. Palu. (2011, May 25). Anal and Oral Human Papillomavirus (HPV) Infection in HIV-Infected Subjects in Northern Italy: A Longitudinal Cohort Study Among Men Who Have Sex with Men. *BMC Infectious Diseases* 11(150).

Pascoe, G., J. McDowell, and L. Bradley-Springer. (2002, August). HIV/AIDS in Dental Care. Mountain Plains AIDS Education and Training Center, www.hivdent.org/_oralmanifestations_/PDF/Dental%20HIV.pdf.

Patel, K., V. Mahima, and R. Prathibha-Rani. (2009, September-December). Oral Histoplasmosis. *Journal of Indian Society of Periodontology* 13(3), 157–159.

Pebody, R. (2012, May 22). NICE Says Sperm Washing Is No Safer Than Effective Treatment and Timed Intercourse. http://www.aidsmap.com/NICE-says-sperm-washing-is-no-safer-than-effective-treatment-and-timed-intercourse/page/2364056/.

Pedezanin, S. Fear of Dentists. (2002; cited 2008, May 17). http://www.essortment.com/all/feardentists_rcos.htm.

Penn, M. *Fighting Heart Disease: Should You Be Pro or Anti Antioxidants?* Cleveland Clinic Heart and Vascular Institute, 2008.

Petrangelo, A. (2013, July 24). Living with HIV: Is Serosorting Safe? http://www.healthline.com/health/hiv-aids/serosorting-safe#Serosorting1.

Picha, G., and J. Raj. (2013, July 26). History of Liposuction. http://www.liposuction4you.com/liposuction_history.htm

Pieribone, D. (2003). The HIV Life Cycle. http://www.thebody.com/content/art14193.html#latency.

Powderly, W.G. (1998). Effect of Opportunistic Illness on Risk of Death in HIV Disease. *Journal of the American Medical Association* 279(18), 1500.

Project Inform. (2015, March 10). New HIV Maturation Inhibitor BMS-955176 Appears Safe and Potent. The 22nd Conference on Retroviruses and Opportunistic Infections (CROI 2015), p. 1.

Project Inform Staff. HIV Treatment Information: Lipodystrophy Syndrome(s). (2001, November 1). http://www.projinf.org/fs/lipo.html.

Psevdos, G. (2007, September). Oral Histoplasmosis. *Consultant* 360, 47(9), 1.

Quan, K. Issues Affecting Patient Education. (2004). http://nursing.about.com/od/patienteducation/a/patienteduc.html.

Rabkin, J. (1994). The Good HIV Patient. In *Good Patients, Good Doctors.* New York: NCM.

Racaniello, V. (2014, September). The Berlin Patient. http://www.virology.ws/2014/09/06/the-berlin-patient/.

Randall, M.C. (2003, December). Support Groups: What They Are and What They Do. *Genetic Health.*

Raymond, D., and H. Rogers. (2016, January 11). Congress Ends Ban on Federal Funding for Needle Exchange Programs. (A. Cornish, interviewer.)

Recer, P. (2002). Education Helps Patient Health. Associated Press.

Reichart, P. (2003). Oral Manifestations in HIV: Fungal and Bacterial Infections; Kaposi's Sarcoma. *Medical Microbiology and Immunology* 192(3), 165–169.

Reiter, G. (1996). The HIV Wasting Syndrome, *AIDS Clinical Care*.

Reznik, D. (2005). Perspective: Oral Manifestations of HIV Disease. In 8th Annual Clinical Conference for the Ryan White CARE Act Clinicians, New Orleans, LA.

Richters, J., and S. Clayton. (2010). The Practical and Symbolic Purpose of Dental Dams in Lesbian Safer Sex Promotion. *Sexual Health*, 103–106.

Rodriquez, M. (2014, February 19). Life Expectancy in Some People with HIV Exceeds Average. http://www.thebody.com/content/73879/life-expectancy-in-some-people-with-hiv-exceeds-av.html.

Rose, L. (2015, April 4). Kaposi Sarcoma Treatment and Management. http://emedicine.medscape.com/article/279734-treatment.

Roxby, A., G. John-Stewart, and C. Behrens. (2014, June 10). Breastfeeding for HIV-Infected Mothers in Resource-Limited Settings. http://www.hivwebstudy.org/cases/resource-limited-setting/breastfeeding-hiv-infected-mothers-resource-limited-settings.

Sanders, A. (1999). HIV-Associated Bacterial Pneumonia. *The AIDS Reader* 9(8), 580–583.

Schimelpfening, N. (2015, March 25). Top 9 Depression Symptoms. http://depression.about.com/od/diagnosis/tp/depsymptoms.htm.

Schwartz, J. (2015, April 22). Healthy Cholesterol Ranges for HDL & LDL. http://www.livestrong.com/article/264792-healthy-cholesterol-ranges-for-hdl-ldl/.

Schwartz, R. (2015, October 25). Kaposi Sarcoma Treatment Protocols. http://emedicine.medscape.com/article/2006845-overview.

Scott, J. What Is a Calorie and Why Should I Care? (2008, March 17; cited 2008, May 18). http://weightloss.about.com/od/nutrition/a/blwhatcal.htm.

Scully, C. (2016, February 16). Noncandidal Fungal Infections of the Mouth. http://emedicine.medscape.com/article/1077685-followup.

Seah, R. (1981, August 1). Stop Diarrhea Naturally. http://www.natural-cancer-cures.com/stop-diarrhea.html.

Sharp, P. M., and B.H. Hahn. (2011). Origins of HIV and the AIDS Pandemic. *Cold Spring Harbor Perspectives in Medicine*, 1–22.

Sheehan, J. (2015, October 11). What Raises Triglyceride Levels? SF Gate, p. 10.

Siegal, H.A., R.S. Falck, R.G. Carlson, and J. Wang. (1995). Reducing HIV Needle Risk Behaviors Among Injection-Drug Users in the Midwest: An Evaluation of the Efficacy of Stand and Enhanced Interventions. *AIDS Education and Prevention* 7(4), 308–319.

Sifris, D., and J. Myhre. (2015, June 30). Hairy Leukoplakia: HIV-Associated Oral Disease. https://www.verywell.com/hairy-leukoplakia-hiv-associated-oral-disease-48956.

Sikkema, K. (2000). Predictors of AIDS-Related Grief Among HIV-Infected Men and Women. In International Conference on AIDS. Durban, South Africa.

Simon, H. (2012, July 10). Sinusitis. http://umm.edu/health/medical/reports/articles/sinusitis

Simple Facts Project Staff. Starting HIV Treatment: New Guidelines and Questions. The Simple Facts Project (2008, April 12; cited 2008, May 19). http://www.atdn.org/simple/guidelines.html.

Singh, N. (2013, May 2). CNS Toxoplasmosis in HIV. http://emedicine.medscape.com/article/1167298-overview#a1.

Skolnik, H., and A. Chernus. (2010). *Nutrient Timing for Peak Performance*. Champaign, IL: Human Kinetics.

Slanetz, L.W., and E.A. Brown. (1949). Studies on the Number of Bacteria in the Mouth and Their Reduction by the Use of Oral Antiseptics. *Journal of Dental Research* 23(3), 313–323.

Small, C., and D. Rosenstreich. (1997, May). Sinusitis in HIV Infection. *Immunology and Allergy Clinics of North America* 17(2), 267–289.

Speakes, L. White House Press Briefing. (1982). Office of the Press Secretary, Washington, D.C.

Spitzer, G. (2014, August 29). The Woman Who Discovered HIV Says a Cure Is Possible. http://www.humanosphere.org/podcasts/2014/08/the-woman-who-discovered-hiv-says-a-cure-is-possible/.

Sreebny, L., and S.S. Schwartz. Treatment of Drug-Induced Xerostomia. (2008; cited 2008, May 16). http://www.drymouth.info/practitioner/treatment.asp.

Stafford, N.D. (1989). Kaposi's Sarcoma of the Head and Neck in Patients with AIDS. *The Journal of Laryngology and Otology* (103), 379–382.

STD-AIDS-Hepatitis. (2008, January 7). Indirect Immunofluorescence testing for HIV-1. http://www.aids.gov.br/en/noticia/indirect-immunofluorescence-testing-hiv1.

Stefan, N., K. Konstantinos, and H.-U. Häring. (2013, July 1). Causes and Metabolic Consequences of Fatty Liver. *Endocrine Reviews* 29(7), 939–960.

Stolarski, C. R. (2015, December). HIV and Oral Healthcare. New Jersey AIDSline, 25–29.

Timpe, J.M., et al. (2007). Hepatitis C Virus Cell-Cell Transmission Hepatoma Cells in the Presence of Neutralizing Antibodies. *Hepatology* (47), 17–24.

Tofferi, J.K. (2006, January). Avascular Necrosis. http://emedicine.medscape.com/article/333364-overview.

Tofferi, J. K. (2015, March 4). Avascular Necrosis. http://emedicine.medscape.com/article/333364-overview.

Torre, D. (2010). Is It Time to Treat HIV Elite Controllers with Combined Antiretroviral Therapy? *Clinical Infectious Diseases* 50(10), 1425.

Tsang, G. Fiber 101: Soluble Fiber vs. Insoluble Fiber. (2005; cited 2005, November). http://www.healthcastle.com/fiber-solubleinsoluble.shtml.

Tyagi, M., and M. Bukrinsky. (2012). Human Immunodeficiency Virus (HIV) Latency: The Major Hurdle in HIV Eradication. *Molecular Medicine*, 1096–1108.

Understanding the Immune System: How It Works. U.S. Department of Health and Human Services. National Institute of Allergy and Infectious Diseases, National Institutes of Health and National Cancer Institute, 2003.

United States Food and Drug Administration. (2013, August 8). Vaccines, Blood & Biologics: Testing for HIV. http://www.fda.gov/BiologicsBloodVaccines/SafetyAvailability/HIVHomeTestKits/ucm126460.htm.

University of California San Francisco. (2002–2015). Hemoglobin and Functions of Iron. http://www.ucsfhealth.org/education/hemoglobin_and_functions_of_iron/.

University of Maryland Medical Center. (2016, May 24). Medical Reference Guide. http://umm.edu/health/medical.

University of Virginia Health Center. (2011, March 16). North America (U.S. and Canada): Policy and Legislation. http://www.medicalcenter.virginia.edu/safetycenter/internetsafetycenterwebpages/policylegislation/northamericapolicyleg.html.

Vernazza, P., et al. (2006). HIV-Discordant Couples and Parenthood: How Are They Dealing with the Risk of Transmission? *AIDS* 20(4), 635–636.

Volkow, N. (2005). What Do We Know About Addiction? *American Journal of Psychology* (162), 1401–1402.

Volkow, N. (2008, August). Methadone: Appropriate Use Provides Valuable Treatment for Pain and Addiction. https://www.drugabuse.gov/about-nida/directors-page/messages-director/2008/08/methadone-appropriate-use-provides-valuable-treatment-pain-addiction.

Von Roenn, J. (2003, June; cited 2007, April 4). Treatment of HIV-Associated Kaposi's Sarcoma. http://hivinsite.ucsf.edu/InSite?page=kb-06-02-04.

Waknine, Y. (2006). Highlights from MMWR: Decline in Adult Smoking Stalls and More. *Morbidity and Mortality Weekly Report* (55), 1145–1168.

Wall Street Journal Staff. (1989, December 12). Americans Awaken to the AIDS Crisis, 1985. *The Wall Street Journal*, B1.

Watson, J. (2008; cited 2008, May 18). Five Lessons on Motivation from a Visit to the Dentist. http://ezinearticles.com/?Five-Lessons-On-Motivation-From-A-Visit-To-The-Dentist&id=116094.

Wilburn, S. Q. (2004, September 30). Needlestick and Sharps Injury Prevention. Online Journal of Issues in Nursing, http://www.nursingworld.org/MainMenuCategories/ANAMarketplace/ANAPeriodicals/OJIN/TableofContents/Volume92004/No3Sept04/InjuryPrevention.html#WHO.

Woolston, C. Finding a Dentist. (2003, February 11; cited 2003, March 4). http://www.yourhealthconnection.com/topic/dentist.

Workowski, K., and S.M. Berman. (2006). *Mortality and Morbidity Weekly Report: Sexually Transmitted Diseases Treatment Guidelines, 2006.* National Center for HIV/AIDS, Viral Hepatitis, STD, and TB Prevention.

World Health Organization. (2004). Hepatitis C. From Global Alert and Response, http://www.who.int/csr/disease/hepatitis/whocdscsrlyo2003/en/index3.html#transmission.

World Health Organization. (2007, November). Psychosocial Support HIV/AIDS. http://www.who.int/hiv/topics/psychosocial/support/en.

Zeratsky, K. (2015, February 5). What Is Vitamin D Toxicity, and Should I Worry About It Since I Take Supplements? http://www.mayoclinic.org/healthy-lifestyle/nutrition-and-healthy-eating/expert-answers/vitamin-d-toxicity/faq-20058108?reDate=22082015.

Zickler, P. (2006). Buprenorphine Plus Behavioral Therapy Is Effective for Adolescents with Opioid Addiction. National Institute on Drug Abuse (NIDA).

Zorilla, C.D. (2008). Women Living with HIV: An Evolving Story. In *11th Annual Clinical Update*. Washington, D.C.: International AIDS Society.

INDEX